Hydration and Fluid Needs during Physical Activity

Hydration and Fluid Needs during Physical Activity

Editors

Douglas J. Casa
Stavros Kavouras

MDPI • Basel • Beijing • Wuhan • Barcelona • Belgrade • Manchester • Tokyo • Cluj • Tianjin

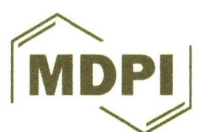

Editors

Douglas J. Casa
University of Connecticut
USA

Stavros Kavouras
Arizona State University
USA

Editorial Office
MDPI
St. Alban-Anlage 66
4052 Basel, Switzerland

This is a reprint of articles from the Special Issue published online in the open access journal *Nutrients* (ISSN 2072-6643) (available at: https://www.mdpi.com/journal/nutrients/special_issues/hydration_fluid).

For citation purposes, cite each article independently as indicated on the article page online and as indicated below:

LastName, A.A.; LastName, B.B.; LastName, C.C. Article Title. *Journal Name* **Year**, *Volume Number*, Page Range.

ISBN 978-3-0365-3747-4 (Hbk)
ISBN 978-3-0365-3748-1 (PDF)

Cover image courtesy of KSI.

© 2022 by the authors. Articles in this book are Open Access and distributed under the Creative Commons Attribution (CC BY) license, which allows users to download, copy and build upon published articles, as long as the author and publisher are properly credited, which ensures maximum dissemination and a wider impact of our publications.

The book as a whole is distributed by MDPI under the terms and conditions of the Creative Commons license CC BY-NC-ND.

Contents

About the Editors ix

Preface to "Hydration and Fluid Needs during Physical Activity" xi

Nicolas Bouscaren, Robin Faricier, Guillaume Y. Millet and Sébastien Racinais
Heat Acclimatization, Cooling Strategies, and Hydration during an Ultra-Trail in Warm and Humid Conditions
Reprinted from: *Nutrients* **2021**, *13*, 1085, doi:10.3390/nu13041085 1

Arpie Haroutounian, Fabiano T. Amorim, Todd A. Astorino, Nazareth Khodiguian, Katharine M. Curtiss, Aaron R. D. Matthews, Michael J. Estrada, Zachary Fennel, Zachary McKenna, Roberto Nava and Ailish C. Sheard
Change in Exercise Performance and Markers of Acute Kidney Injury Following Heat Acclimation with Permissive Dehydration
Reprinted from: *Nutrients* **2021**, *13*, 841, doi:10.3390/nu13030841 15

Catalina Capitán-Jiménez and Luis F. Aragón-Vargas
Awareness of Fluid Losses Does Not Impact Thirst during Exercise in the Heat: A Double-Blind, Cross-Over Study
Reprinted from: *Nutrients* **2021**, *13*, 4357, doi:10.3390/nu13124357 29

Ian Rollo, Rebecca K. Randell, Lindsay Baker, Javier Yanguas Leyes, Daniel Medina Leal, Antonia Lizarraga, Jordi Mesalles, Asker E. Jeukendrup, Lewis J. James and James M. Carter
Fluid Balance, Sweat Na$^+$ Losses, and Carbohydrate Intake of Elite Male Soccer Players in Response to Low and High Training Intensities in Cool and Hot Environments
Reprinted from: *Nutrients* **2021**, *13*, 401, doi:10.3390/nu13020401 37

Juthamard Surapongchai, Vitoon Saengsirisuwan, Ian Rollo, Rebecca K. Randell, Kanpiraya Nithitsuttibuta, Patarawadee Sainiyom, Clarence Hong Wei Leow and Jason Kai Wei Lee
Hydration Status, Fluid Intake, Sweat Rate, and Sweat Sodium Concentration in Recreational Tropical Native Runners
Reprinted from: *Nutrients* **2021**, *13*, 1374, doi:10.3390/nu13041374 49

Joanna Kamińska, Tomasz Podgórski, Krzysztof Rachwalski and Maciej Pawlak
Does the Minerals Content and Osmolarity of the Fluids Taken during Exercise by Female Field Hockey Players Influence on the Indicators of Water-Electrolyte and Acid-Basic Balance?
Reprinted from: *Nutrients* **2021**, *13*, 505, doi:10.3390/nu13020505 61

Lawrence E. Armstrong
Rehydration during Endurance Exercise: Challenges, Research, Options, Methods
Reprinted from: *Nutrients* **2021**, *13*, 887, doi:10.3390/nu13030887 73

JohnEric W. Smith, Marissa L. Bello and Ffion G. Price
A Case-Series Observation of Sweat Rate Variability in Endurance-Trained Athletes
Reprinted from: *Nutrients* **2021**, *13*, 1807, doi:10.3390/nu13061807 95

Alice E. Disher, Kelly L. Stewart, Aaron J. E. Bach and Ian B. Stewart
Contribution of Dietary Composition on Water Turnover Rates in Active and Sedentary Men
Reprinted from: *Nutrients* **2021**, *13*, 2124, doi:10.3390/nu13062124 107

Michael R. Szymanski, Gabrielle E. W. Giersch, Margaret C. Morrissey, Courteney L. Benjamin, Yasuki Sekiguchi, Ciara N. Manning, Rebecca L. Stearns and Douglas J. Casa
Availability of a Flavored Beverage and Impact on Children's Hydration Status, Sleep, and Mood
Reprinted from: *Nutrients* **2021**, *13*, 1757, doi:10.3390/nu13061757 . . . . **119**

Susan Yeargin, Toni M. Torres-McGehee, Dawn Emerson, Jessica Koller and John Dickinson
Hydration, Eating Attitudes and Behaviors in Age and Weight-Restricted Youth American Football Players
Reprinted from: *Nutrients* **2021**, *13*, 2565, doi:10.3390/nu13082565 . . . . **129**

About the Editors

Douglas J. Casa

Interests: hydration; exercise in heat; thermoregulation; heat stroke; maximizing performance in the heat.

Stavros Kavouras

Interests: water intake and glucose homeostasis; hydration and childhood obesity; fluid and electrolyte balance during exercise; hydration assessment and biomarkers; hydration and cardiovascular health.

Preface to "Hydration and Fluid Needs during Physical Activity"

Dear colleagues,

We are excited to announce a Special Issue in the journal Nutrients that focuses on hydration during physical activity. This Special Issue specifically addresses a variety of hydration topics related to performance, health, heat exposure, safety, recovery, and physiology, as well as other factors that are influenced when fluid balance is altered during physical activity. We have brought together hydration experts from around the globe, who have contributed their recent data to the collection of articles in this Special Issue. We have incorporated outside-the-box concepts, ideas, methodologies, and questions to invigorate the discussion of this vital topic, which has such a huge impact on hundreds of millions of laborers, soldiers, athletes, and recreationally active individuals around the world.

Douglas J. Casa and Stavros Kavouras
Editors

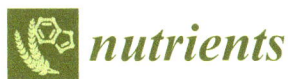

Article

Heat Acclimatization, Cooling Strategies, and Hydration during an Ultra-Trail in Warm and Humid Conditions

Nicolas Bouscaren [1,2,*], Robin Faricier [2], Guillaume Y. Millet [2,3,†] and Sébastien Racinais [4,†]

1. Inserm CIC1410, CHU Réunion, 97448 Saint Pierre, France
2. Inter-University Laboratory of Human Movement Biology, UJM-Saint-Etienne, Univ Lyon, EA 7424, 42023 Saint-Etienne, France; robinfaricier@live.fr (R.F.); guillaume.millet@univ-st-etienne.fr (G.Y.M.)
3. Institut Universitaire de France (IUF), 75231 Paris, France
4. Research and Scientific Support Department, Aspetar Orthopedic and Sports Medicine Hospital, Doha 29222, Qatar; Sebastien.Racinais@aspetar.com
* Correspondence: nicolas.bouscaren@chu-reunion.fr; Tel.: +33-262-719-830
† These authors contributed equally to this work.

Abstract: The aim of this study was to assess the history of exertional heat illness (EHI), heat preparation, cooling strategies, heat related symptoms, and hydration during an ultra-endurance running event in a warm and humid environment. This survey-based study was open to all people who participated in one of the three ultra-endurance races of the Grand Raid de la Réunion. Ambient temperature and relative humidity were 18.6 ± 5.7 °C (max = 29.7 °C) and $74 \pm 17\%$, respectively. A total of 3317 runners (56% of the total eligible population) participated in the study. Overall, 78% of the runners declared a history of heat-related symptoms while training or competing, and 1.9% reported a previous diagnosis of EHI. Only 24.3% of study participants living in temperate climates declared having trained in the heat before the races, and 45.1% of all respondents reported a cooling strategy during the races. Three quarter of all participants declared a hydration strategy. The planned hydration volume was 663 ± 240 mL/h. Fifty-nine percent of the runners had enriched their food or drink with sodium during the race. The present study shows that ultra-endurance runners have a wide variability of hydration and heat preparation strategies. Understandings of heat stress repercussions in ultra-endurance running need to be improved by specific field research.

Keywords: hot temperature; hydration; dehydration; electrolyte balance; body temperature regulation; acclimatization; ultra-endurance running; running

Citation: Bouscaren, N.; Faricier, R.; Millet, G.Y.; Racinais, S. Heat Acclimatization, Cooling Strategies, and Hydration during an Ultra-Trail in Warm and Humid Conditions. *Nutrients* 2021, *13*, 1085. https://doi.org/10.3390/nu13041085

Academic Editor: William M. Adams

Received: 17 February 2021
Accepted: 24 March 2021
Published: 26 March 2021

Publisher's Note: MDPI stays neutral with regard to jurisdictional claims in published maps and institutional affiliations.

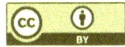

Copyright: © 2021 by the authors. Licensee MDPI, Basel, Switzerland. This article is an open access article distributed under the terms and conditions of the Creative Commons Attribution (CC BY) license (https://creativecommons.org/licenses/by/4.0/).

1. Introduction

Hot and humid ambient conditions impair prolonged exercise capacity and may favor exertional heat illness (EHI) [1,2]. Its most severe form, exertional heat stroke (EHS), is characterized by a core body temperature above 40.5 °C associated with central nervous system dysfunction (delirium, convulsions, coma) [3,4]. EHS is considered the second most common cause of sport- and exercise-related sudden death, after cardiac conditions [5]. Thus, several guidelines regarding training and competing in the heat have been published [6,7]. These guidelines are mostly based on laboratory studies [8] and are limited to running events up to the marathon distance. In other words, they may not apply to ultra-endurance sport, defined in the present paper as any event longer than 6 h [9,1]. In ultra-endurance sports, the thermoregulation and hydration challenges are different compared to shorter exercises due to the moderate intensity but prolonged duration, sometimes associated with exotic destinations, hot or warm environments (desert, tropical climate), and with high prevalence of digestive disorders and pathological processes in various organs such as skeletal muscles, heart, kidneys, and immune and endocrine systems [9–11]. Because of these specificities, the transposition of current knowledge and guidelines for road-races up to marathon toward ultra-endurance running is hazardous [9,10,12].

With the growing popularity of ultra-endurance events, attention to the unique needs of this population becomes increasingly important [13]. Only a few studies have focused on the influence of heat on performance [14], exercise-associated hyponatremia [15,16], or hydration requirements [17–19] in ultra-endurance events. Areas of uncertainty remain regarding thermoregulatory function, EHI prevalence, and health impairment during ultra-endurance running events in warm or hot conditions [1,13,19]. Moreover, despite the well-accepted benefits of heat acclimatization and cooling strategies before running in hot and humid conditions [6,20], it remains unknown whether ultra-endurance runners follow those guidelines from classical endurance activities.

Moreover, debates continue as to how endurance athletes should hydrate during exercise, i.e., ad libitum/drinking to thirst vs. pre-programmed drinking schedule [21]. For Kenefick et al. [21], drinking to thirst is more applicable for short-duration endurance exercise (<90 min), whereas a programmed drinking strategy should be tailored to prevent body mass losses or gains of $\pm$ 2% during activities longer than 2 h in duration, especially if they take place in warm or hot environments. For Hoffman et al. [12], hydration guidelines suitable for short periods of exercise in classical endurance events are not appropriate for ultra-endurance activities and may even cause harm. Hyperhydration can potentially cause the serious complication of exercise associated hyponatremia, so ultra-endurance athletes have been advised to avoid drinking beyond the dictate to thirst [12]. In addition, while the sodium consumed with a typical race diet appears to be adequate to replace losses and avoid salt-depletion in ultra-endurance [22,23], hydration guidelines recommend ingestion of sodium during endurance exercise, and use of supplementation has been a common practice among ultra-endurance athletes [24].

Given the lack of information about heat mitigation strategies in ultra-endurance runners before a race in a tropical environment and the controversies about hydration and sodium supplementation during endurance exercise, the aim of the current study was to survey heat preparation, cooling strategies, and heat-related symptoms (HRS) and to focus on hydration and sodium intake during an ultra-endurance running event in warm and humid environment.

2. Materials and Methods

2.1. Study Design

This survey-based cross-sectional study was open to all people who participated in one of the three races of the 2019 edition of the Grand Raid de la Réunion. A survey was distributed before and after the race. E-versions were transmitted by the organizing committee through a mailing-list. A hard copy of the pre-race survey was also available at race-bib collection.

2.2. Ethics Approval

This study was approved by the Saint-Etienne University Hospital ethics committee (#IRBN 572019/CHUSTE) and registered in ClinicalTrials.gov (#NCT04136925). The data were collected, recorded, and stored after obtained consent from the research subjects and were included in the register of processing activities of the Réunion Island University Hospital Center.

2.3. Characteristics of the Races

The event was held in Réunion Island (a tropical island in the Indian Ocean) and included three races: *La Diagonale des Fous* (DDF; 2900 runners, 165 km, 9576 m of positive and negative elevation, 2019 finish time range (23:33:45–66:04:00)); *Le Trail de Bourbon* (TDB; 1600 runners, 111 km, 6433 m elevation, (15:34:56–41:54:16)); and *La Mascareignes* (MAS; 1700 runners, 65 km, 3505 m elevation, (07:43:55–20:23:19)). Environmental conditions measured across 8 weather stations distributed along the three running courses reported a temperature of 18.6 $\pm$ 5.7 °C (range: 3.6 to 29.7 °C), a relative humidity of 74 $\pm$ 17%

(5 to 100%), a dew point of 13.0 ± 5.9 °C (−24.7 to 23.4 °C), and a solar radiation of 87 ± 116 °J/cm² (0 to 402 °J/cm²).

2.4. Participants

A total of 3317 runners participated in the study, representing 56% of the total eligible population. Sixty-nine percent (n = 2286) of study participants completed the pre-race survey, and 62% (n = 2050) completed the post-race survey. Overall, 1763 respondents took part in the 165-km race, 882 in the 65-km race, and 665 in the 111-km race; 83% of the responders (both pre- and post-race survey) were finishers. The sex ratio was 5:1 for men, and the mean age of runners was 42.2 years (representative of the starters). The climate of residence was temperate or continental for 55% of runners, and hot (tropical or dry) for 45% of runners. The demographic, morphological, and training characteristics of the participants are presented in Table 1.

Table 1. Characteristics of study participants in the Grand Raid de la Réunion runners by total sample and according to the race.

Variables	Total	La Mascareignes	Le Trail De Bourbon	La Diagonale Des Fous
Demographic characteristics				
Sex				
Men	2601 (83.2)	630 (74.5) #	498 (78.7) $	1468 (89.5) *
Women	525 (16.8)	216 (25.5)	135 (21.3)	173 (10.5) *
Age (years)	42 (35–50)	38 (32–46) #	41 (33–50) $	44 (38–50) *
Place of residence				
Réunion Island	1605 (52.0)	596 (71.0)	420 (66.9) $	589 (36.4) *
Metropolitan France	1310 (42.5)	208 (24.8)	179 (28.5)	923 (57.0)
Other country	171 (5.5)	35 (4.2)	29 (4.6)	107 (6.6)
Living in a tropical climate	1688 (54.4)	611 (72.7)	440 (70.1) $	635 (39.1) *
Morphological characteristics				
Men				
Mass (kg)	71 (66–76)	72 (66–77)	71 (66–76)	71 (66–75)
Height (cm)	176 (172–181)	176 (172–181)	176 (172–181)	176 (172–181)
BMI (kg/m2)	22.8 (21.5–24.2)	22.9 (21.5–24.3)	22.6 (21.4–24.2)	22.7 (21.5–24.0)
Women				
Mass (kg)	56 (52–61)	56 (52–62)	56 (52–62)	56 (52–60)
Height (cm)	165 (160–170)	165 (160–170)	165 (160–170)	164 (160–168)
BMI (kg/m2)	20.7 (19.6–22.0)	20.8 (19.5–22.2)	20.7 (19.3–22.2)	20.7 (19.8–21.7)
Training characteristics				
Trail running experience (yr)	5 (3–10)	3 (1–6) #	5 (3–9) $	6 (4–10) *
Number of ultra-races >60 km ran throughout career (n)	5 (2–10)	1 (0–3) #	3 (2–7) $	8 (4–13) *
Yearly number of ultra-races >60 km (n/yr)	1 (0.4–1.5)	0.1 (0–0.7) #	0.9 (0.5–1.3) $	1.3 (0.8–2.0) *
Average weekly training (over the 6-month period before the race)				
Duration (h)	8 (5–10)	6 (4–8) #	7 (5–10) $	8 (6–12) *
Distance (km)	50 (30–60)	40 (25–50) #	40 (30–50) $	50 (40–70) *
Ascent (m)	1200 (700–2000)	1000 (500–1500) #	1000 (700–2000) $	1500 (900–2000) *

Categorical variables are expressed as n (percentages) and quantitative variables as medians (Q1–Q3). Percentages are calculated on the number of respondents for each variable. BMI = Body Mass Index. * Comparisons between La Diagonale des Fous (DDF) vs. La Mascareignes (MAS), $ comparisons between DDF vs. Le Trail de Bourbon (TDB), # comparisons between MAS vs. TDB. *, $, # significant difference after Bonferroni correction.

2.5. Survey

The pre-race survey (Supplementary S1) contained questions on demographic characteristics and on trail-running and training experience, followed by specific questions on trail-running experience in hot environments, medical history of heat symptoms and heat illness before this race, and heat acclimatization before the race, and then by questions on planned hydration and cooling strategies. Cooling strategy was defined as any method used for reducing or preventing excessive heat storage during exercise. Only mid-cooling (i.e., cooling during the races) strategies used by runners were assessed. To help the runners answering, the main cooling methods were provided in the questionnaire (Supplementary S1). The post-race survey (Supplementary S2) looked at the impact of environmental conditions on performance, the occurrence of HRS during the race, and questions on effective hydration during the race. Planned hydration was asked in pre-race survey by "How amount of fluid do you plan to drink during the race? (in mL/h)", and effective hydration was asked in post-race survey by "What amount of fluid did you drink during the race (in mL/h)?" (Supplementaries S1 and S2). Data on runners (i.e., withdrawal status and finish time) were provided by the organizing committee of the Grand Raid de la Réunion.

2.6. Statistical Analyses

Qualitative variables were expressed as numbers and percentages, and quantitative variables were expressed as medians (Q1–Q3) or means ± SD. Univariate analyses were performed using Pearson's chi-squared test for categorical variables, and the Student's t-test or the Mann–Whitney U test for quantitative variables as appropriate. The Kruskal–Wallis test and the Wilcoxon rank-sum test were performed to compare fluid volume consumption between the races. The significance level was set to 5%. Bonferroni correction was applied to multiple comparisons. All analyses were performed using Stata V13 software (StataCorp LP, College Station, TX, USA).

3. Results

3.1. Medical History of Heat Related Illness before This Race

Before this race, 78% of participants reported a history of HRS; this value was higher in men than women (79.9% vs. 70.2%, $p < 0.001$), and higher in runners living in hot climates (HCR) than runners living in temperate climates (TCR) (80.5% vs. 75.3%, $p = 0.003$). A higher prevalence of a history of muscle cramps was found in men compared to women and in HCR compared to TCR ($p < 0.001$) (Table 2). A total of 44 (1.9%) runners reported a previous diagnosis of EHI; of these, 18 (0.8%) had been hospitalized or had visited the emergency room and 4 (0.2%) had received intensive care. A higher prevalence of heat-related hospitalization was found in TCR compared to HCR ($p = 0.021$). No difference was found according to sex (Table 2).

3.2. Heat Training and Acclimatization

About one-quarter (24.3%) of the 1033 TCR declared having trained in the heat. This value was similar between men and women (21.8% vs. 24.8%, $p = 0.427$) independently across the three races ($p = 0.599$). Most of these runners (98.4%) used natural heat (length of preparation: 15 (10–30) days) while only five runners used a climatic chamber (length of preparation: 6 (3–9.5) days). Among TCR, 56.8% declared having voluntarily scheduled an early arrival on the island to acclimatize to local environmental conditions (outside a holiday context), a proportion that was higher in women (65.2%) than men (55.2%, $p = 0.022$). However, the time to start of the race was only 4 (3–6) days with 6.8% of runners landing the day before the start of the race and 86.7% landing within 7 days before the race. No significant difference in arrival times before the race was found between TCR finishers and TCR non-finishers (4 (3–6) vs. 5 (3–6), respectively, $p = 0.163$).

Table 2. Previous history of symptoms and diagnosis of heat illness in the Grand Raid de la Réunion runners by total sample and according to sex and climate of residence.

Variables	Total (n = 2286)	Women (n = 410)	Men (n = 1876)	Hot Climate (n = 1250)	Temperate Climate (n = 1033)
History of heat-related symptoms	1771 (78.2)	287 (70.2)	1484 (79.9) *	997 (80.5) *	771 (75.3)
Fatigue/performance decrease	1318 (58.2)	226 (55.3)	1092 (58.8)	723 (58.4)	593 (57.9)
Muscle cramps	852 (37.6)	92 (22.5)	760 (40.9) *	551 (44.5) *	298 (29.1)
Digestive disorders	361 (15.9)	55 (13.5)	306 (16.5)	170 (13.7) *	191 (18.7)
Severe headache	98 (4.3)	25 (6.1)	73 (3.9)	65 (5.3)	33 (3.2)
Collapse	61 (2.7)	12 (2.9)	49 (2.6)	29 (2.3)	32 (3.1)
Other	24 (1.1)	6 (1.5)	18 (1.0)	12 (1.0)	12 (1.2)
History of heat illness diagnosis	43 (1.9)	4 (1.0)	39 (2.1)	20 (1.6)	23 (2.2)
Dehydration	24 (1.1)	0	24 (1.3)	9 (0.7)	15 (1.5)
Hyponatremia	3 (0.1)	2 (0.5)	1 (0.05)	0	3 (0.3)
Heat exhaustion	6 (0.3)	0	6 (0.3)	3 (0.2)	3 (0.3)
Heat stroke	14 (0.6)	2 (0.5)	12 (0.6)	6 (0.5)	8 (0.8)
Other	6 (0.3)	0	6 (0.3)	4 (0.3)	2 (0.2)
Hospitalization	18 (0.8)	4 (1.0)	14 (0.8)	5 (0.4)	13 (1.3) *
Intensive Care Unit hospitalization	4 (0.2)	1 (0.2)	3 (0.2)	1 (0.1)	3 (0.3)

Data are expressed as n (percentages). All * refer to comparisons between (1) women vs. men, or (2) runners from hot climates vs. runners from temperate climates. Percentages are calculated on the number of respondents for each variable. * Significant difference after Bonferroni correction.

3.3. Cooling Strategy

A cooling strategy during the race was reported by 45.1% of runners with no difference according to sex ($p = 0.107$) or climate of residence ($p = 0.569$) (Table).

Table 3. Planned hydration and per-cooling strategies in the Grand Raid de la Réunion runners by total sample and according to sex and climate of residence.

Variables	Total (n = 2286)	Women (n = 410)	Men (n = 1876)	Hot Climate (n = 1250)	Temperate Climate (n = 1033)
Planned cooling strategy	880 (45.1)	122 (40.8)	681 (45.9)	422 (45.8)	374 (44.4)
Stop/rest in the shade	379 (19.4)	54 (18.1)	292 (19.7)	200 (21.7)	146 (17.3)
Wet sponge	232 (11.9)	34 (11.4)	179 (12.1)	108 (11.7)	104 (12.4)
Leg immersion in cold water (creek, river)	131 (6.7)	25 (8.4)	96 (6.5)	69 (7.5)	50 (5.9)
Shower/whole body immersion	71 (3.6)	7 (2.3)	53 (3.6)	35 (3.8)	24 (2.9)
Head/neck cooling	327 (16.8)	52 (17.4)	252 (17.0)	136 (14.8)	164 (19.5)
Cooling of other body area	50 (2.3)	7 (2.3)	57 (3.8)	24 (2.6)	39 (4.6)
Cold towel	80 (4.1)	7 (2.3)	64 (4.3)	44 (4.8)	26 (3.1)
Hat, cap, etc.	239 (12.3)	36 (12.0)	184 (12.4)	86 (9.3)	131 (15.6) *
Neck collar	55 (2.8)	10 (3.3)	44 (3.0)	26 (2.8)	26 (3.1)
Ice slurry/water ingestion	33 (1.7)	6 (2.0)	24 (1.6)	24 (2.6) *	5 (0.6)
Ice vest	5 (0.3)	0	5 (0.3)	3 (0.3)	1 (0.1)
Other	23 (1.2)	2 (0.7)	18 (1.2)	12 (1.3)	8 (1.0)
Planned fluid consumption					
Pure Water	1688 (75.3)	299 (74.2)	1389 (75.5)	968 (78.4) *	720 (71.4)
Sodium-enriched water	701 (31.3)	96 (23.8)	605 (32.9) *	350 (28.3)	351 (34.8) *
Homemade preparation	306 (13.6)	66 (16.4)	240 (13.0)	207 (16.8) *	99 (9.8)
Exercise drink	1341 (59.8)	222 (55.1)	1119 (60.8)	733 (59.4)	608 (60.3)
Other	416 (18.6)	80 (19.9)	336 (18.3)	242 (19.6)	174 (17.3)
Pure water alone (no other beverage)	237 (10.6)	44 (10.9)	193 (10.5)	121 (9.8)	116 (11.5)

Data are expressed as n (percentages). All * refer to comparisons between (1) women vs. men, or (2) runners from hot climates vs. runners from temperate climates. Percentages are calculated on the number of respondents for each variable. * Significant difference after Bonferroni correction.

3.4. Heat Related Symptoms during the Races

The post-race survey revealed that 23.8% of runners suffered from the heat during the race; this value was similar according to sexes ($p = 0.898$) but higher in HCR than TCR (25.8% vs. 19.9%, $p = 0.003$). These findings were consistent across the three races. A similar proportion of runners (20.2%) thought that the heat had negatively impacted their performance, without reaching the level of significance between HCR and TCR ($p = 0.078$). Up to 54.6% of the runners reported at least one HRS; this value was higher in men than in women (56.5% vs. 46.8%, $p = 0.002$) but did not vary according to climate of residence ($p = 0.603$). Runners declared the following HRS: muscle cramping (43.4%), digestive disorder (14.3%), collapse (1.2%), and severe headache (0.9%). A detailed list of HRS according to sex is provided in Figure 1.

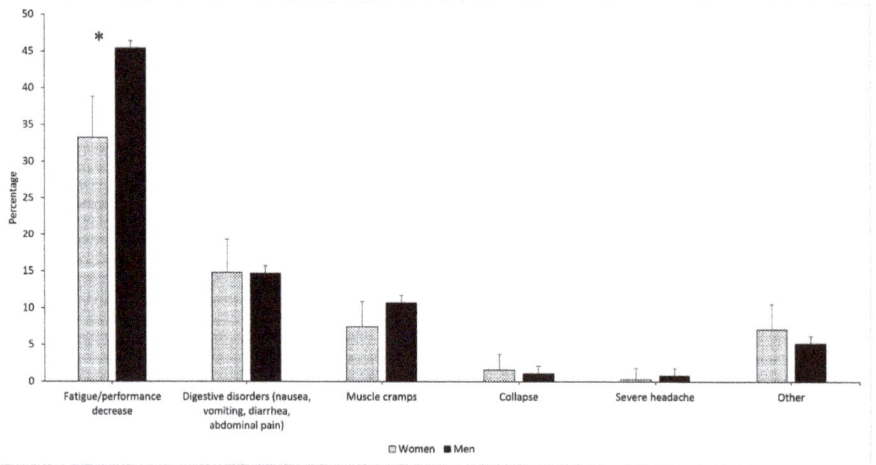

Figure 1. Heat-related symptoms experienced during the race by Grand Raid de la Réunion runners according to sex. * Significant difference between men and women.

3.5. Hydration

The hydration rate planned by runners was 663 ± 240 mL/h (corresponding to 9.7 ± 3.7 mL/kg/h) for the whole population (686 ± 237 mL/h for MAS vs. 640 ± 235 mL/h for TDB vs. 661 ± 242 mL/h for DDF ($p = 0.018$)). This rate was 624 ± 229 mL/h for women vs. 671 ± 241 mL/h for men ($p = 0.002$) (see repartition per race in Figure 2A), and 635 ± 236 mL/h for non-finishers vs. 671 ± 240 mL/h for finishers ($p = 0.009$). No differences in planned hydration volume were found according to climate of residence ($p = 0.569$). More men than women planned to drink sodium-enriched water (33 vs. 24%, $p < 0.001$) (Table 3). The consumption of pure water or homemade preparation was more prevalent in HCR ($p < 0.001$), whereas the consumption of sodium-enriched water was more prevalent in TCR ($p < 0.001$). Ten percent of runners planned to drink only pure water during the races, namely 13.5% of MAS runners vs. 11.0% of TDB runners vs. 9.0% of DDF runners ($p = 0.013$). Repartition of beverage composition extrapolated on a 1-L bottle is illustrated in Figure 2C. Qualitative analysis of the variables "homemade preparation" and "other kind of beverage" found that 24.0% of runners planned to add carbohydrates to their beverage, 12.6% planned to consume sparkling beverages, and 11.9% planned to consume soda drinks.

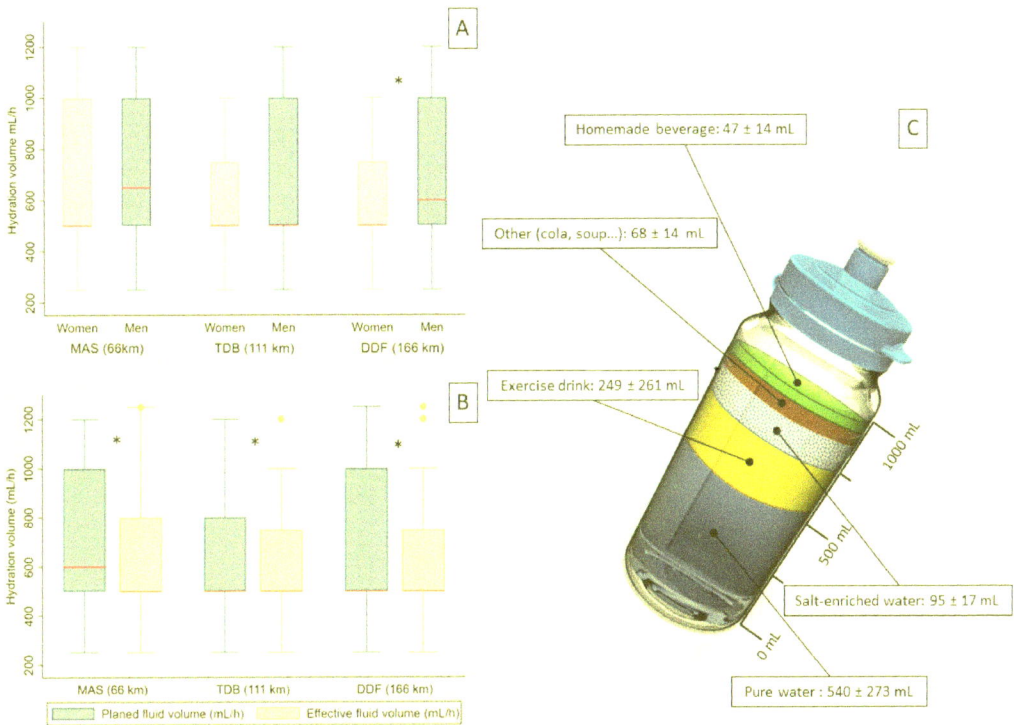

Figure 2. Hydration strategies of runners of the "Grand Raid de la Réunion" 2019 edition. MAS: *La Mascareignes*, TDB: *Le Trail de Bourbon*, DDF: *La Diagonale des Fous*. (**A**) Hydration volume in mL/h according to race and sex. * Significant difference between men and women. (**B**) Planned and effective hydration volume in mL/h reported by runners according to race. * Significant difference between planned and effective hydration volume. (**C**) Distribution of beverage types extrapolated on a 1-L bottle. Data are presented in milliliters (mL) with mean ± SD.

Overall, 77.0% of runners declared having a hydration strategy; this value was higher in HCR than TCR (79.9% vs. 74.9%, $p = 0.013$), but did not vary according to sex ($p = 0.518$). Drinking to thirst was declared by 39.2% of runners. Other factors determining runners' hydration were color of urines (10.9%), and maximum tolerated hydration (6.4%). The value of hydration volume reported post-race was 61 ± 244 mL/h lower than the value planned by the runners pre-race ($p < 0.0001$); this difference was consistent across the three races (Figure B). According to the post-race survey, 80.3% of runners considered their hydration to be sufficient; this value was lower in women than men (73.9% vs. 81.5%, respectively, $p = 0.002$) but did not vary according to climate of residence ($p = 0.301$). Moreover, 58.8% of the runners added sodium to their food or beverage during the race; this value was higher in HCR than TCR (62.9% vs. 53.8%, $p < 0.001$) but did not vary according to sex difference ($p = 0.585$). The proportion of runners (51.8%) who ate soup during the race was similar between HCR and TCR.

4. Discussion

The main results of the present study are that (i) although 78% of ultra-endurance runners had a previous history of HRS, 1.9% declared a medical history of EHI; (ii) only one quarter of TCR reported having specifically trained in the heat, yet the prevalence of self-declared negative impact of environmental conditions in performance (20%) and HRS incidence (54.6%) was not higher for TCR compared to HCR; (iii) three quarter of all participants had a hydration strategy, with thirst representing a hydration signal for 39% of them, and 59% of runners added sodium to their food or beverage during the race. To our knowledge, this is the first study describing the heat mitigation strategies in ultra-endurance runners before a race in a tropical environment.

4.1. History of Heat-Related Symptoms and Exertional Heat Illness

Three-quarters of participants reported a history of HRS before this race, which is higher than what has been reported by elite athletes (48%) and elite cyclists (57%) [25,26]. Conversely, forty-four runners (2%) of the athletes participating in the present study reported a history of EHI, leading to hospitalization or emergency consulting in 18 (0.8%) of them. This prevalence is lower than in previous cross-sectional study in elite athletes (16% in road cycling [26] and 9% in athletics [25]). This relatively low EHI prevalence in ultra-endurance running compared to other sports must be confirmed by prospective epidemiological studies but can partially be explained by the fact that exercise intensity is at least as important as environmental conditions for increasing core temperature [19,26]. Another explanation can be found in the "flush model" developed by Millet [27]. In his holistic model, the author suggests that elite athletes (who are very rare in ultra-trail pelotons) could finish the race with a lower security reserve (i.e., a reserve allowing one to prevent physiological damage) and therefore could be more exposed to EHI in hot and humid environments than amateur ultra-endurance runners [27]. Finally, a relative low prevalence of EHI compared to HRS declared by runners could be related to an under-diagnosis of the true rate of EHI [28]. Given the frequent failure to measure core body temperature during races, it is plausible that some events could be erroneously attributed to cardiac conditions based on incidental pathological findings, whereas heat stroke was the real etiology. A previous study suggested that serious cardiac events were outnumbered by heat stroke events by a factor of 10 during endurance sport [29].

4.2. Heat Training and Acclimatization

Heat acclimatization is considered as the most important countermeasure to protect the health of athletes and to enhance their performance in hot conditions [6,30]. Ideally, the heat acclimatization period should pass 2 weeks in order to maximize all benefits [6]. In our study, only one-quarter of TCR reported having trained in the heat (mostly in natural environments) before the event, with an average training duration of 15 days. This percentage is higher than that observed in the high-performance athletes who participated in the 2015 IAAF Worlds Athletics Championships held in Beijing (15%) [25]. The comparison with the Worlds Athletics Championships study must however be made with caution because this study included track and field athletes for which heat acclimatization is less important [6]. Considering the repercussions of heat stress on endurance performance [14,31,32], and given the fact that heat acclimatization can reduce the likelihood of heat illness [20], one may wonder why so few runners in our study acclimatized before the event. We suggest two possible explanations for this. First, this may be due a lack of awareness of the potential risks in this population due to the scarcity of epidemiological data on the prevalence of EHI in ultra-endurance running and to the absence of guidelines and recommendations for ultra-endurance runners [13]. Second, ultra-endurance runners are mostly amateurs with a limited possibility to organize training camps. In our study, 42% of the runners who had trained in the heat before the event reported a training duration less than 14 days. Half of our eligible population was made up of runners from metropolitan France, where the climate is temperate (mean temperature in October 2019 was 15.1 °C), making optimal heat-acclimatization difficult. The time required to achieve optimal acclimatization likely varies, but a total period of 2 weeks has been shown to facilitate maximal adaptations [6,33,34]. In our study, the time to start of the race was only 4 days. In the present study, no significant difference in arrival times before the race was found between TCR finishers and TCR non-finishers ($p = 0.163$).

4.3. Cooling Strategy

While several reviews concluded that cooling can increase prolonged exercise capacity in hot conditions [,], only 45% of ultra-endurance runners in our study used cooling strategies during the race. This proportion is lower than mid-cooling strategy using prevalence (98%) found in elite road race athletes during the Doha 2019 IAAF World Athletics Championships [ ]. In our study, runners used mostly external cooling strategies, namely natural cooling strategies (leg (7%) or whole-body (4%) immersion in creeks or rivers, resting in the shade (19%)) and classic strategies (wet sponge (12%), head/neck cooling (17%), hat, cap (12%), cold towel (4%), neck collar (3%)).

4.4. Heat Related Symptoms during the Races

During the races, 24% of runners declared having suffered from the heat, and only 20% stated that the heat had negatively impacted their performance. This relative low prevalence of perceived heat repercussions may be partly due to the relatively mild conditions that prevailed during this edition of the Grand Raid de la Réunion, with temperatures not exceeding 30 °C (range 3.6 to 29.7 °C) and humidity remaining at usual levels (75%). This was in fact the coolest edition of the last 6 years (range 5.8–32.3 °C). Importantly, only 61 non-finishers answered the post-race survey (accounting for 3% of all completed post-race survey), which contained questions on HRS during the race. Considering that the proportion of non-finisher of the three races of the 2019 edition was 28%, heat repercussions during races were most probably underestimated. In future studies, data should be collected from the onsite medical team and from local hospitals to determine the prevalence of EHI during the race. Up to 55% of the runners reported at least one HRS, which is surprising given that only 20% of the runners stated that the heat had negatively impacted their performance. The reasons are unclear. This gap may be explained by the fact that respondents reporting symptoms were not due to the heat but to other issues (injuries, sleep deprivation, etc.), even though the survey question was explicitly about HRS. It is also possible that runners had symptoms but considered that it did not limit their performance (i.e., they considered to be limited by other factors). This may be further exacerbated by declarative bias, i.e., runners would appear strong and declare symptoms without mentioning it was influencing their performance. Although only a quarter of athletes of TCR reported having trained specifically in the heat, similar prevalence of negative impact of environmental conditions in performance (~20%) and HRS incidence (55%) during races were declared according to climate of residence. Moreover, a higher percentage of HCR declared having suffered from the heat (25.8% vs. 19.9%, $p = 0.003$). This unexpected difference could be partly explained by the date of the race and the importance of seasonal acclimatization. The race took place in mid-October, just after the end of summer for the inhabitants of the northern hemisphere, but just before the start of the hot season (November) for local residents (mean temperature in October 2019 in Réunion Island was 22 °C). Although temperatures in France were only 15 °C at the time of the race, the temperature in the month preceding the events could rise to above 25 °C, allowing the TCR runners to repeatedly train in warm environments. Residing in a hot climate may not confer an advantage if one has not been yet exposed to heat for many months, i.e., has not benefited from seasonal acclimatization of a hot season as was the case from the runners from La Réunion, i.e., the vast majority of our HCR population [ ]. This is critical, as seasonal acclimatization is important in protecting athletes' health when practicing in the heat. Indeed, it has been shown that the risk of heat related collapse was higher at the beginning than the middle of the summer when athletes had not yet acquired natural acclimatization to heat [ ]. Moreover, a recent study of analysis of heat illness in the Beach Volleyball World Tour showed that there were more medical time-outs related to the heat during competition in Asia in the winter when northern hemisphere players do not benefit anymore from seasonal acclimation [ ].

4.5. Hydration

Data on hydration strategies during ultra-endurance running remain scarce [13]. In our study, 77.0% of runners declared having a hydration strategy, with a planned hydration rate of 663 mL/h (corresponding to 9.7 ± 3.7 mL/kg/h), with a higher hydration rate in shorter races: 686 ± 237 mL/h for MAS (65 km) vs. 640 ± 235 mL/h for TDB (111 km) vs. 661 ± 242 mL/h for DDF (165 km) ($p = 0.018$). These results are in line with recent publications in ultra-endurance running reporting a mean hydration volume of 685 [38] and 732 mL/h [39]. Past consensus statements recommended minimizing fluid deficit; however, debates continue as to how athletes should hydrate during exercise, i.e., ad libitum vs. pre-programmed drinking schedule [18]. The typical hydration guidelines to avoid more than 2% body mass loss may not apply in ultra-endurance activities [12]. In our sample, thirst was the factor determining hydration for only 39% of runners; the other factors were color of urine for 11% and maximum tolerated hydration for 6% of the runners. Recent considerations of hydration concluded that ultra-endurance runners should be cautious to avoid drinking beyond the dictate of thirst and taking in excessive sodium during prolonged exercises [12]. Whilst hyperhydration can lead to exercise associated hyponatremia, hypohydration during exercise in hot ambient conditions can increase the risk of developing EHI [40]. Moreover, pronounced dehydration associated with influx of muscle protein (myoglobin) caused by muscle damage may lead to kidney damage. The prevalence of an acute kidney insult in ultra-marathon running is nearly 45% of all runners [41].

A wide range of hydration strategies was observed in our population. Most runners (75.3%) had planned to drink water; 59.8% had planned to consume exercise drinks, almost 60% had planned to consume sodium-enriched water or food, 24% had planned to consume carbohydrate-enriched water or food, and 10% of the runners declared drinking exclusively pure water during the race. Hydration and nutrition recommendations commonly prescribe sodium and carbohydrate ingestion during prolonged endurance exercise in the heat [42]. However, sodium supplementation should not be aimed at replacing all losses and should not be excessive during ultra-endurance activities, as sodium consumption in the typical race diet of ultra-endurance runners appears to be adequate [12].

In our study, the heterogeneity of hydration practices is reflected in the extreme diversity of products that were added to homemade preparations by runners: coffee or tea, fruit juice, spices, milk, plants or herbs, proteins, amino acid supplements, etc. Of note, the challenges of endurance sports include the potential for large variations in ambient conditions during a single event, and practical considerations include the availability of nutrition supplies at aid stations, the difficulties of ingestion during exercise, and the interaction with gastrointestinal comfort/function [42]. Specific recommendations are needed regarding hydration volume and drink content during ultra-endurance running adapted to (i) individual tastes and avoidance of loss of appetence, and (ii) the practical considerations associated with each race (autonomy or semi-autonomy).

4.6. Study Strengths and Limitations

The low rate of response to the post-race survey among non-finishers may have biased our analysis of the effects of hot and humid conditions on ultra-endurance running. As this study is a survey-based study, it is subject to the declarative bias of athletes. It remains possible that despite the specify of the questions regarding HRS and HRI, some runners attributed to heat some conditions being not heat-related. Comparisons of prevalence made with the prevalence of other disciplines or other papers should therefore be considered with caution due to the lack of clinical data in our study to confirm the self-assessment of the runners. However, our study provides a relevant estimation of the burden of EHI self-reported in ultra-endurance running, a discipline poorly investigated. Nevertheless, a major strength of the present study is its total sample size ($n = 3317$) and representativeness, as 56% of the total eligible population was included in at least one of the two surveys (pre- and post-race surveys). Environmental conditions during the race were not extreme due to relatively low temperatures; since runners did not know ahead of time what environmental conditions would be like, our findings concerning the strategies they employed (as declared on the pre-race survey) can be considered as representative of the population.

5. Conclusions

The present study shows that ultra-endurance runners have a wide variability of hydration and heat preparation strategies. However, although consensus recommendations on training and competing in the heat are only partially adopted by ultra-endurance runners, prevalence of EHI remains low in ultra-endurance, probably because exercise intensity is a more potent parameter for increasing body temperature than environmental parameters. Being native as a resident of tropical country seems not to confer an advantage in reducing the negative impact of heat on performance and HRS incidence if the athletes have not been exposed to heat in the weeks preceding the race (i.e., no seasonal acclimatization). In our study, 3/4 of runners declared having a hydration strategy, with a planned hydration volume of about 650 mL/h. Thirst represented the hydration signal for 40% of ultra-endurance runners, and 60% of them added sodium to their food or beverage. Recent considerations recommending that ultra-endurance runners should be cautioned to avoid drinking beyond the dictate of thirst and taking in excessive sodium during prolonged exercises are only partially respected. Understandings of heat stress repercussions in ultra-endurance running need to be improve by specific field research.

6. Practical Implications

- Information of the ultra-endurance runners about benefits of heat acclimatization and cooling strategies before running in hot and humid conditions is needed.
- Prevalence of EHI remains low in ultra-endurance based on declarative evaluation in this study. However, prospective studies with clinical assessment of EHI (core temperature, symptoms) to better estimate the burden of heat stress in ultra-endurance disciplines are needed.
- The importance of hydration requirements in hot and humid conditions in ultra-endurance running needs to be kept in mind.

Supplementary Materials: The following are available online at https://www.mdpi.com/article/10.3390/nu13041085/s1, Supplementary S1: Pre-race survey (French version), Supplementary S2: Post-race survey (French version).

Author Contributions: Conceptualization, N.B., G.Y.M. and S.R.; methodology, N.B., G.Y.M. and S.R.; formal analysis, N.B. and R.F.; investigation, N.B.; data curation, N.B. and R.F.; writing—original draft preparation, N.B.; writing—review and editing, N.B., G.Y.M. and S.R.; supervision, G.Y.M. and S.R. All authors have read and agreed to the published version of the manuscript.

Funding: This research received no external funding.

Institutional Review Board Statement: This study was approved by the Saint-Etienne University Hospital ethics committee (#IRBN 572019/CHUSTE) and registered in https://www.clinicaltrials.gov/ct2/show/NC T04136925 (accessed on 25 March 2021). The data were collected, recorded, and stored after obtained consent from the research subjects and were included in the register of processing activities of the Réunion Island University Hospital Center.

Informed Consent Statement: Informed consent was obtained from all subjects involved in the study.

Data Availability Statement: The data presented in this study are available on reasonable request from the corresponding author.

Acknowledgments: This study was supported by the Réunion Island University Hospital Center. The author would like to thank Arianne Dorval for proofreading the manuscript as well as all the medical students of the Réunion Island University Hospital Center who participated in data collection.

Conflicts of Interest: The authors declare no conflict of interest.

References

1. Gamage, P.J.; Fortington, L.V.; Finch, C.F. Epidemiology of Exertional Heat Illnesses in Organised Sports: A Systematic Review. *J. Sci. Med. Sport* **2020**, *23*, 701–709. [CrossRef]
2. Filep, E.M.; Murata, Y.; Endres, B.D.; Kim, G.; Stearns, R.L.; Casa, D.J. Exertional Heat Stroke, Modality Cooling Rate, and Survival Outcomes: A Systematic Review. *Medicina* **2020**, *56*, 589. [CrossRef] [PubMed]
3. Bouchama, A.; Knochel, J.P. Heat Stroke. *N. Engl. J. Med.* **2002**, *346*, 1978–1988. [CrossRef]
4. Leon, L.R.; Bouchama, A. Heat Stroke. *Compr. Physiol.* **2015**, *5*, 611–647. [CrossRef] [PubMed]
5. Racinais, S.; Alhammoud, M.; Nasir, N.; Bahr, R. Epidemiology and Risk Factors for Heat Illness: 11 Years of Heat Stress Monitoring Programme Data from the FIVB Beach Volleyball World Tour. *Br. J. Sports Med.* **2020**. [CrossRef] [PubMed]
6. Racinais, S.; Alonso, J.M.; Coutts, A.J.; Flouris, A.D.; Girard, O.; González-Alonso, J.; Hausswirth, C.; Jay, O.; Lee, J.K.W.; Mitchell, N.; et al. Consensus Recommendations on Training and Competing in the Heat. *Br. J. Sports Med.* **2015**, *49*, 1164–1173. [CrossRef]
7. Bergeron, M.F.; Bahr, R.; Bärtsch, P.; Bourdon, L.; Calbet, J.A.L.; Carlsen, K.H.; Castagna, O.; González-Alonso, J.; Lundby, C.; Maughan, R.J.; et al. International Olympic Committee Consensus Statement on Thermoregulatory and Altitude Challenges for High-Level Athletes. *Br. J. Sports Med.* **2012**, *46*, 770–779. [CrossRef]
8. Cheuvront, S.N.; Haymes, E.M. Thermoregulation and Marathon Running: Biological and Environmental Influences. *Sports Med.* **2001**, *31*, 743–762. [CrossRef]
9. Bergeron, M.F. Heat Stress and Thermal Strain Challenges in Running. *J. Orthop. Sports Phys. Ther.* **2014**, *44*, 831–838. [CrossRef]
10. Bouscaren, N.; Millet, G.Y.; Racinais, S. Heat Stress Challenges in Marathon vs. Ultra-Endurance Running. *Front. Sports Act. Living* **2019**, *1*, 59. [CrossRef]
11. Knechtle, B.; Nikolaidis, P.T. Physiology and Pathophysiology in Ultra-Marathon Running. *Front. Physiol.* **2018**, *9*, 634. [CrossRef]
12. Hoffman, M.; Stellingwerff, T.; Costa, R.J.S. Considerations for Ultra-Endurance Activities: Part 2—Hydration. *Res. Sports Med.* **2019**, *27*, 182–194. [CrossRef]
13. Hoffman, M.D. State of the Science on Ultramarathon Running After a Half Century: A Systematic Analysis and Commentary. *Int. J. Sports Physiol. Perform.* **2020**, *15*, 1052–1056. [CrossRef]
14. Parise, C.A.; Hoffman, M.D. Influence of Temperature and Performance Level on Pacing a 161 Km Trail Ultramarathon. *Int. J. Sports Physiol. Perform.* **2011**, *6*, 243–251. [CrossRef]
15. Knechtle, B.; Gnädinger, M.; Knechtle, P.; Imoberdorf, R.; Kohler, G.; Ballmer, P.; Rosemann, T.; Senn, O. Prevalence of Exercise-Associated Hyponatremia in Male Ultraendurance Athletes. *Clin. J. Sport Med. Off. J. Can. Acad. Sport Med.* **2011**, *21*, 226–232. [CrossRef]
16. Seal, A.D.; Anastasiou, C.A.; Skenderi, K.P.; Echegaray, M.; Yiannakouris, N.; Tsekouras, Y.E.; Matalas, A.L.; Yannakoulia, M.; Pechlivani, F.; Kavouras, S.A. Incidence of Hyponatremia During a Continuous 246-Km Ultramarathon Running Race. *Front. Nutr.* **2019**, *6*, 161. [CrossRef] [PubMed]
17. Rehrer, N.J. Fluid and Electrolyte Balance in Ultra-Endurance Sport. *Sports Med.* **2001**, *31*, 701–715. [CrossRef]
18. Goulet, E.D.B.; Hoffman, M.D. Impact of Ad Libitum Versus Programmed Drinking on Endurance Performance: A Systematic Review with Meta-Analysis. *Sports Med.* **2019**, *49*, 221–232. [CrossRef] [PubMed]
19. Valentino, T.R.; Stuempfle, K.J.; Kern, M.; Hoffman, M.D. The Influence of Hydration on Thermoregulation During a 161-Km Ultramarathon. *Wilderness Environ. Med.* **2015**, *26*, e3. [CrossRef]
20. Racinais, S.; Casa, D.; Brocherie, F.; Ihsan, M. Translating Science Into Practice: The Perspective of the Doha 2019 IAAF World Championships in the Heat. *Front. Sports Act. Living* **2019**, *1*, 39. [CrossRef] [PubMed]
21. Kenefick, R.W. Drinking Strategies: Planned Drinking Versus Drinking to Thirst. *Sports Med.* **2018**, *48*, 31–37. [CrossRef] [PubMed]
22. Casa, D.J.; DeMartini, J.K.; Bergeron, M.F.; Csillan, D.; Eichner, E.R.; Lopez, R.M.; Ferrara, M.S.; Miller, K.C.; O'Connor, F.; Sawka, M.N.; et al. National Athletic Trainers' Association Position Statement: Exertional Heat Illnesses. *J. Athl. Train.* **2015**, *50*, 986–1000. [CrossRef]
23. Hoffman, M.D.; Stuempfle, K.J. Is Sodium Supplementation Necessary to Avoid Dehydration During Prolonged Exercise in the Heat? *J. Strength Cond. Res.* **2016**, *30*, 615–620. [CrossRef]
24. Hoffman, M.D.; Stuempfle, K.J. Hydration Strategies, Weight Change and Performance in a 161 Km Ultramarathon. *Res. Sports Med.* **2014**, *22*, 213–225. [CrossRef]
25. Périard, J.D.; Racinais, S.; Timpka, T.; Dahlström, Ö.; Spreco, A.; Jacobsson, J.; Bargoria, V.; Halje, K.; Alonso, J.-M. Strategies and Factors Associated with Preparing for Competing in the Heat: A Cohort Study at the 2015 IAAF World Athletics Championships. *Br. J. Sports Med.* **2017**, *51*, 264–270. [CrossRef]
26. Racinais, S.; Moussay, S.; Nichols, D.; Travers, G.; Belfekih, T.; Schumacher, Y.O.; Periard, J.D. Core Temperature up to 41.5 °C during the UCI Road Cycling World Championships in the Heat. *Br. J. Sports Med.* **2019**, *53*, 426–429. [CrossRef]
27. Millet, G.Y. Can Neuromuscular Fatigue Explain Running Strategies and Performance in Ultra-Marathons? *Sports Med.* **2011**, *41*, 489–506. [CrossRef]
28. Driscoll, T.R.; Cripps, R.; Brotherhood, J.R. Heat-Related Injuries Resulting in Hospitalisation in Australian Sport. *J. Sci. Med. Sport* **2008**, *11*, 40–47. [CrossRef] [PubMed]
29. Yankelson, L.; Sadeh, B.; Gershovitz, L.; Werthein, J.; Heller, K.; Halpern, P.; Halkin, A.; Adler, A.; Steinvil, A.; Viskin, S. Life-Threatening Events during Endurance Sports: Is Heat Stroke More Prevalent than Arrhythmic Death? *J. Am. Coll. Cardiol.* **2014**, *64*, 463–469. [CrossRef] [PubMed]

30. Périard, J.D.; Racinais, S.; Sawka, M.N. Adaptations and Mechanisms of Human Heat Acclimation: Applications for Competitive Athletes and Sports. *Scand. J. Med. Sci. Sports* **2015**, *25* (Suppl. 1), 20–38.
31. Guy, J.H.; Deakin, G.B.; Edwards, A.M.; Miller, C.M.; Pyne, D.B. Adaptation to Hot Environmental Conditions: An Exploration of the Performance Basis, Procedures and Future Directions to Optimise Opportunities for Elite Athletes. *Sports Med.* **2015**, *45*, 303–311.
32. Ely, M.R.; Cheuvront, S.N.; Roberts, W.O.; Montain, S.J. Impact of Weather on Marathon-Running Performance. *Med. Sci. Sports Exerc.* **2007**, *39*, 487–493.
33. Racinais, S.; Périard, J.D.; Karlsen, A.; Nybo, L. Effect of Heat and Heat Acclimatization on Cycling Time Trial Performance and Pacing. *Med. Sci. Sports Exerc.* **2015**, *47*, 601–606.
34. Tyler, C.J.; Sunderland, C.; Cheung, S.S. The Effect of Cooling Prior to and during Exercise on Exercise Performance and Capacity in the Heat: A Meta-Analysis. *Br. J. Sports Med.* **2015**, *49*, 7–13.
35. Bongers, C.C.W.G.; Thijssen, D.H.J.; Veltmeijer, M.T.W.; Hopman, M.T.E.; Eijsvogels, T.M.H. Precooling and Percooling (Cooling during Exercise) Both Improve Performance in the Heat: A Meta-Analytical Review. *Br. J. Sports Med.* **2015**, *49*, 377–384.
36. Racinais, S.; Ihsan, M.; Taylor, L.; Cardinale, M.; Adami, P.E.; Alonso, J.M.; Bouscaren, N.; Buitrago, S.; Esh, C.J.; Gomez-Ezeiza, J.; et al. Hydration and Cooling in Elite Athletes: Relationship with Performance, Body Mass Loss and Body Temperatures during the Doha 2019 IAAF World Athletics Championships. *Br. J. Sports Med.* **2021**.
37. Gosling, C.M.; Gabbe, B.J.; McGivern, J.; Forbes, A.B. The Incidence of Heat Casualties in Sprint Triathlon: The Tale of Two Melbourne Race Events. *J. Sci. Med. Sport* **2008**, *11*, 52–57.
38. Lavoué, C.; Siracusa, J.; Chalchat, É.; Bourrilhon, C.; Charlot, K. Analysis of Food and Fluid Intake in Elite Ultra-Endurance Runners during a 24-h World Championship. *J. Int. Soc. Sports Nutr.* **2020**, *17*, 36.
39. Costa, R.J.; Teixeira, A.; Rama, L.; Swancott, A.J.; Hardy, L.D.; Lee, B.; Camões-Costa, V.; Gill, S.; Waterman, J.P.; Freeth, E.C.; et al. Water and Sodium Intake Habits and Status of Ultra-Endurance Runners during a Multi-Stage Ultra-Marathon Conducted in a Hot Ambient Environment: An Observational Field Based Study. *Nutr. J.* **2013**, *12*, 13.
40. Sawka, M.N.; Cheuvront, S.N.; Kenefick, R.W. Hypohydration and Human Performance: Impact of Environment and Physiological Mechanisms. *Sports Med.* **2015**, *45* (Suppl. 1), 51–60.
41. Lipman, G.S.; Shea, K.; Christensen, M.; Phillips, C.; Burns, P.; Higbee, R.; Koskenoja, V.; Eifling, K.; Krabak, B.J. Ibuprofen versus Placebo Effect on Acute Kidney Injury in Ultramarathons: A Randomised Controlled Trial. *Emerg. Med. J. EMJ* **2017**, *34*, 637–642.
42. McCubbin, A.J.; Allanson, B.A.; Caldwell Odgers, J.N.; Cort, M.M.; Costa, R.J.S.; Cox, G.R.; Crawshay, S.T.; Desbrow, B.; Freney, E.G.; Gaskell, S.K.; et al. Sports Dietitians Australia Position Statement: Nutrition for Exercise in Hot Environments. *Int. J. Sport Nutr. Exerc. Metab.* **2020**, *30*, 83–98.

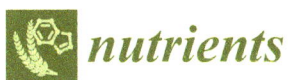

Article

Change in Exercise Performance and Markers of Acute Kidney Injury Following Heat Acclimation with Permissive Dehydration

Arpie Haroutounian [1], Fabiano T. Amorim [2], Todd A. Astorino [3], Nazareth Khodiguian [1], Katharine M. Curtiss [1], Aaron R. D. Matthews [1], Michael J. Estrada [1], Zachary Fennel [2], Zachary McKenna [2], Roberto Nava [2] and Ailish C. Sheard [1,*]

[1] School of Kinesiology, Nutrition, and Food Science, California State University Los Angeles, Los Angeles, CA 90032, USA; aharout4@calstatela.edu (A.H.); nkhodig@exchange.calstatela.edu (N.K.); kcurtiss2019@gmail.com (K.M.C.); amatth10@calstatela.edu (A.R.D.M.); m.estrada9208@gmail.com (M.J.E.)

[2] Department of Health, Exercise, and Sports Sciences, University of New Mexico, Albuquerque, NM 87131, USA; amorim@unm.edu (F.T.A.); zfennel@unm.edu (Z.F.); zmckenna@unm.edu (Z.M.); rnavabjj@unm.edu (R.N.)

[3] Department of Kinesiology, California State University San Marcos, San Marcos, CA 92096, USA; astorino@csusm.edu

* Correspondence: asheard@calstatela.edu; Tel.: +1-323-343-5334

Citation: Haroutounian, A.; Amorim, F.T.; Astorino, T.A.; Khodiguian, N.; Curtiss, K.M.; Matthews, A.R.D.; Estrada, M.J.; Fennel, Z.; McKenna, Z.; Nava, R.; et al. Change in Exercise Performance and Markers of Acute Kidney Injury Following Heat Acclimation with Permissive Dehydration. *Nutrients* 2021, 13, 841. https://doi.org/10.3390/nu13030841

Academic Editors: Douglas J. Casa and Stavros Kavouras

Received: 25 January 2021
Accepted: 25 February 2021
Published: 4 March 2021

Publisher's Note: MDPI stays neutral with regard to jurisdictional claims in published maps and institutional affiliations.

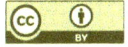

Copyright: © 2021 by the authors. Licensee MDPI, Basel, Switzerland. This article is an open access article distributed under the terms and conditions of the Creative Commons Attribution (CC BY) license (https://creativecommons.org/licenses/by/4.0/).

Abstract: Implementing permissive dehydration (DEH) during short-term heat acclimation (HA) may accelerate adaptations to the heat. However, HA with DEH may augment risk for acute kidney injury (AKI). This study investigated the effect of HA with permissive DEH on time-trial performance and markers of AKI. Fourteen moderately trained men (age and VO_{2max} = 25 ± 0.5 yr and 51.6 ± 1.8 mL·kg^{-1}·min^{-1}) were randomly assigned to DEH or euhydration (EUH). Time-trial performance and VO_{2max} were assessed in a temperate environment before and after 7 d of HA. Heat acclimation consisted of 90 min of cycling in an environmental chamber (40 °C, 35% RH). Neutrophil gelatinase-associated lipocalin (NGAL) and kidney injury molecule-1 (KIM-1) were assessed pre- and post-exercise on day 1 and day 7 of HA. Following HA, VO_{2max} did not change in either group (p = 0.099); however, time-trial performance significantly improved (3%, p < 0.01) with no difference between groups (p = 0.485). Compared to pre-exercise, NGAL was not significantly different following day 1 and 7 of HA (p = 0.113) with no difference between groups (p = 0.667). There was a significant increase in KIM-1 following day 1 and 7 of HA (p = 0.002) with no difference between groups (p = 0.307). Heat acclimation paired with permissive DEH does not amplify improvements in VO_{2max} or time-trial performance in a temperate environment versus EUH and does not increase markers of AKI.

Keywords: heat acclimation; dehydration; kidney injury; performance

1. Introduction

Heat acclimation allows athletes, military personnel, and occupational workers to adapt to heat stress by enhancing performance and thermal tolerance to future heat exposure [1,2] and reducing the risk of heat illness [ ]. For example, heat acclimation significantly increases exercise performance when exercise is performed in a hot environment [,]; however, it is unclear whether heat acclimation improves exercise performance and VO_{2max} in a cool or temperate environment [,]. The process of heat acclimation involves various whole-body [,] and cellular changes [ ] which are dependent on the frequency, duration, and level of thermal strain of the protocol [,]. It is reported that reductions in core and skin temperature typically occur by the fifth day [,], while increases in sweat rate usually develop by the tenth day of heat acclimation [,]. In addition, reduced heart rate and increased plasma volume (PV) occur within the first

3–6 days of heat acclimation [10,11,13,14]. In fact, 75–80% of these whole-body physiological changes occur within 4–7 days of heat acclimation [14–16]. However, the traditional 10–14-day timeframe implemented to elicit heat acclimation [7,17–19] may be too time consuming and impractical to employ in non-laboratory settings [13,20]. Furthermore, it has been suggested that implementing permissive dehydration during short-term heat acclimation, which is defined as restricting fluid intake during exercise to a point of modest dehydration (2–3% total body water loss), may accelerate adaptations to the heat [6].

Repeated fluid restriction during heat acclimation may expedite the onset of physiological changes because of the interrelationship between heat strain and dehydration [21–23]. For example, permissive dehydration during five consecutive days of heat acclimation in trained athletes increases sweat rate and electrolyte retention, expands PV, and accelerates cardiovascular and thermoregulatory adaptations similar to longer duration heat acclimation [6,20,24]. Also, the implementation of a heat acclimation and permissive dehydration protocol significantly increased lactate threshold and power output during a 20-km time-trial (TT) [20], and improved peak power output (PPO) during a VO_{2max} test in a temperate environment [13,20]. However, Neal et al. [13] concluded that heat acclimation paired with permissive dehydration did not lead to superior adaptations compared to euhydration. Consequently, the practicality and ergogenic potential of heat acclimation and permissive dehydration in accelerating adaptations or improving performance in a temperate environment is less clear and warrants further investigation.

Repeated exposure to heat stress and dehydration has been suggested to result in chronic kidney disease. Wesseling et al. [25] reported a marked prevalence of chronic kidney disease in male outdoor workers chronically exposed to dehydration and heavy physical exertion. In the context of endurance exercise, recent studies suggest an increase in early markers of acute kidney injury (AKI) when exercise is repeatedly performed in hot environments [26–28]. For example, markers of AKI such as plasma neutrophil gelatinase-associated lipocalin (NGAL) is significantly elevated with increasing ambient and core temperature (T_c) and in response to dehydration in firefighters [29]. Urinary NGAL is significantly expressed in injured epithelial cells and urinary increases may indicate renal tubular damage [30]. In addition, others have shown elevated levels of kidney injury molecule-1 (KIM-1) during an ultra-distance run and following a marathon [31,32]. Kidney injury molecule-1 is a glycoprotein not expressed in healthy kidneys [33] but increases in urinary KIM-1 may indicate proximal tubule injury [34]. Despite this evidence relating to exercise, heat exposure, and increases in markers of AKI, only a few studies have explored the effect of heat acclimation/acclimatization on AKI [27,28,35,36]. In addition, it is not known if heat acclimation paired with permissive dehydration may exacerbate AKI.

Thus, the purpose of this study was to investigate the effect of moderate-term heat acclimation (7 days) with permissive dehydration on changes in exercise performance and VO_{2max} in a temperate environment in moderately trained men. A secondary purpose was to assess markers of AKI following heat acclimation and permissive dehydration. It was hypothesized that 7 days of heat acclimation paired with permissive dehydration would improve VO_{2max} and exercise performance in a temperate environment when compared to euhydration; however, this protocol would have a deleterious effect on kidney function represented by elevations in markers of AKI compared to a euhydrated state. The results of the present study will elucidate whether heat acclimation paired with permissive dehydration is efficacious in increasing endurance performance for individuals competing in a temperate environment and whether it is a safe strategy in regard to markers of kidney injury.

2. Materials and Methods

2.1. Participants

Fourteen healthy, moderately trained men were randomly assigned to either the dehydration (DEH) (*n* = 7) or euhydration (EUH) (*n* = 7) condition. All participants were engaged in moderate-to-vigorous cycling, running, and/or resistance training an average of

5 d/wk within the last year but were not competitive athletes. The participants completed a health history questionnaire to determine that they were free of cardiovascular and metabolic disease and have no current musculoskeletal injury. Written informed consent was obtained from all participants involved in the study, and procedures were approved by the California State University, Los Angeles Institutional Review Board (1066319-5).

2.2. Experimental Design

All testing was conducted in Los Angeles, CA during January–May (average ambient temperature and humidity were equal to 16 °C and 65% RH, respectively) to ensure that subjects were not naturally heat acclimatized. Preliminary testing consisted of completion of a VO_{2max} test, two familiarization 16-km TTs, and one 16-km TT in a temperate environment (22 °C; 40% RH) followed by a heat-tolerance test in a hot and dry environment (40 °C; 30% RH). One week after preliminary testing, subjects began the 7-d heat acclimation protocol in either a EUH or DEH condition. All post-testing including assessment of VO_{2max}, 16-km TT, and the heat-tolerance test, was conducted following day 7 of heat acclimation, and each trial was separated by at least 24 h. The experimental procedures are summarized in Figure 1.

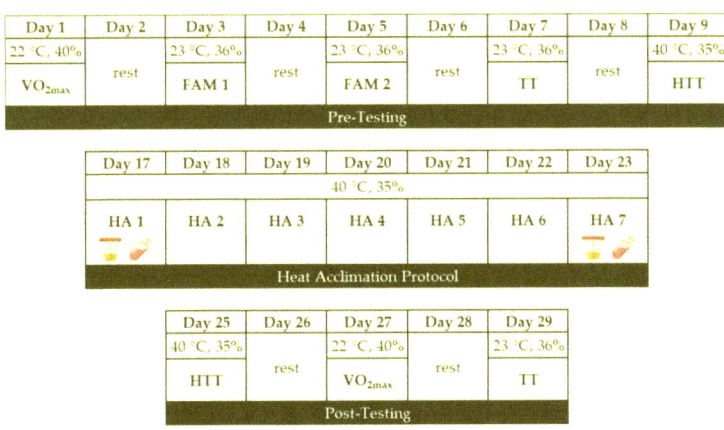

Figure 1. Experimental protocol undertaken by the participants. VO_{2max}, maximal oxygen consumption; FAM, familiarization 16-km cycling time-trial; TT, 16-km cycling time-trial; HTT, heat tolerance test; HA, heat acclimation; urine collection and blood draw before and after the HA session.

All trials occurred at the same time of day, and training logs were completed by each participant prior to all visits. Participants were asked to refrain from strenuous aerobic or resistance training exercise and alcohol ingestion 24 h prior to testing. All participants were instructed to continue their regular training regimen throughout the study, and during heat acclimation they were asked to refrain from any additional lower-body exercise during the seven consecutive days. Prior to all trials, participants provided a urine sample to assess urine specific gravity (USG) (Atago 4410 Digital USG Refractometer, Atago USA Inc, Bellevue, WA, USA) which was used to determine hydration status. If participants were not well hydrated (USG $\geq$ 1.020 g/mL) upon arrival to the laboratory, they were asked to consume 500 mL of water, followed by a second USG assessment 30 min later. Nude body weight was assessed prior to each test after voiding using an electronic scale (Model 220, Seca, Danville, VA, USA).

2.3. Experimental Procedures

2.3.1. Maximal Oxygen Consumption

To determine VO_{2max}, participants cycled on an electronically-braked cycle ergometer (Velotron DynaFit Pro, RacerMate, Spearfish, SD) at 60 W for two minutes and work rate increased 30 W every minute until volitional fatigue. Heart rate (HR) was monitored continuously via telemetry (Polar Electro, model FS1, Woodbury, NY, USA), and rating of perceived exertion (RPE) was measured every minute using a 6–20 scale [37]. Breath-by-breath gas exchange data were continuously measured (Cosmed, Quark CPET, Rome, Italy) and VO_{2max} was recorded as the highest average value over any 15-s period. Ten minutes following the incremental test, a VO_{2max} verification test was performed at a constant load of 105% of the peak power output achieved during the incremental VO_{2max} test until the subject attained volitional fatigue [38,39]. This test was used to confirm attainment of VO_{2max} if the verification VO_{2max} was no more than 5.5% higher than the incremental value [40].

2.3.2. Cycling Time-Trial

Participants completed a total of four 16-km TTs, two of which were categorized as familiarization trials, all separated by a minimum of 24 h. The TT began with a 10-min warm-up at 75 W followed by a 16 km TT (flat course; Velotron RacerMate 3-D Software, Quarq, Spearfish, SD) in a temperate environment (23 °C; 36% RH). Two familiarization trials were performed to minimize any learning effect. Participants were given verbal encouragement and were aware of the distance covered throughout the TT but were blinded to total time, power output, and HR. Heart rate and RPE were measured every 1.6 km, and water was provided ad libitum. The intraclass correlation coefficient and coefficient of variation (CV) for 16-km performance time were equal to 0.87% and 1.84%, respectively. The CV between familiarization trials is similar to values reported in previous studies [19,20,41,42].

2.3.3. Heat Tolerance Test

Participants arrived at the lab after an overnight fast and ingested a standardized breakfast (unfrosted blueberry or strawberry Pop Tart) which contained 210 kcal (5 g fat, 37 g carbohydrate, and 2 g protein) immediately prior to entering the hot room. Subsequently, participants cycled for 60 min in a hot and dry environment (40 °C, 35% RH) at 35% PPO. Every 15 minutes, 250 mL of room temperature water (23 °C) was ingested to replace fluid loss with a total of 1000 mL consumed during the heat tolerance test [6,13]. Core temperature was measured using a rectal thermistor (Model 4TH, Telly Thermometer, Yellow Springs, OH, USA) which was inserted 8–10 cm beyond the anal sphincter. Core temperature, HR, thermal sensation (using a 7-point scale), and RPE were recorded every 5 min. Prior to and following the heat tolerance test, USG and dry nude body were recorded to determine hydration status and whole-body sweat rate, respectively.

2.3.4. Heat Acclimation Protocol

One week after the heat tolerance test, participants initiated the 7-d heat acclimation protocol. Immediately prior to exercise, participants consumed the same standardized breakfast as described above. Participants cycled on a cycle ergometer (Monark Ergomedic 828E, Varberg, Sweden) for 90 min in a hot and dry environment (40 °C, 35% RH). A controlled hyperthermia protocol was implemented, and T_c was maintained within a range of 38.5–38.7 °C [20]. Participants were asked to select a workload eliciting a RPE of 15 which was maintained by adjusting either resistance or cycling cadence until a T_c of 38.3 °C was attained, at which point workload was adjusted by the researchers for the remainder of the 90 min protocol to ensure that the target T_c was maintained. Participants assigned to the EUH group consumed 1750 mL of room temperature water (23 °C) in 250 mL boluses at rest and every 15 min during each heat acclimation trial [6,13]; in contrast, individuals assigned to the permissive DEH group were not allowed to consume water during the 90 min heat acclimation bout in order to promote dehydration. Core temperature, HR, thermal sensation, and RPE were recorded every 5 min. Upon session completion, dry nude body weight and urine volume were recorded.

2.3.5. Blood Sampling

Pre-and post-exercise on day 1 and 7 of heat acclimation, blood samples were drawn from the antecubital vein after 20 min of seated rest using a sterile winged push button needle and placed into sterile vacutainers containing 18 mg EDTA (Becton, Dickinson and Company, Franklin Lakes, NJ, USA). Hematocrit (Hct) was measured in triplicate by centrifuging three micro-hematocrit capillary tubes (Fisher Scientific, Pittsburg, PA) at 12,000 rpm for 5 min. Hematocrit was then determined by placing the centrifuged tubes into a micro-hematocrit capillary tube reader (Lancer, Spiracrit, St. Louis, MO, USA). The Hct was corrected by 0.96 for trapped plasma. Hemoglobin (Hb) concentration was analyzed using the HemoCue 201$^+$ Analyzer (Brea, CA, USA) and measured in triplicate. Plasma volume expansion from day 1 and day 7 of heat acclimation was calculated using pre-exercise Hct and Hb measurements [ ]. A 250 µL aliquot sample of plasma was analyzed in triplicate via freezing point depression using an osmometer (Advance Instruments, Inc., The Advanced Osmometer, Model, 3D3, Norwood, MA, USA).

2.3.6. Assessment of Hydration Level and Markers of Kidney Function

The urine sample was collected in sterile polypropylene tubes pre-and post-exercise on day 1 and day 7 of heat acclimation. Urine KIM-1 (#ADI-900-226-0001, Enzo Life Sciences, Farmingdale, NY, USA) and NGAL (#BPD-KIT-036, BioPorto Diagnostics, Needham, MA, USA) were measured using commercially available enzyme-linked immunosorbent assays. All measurements were performed in duplicate with intra-assay CVs of 10.8% for KIM-1 and 6.8% for NGAL, respectively.

2.4. Statistical Analyses

All data are expressed as mean ± SD and were analyzed using IBM SPSS Version 25 (Armonk, NY, USA). Independent t-tests were used to examine differences in baseline values between groups. Normality for all variables was determined using the Shapiro-Wilks test. To identify differences in VO_{2max}, TT performance, power output, HR, T_c, sweat rate, PV expansion, RPE, and thermal sensation, a repeated measures ANOVA was used, with group (EUH vs. DEH) as the between-subjects variable and time (pre-post) as the within-subjects variable. Similarly, a repeated measures ANOVA was used to assess changes in USG, urine osmolality, NGAL, and KIM-1 from day 1 to day 7 of heat acclimation. The Greenhouse-Geisser statistic was used if the assumption of sphericity was not met. If a significant F ratio was obtained, a Tukey's post-hoc test was used to identify differences between means. Cohen's d was used as a measure of effect size. Statistical significance was set at $p < 0.05$. An a priori power analysis was conducted to examine the within-subjects change in TT performance from pre-to-post-heat acclimation. A sample size of twelve subjects ($n = 6$ per group) would provide sufficient power at an alpha level of 0.05 and power of 0.80.

3. Results

3.1. Heat Acclimation

There were no differences ($p > 0.05$) in any parameter between groups at baseline (Table). Changes in thermal strain from day 1 to day 7 of heat acclimation are shown in Table . Resting HR and T_c decreased from day 1 to day 7 of heat acclimation in both groups ($p = 0.005$ and $p = 0.007$, respectively), but there was no difference between groups ($p = 1.00$). A significant main effect for time was found for sweat rate from day 1 versus day 7 ($p = 0.002$) in both groups, but no interaction was observed ($p = 0.293$). Exercise time to attain T_c equal to 38.5 °C was significantly longer by day 7 in both groups ($p = 0.012$) but did not differ between groups ($p = 0.157$). Target T_c was well-maintained throughout heat acclimation with no T_c differences in either group ($p = 0.804$). There was no significant main effect for average HR from day 1 to day 7 ($p = 0.067$) and no differences were observed between groups ($p = 0.44$). The EUH group lost <1% body weight during heat acclimation from pre-post exercise on day 1 and day 7, while the DEH group lost 2.2% body weight on day 1 and 2.6% on day 7. Seven days of heat acclimation resulted in a significant PV expansion (Table 2) equal to 16% in the EUH group and 9% in DEH group ($p < 0.05$), but there was no difference between groups ($p = 0.156$). There was a significant reduction in Hct and Hb in both groups from day 1 to day 7 of heat acclimation ($p = 0.001$; $p < 0.001$), but no interaction between groups was observed ($p = 0.277$; $p = 0.271$).

Table 1. Physical characteristics of participants (mean ± SD).

Group	Age (yr)	Body Height (cm)	Body Weight (kg)	VO$_{2max}$ (mL × kg^{-1} × min^{-1})	VO$_{2max}$ (L × min^{-1})
EUH	25 ± 2	174.3 ± 3.8	77.9 ± 6.7	52.9 ± 7.1	4.2 ± 0.9
DEH	26 ± 7	172.4 ± 8.8	74.1 ± 11.2	50.3 ± 8.5	3.7 ± 0.3
p-value	0.813	0.612	0.453	0.554	0.213

EUH, euhydrated; DEH, dehydrated.

Table 2. Cardiovascular and thermoregulatory changes on day 1 and day 7 of heat acclimation (mean ± SD).

Parameter	EUH		DEH	
	Day 1	Day 7	Day 1	Day 7
Resting HR (b × min^{-1})	59 ± 9	54 ± 10	58 ± 7	53 ± 6
Resting T$_c$ (°C)	37.2 ± 0.2	37.0 ± 0.2	37.0 ± 0.3	36.9 ± 0.3
BW loss (%)	−0.6 ± 0.3	−0.8 ± 0.4	−2.2 ± 0.8	−2.6 ± 0.5
Sweat rate (L × h^{-1})	1.78 ± 0.18	2.01 ± 0.28	1.59 ± 0.27	1.72 ± 0.28
Average HR (b × min^{-1})	150 ± 15	148 ± 18	150 ± 7	145 ± 5
T$_c$ final 60 (°C)	38.7 ± 0.2	38.6 ± 0.1	38.7 ± 0.2	38.6 ± 0.1
Time to 38.5 °C (min)	30 ± 5.1	34 ± 5.4	29 ± 9.4	40 ± 12.8
Hct (%)	46.7 ± 0.9	43.3 ± 2.7	44.6 ± 3.1	42.6 ± 2.9
Hb (g/dL)	15.8 ± 0.6	14.5 ± 0.9	14.9 ± 0.8	14.2 ± 0.8
PV expansion (%)		16.5 ± 12.0		9.2 ± 4.0

EUH, euhydrated; DEH, dehydrated; HR, heart rate; T$_c$, core temperature; BW, body weight; Hct, hematocrit; Hb, hemoglobin; PV, plasma volume.

3.2. Heat Tolerance

Only six participants in the EUH group and six participants in the DEH group performed the heat-tolerance test and the changes in physiological responses are shown in Table 3. End-exercise HR during the heat tolerance test was significantly reduced in both groups following 7 days of HA ($p = 0.026$). End-exercise HR decreased following heat acclimation in both groups (EUH 163 ± 13 b × min^{-1} to 152 ± 14 b × min^{-1}; DEH 166 ± 9 b × min^{-1} to 143 ± 9 b × min^{-1}). Tukey's post-hoc test revealed a greater reduction in end-exercise HR in the DEH group ($p = < 0.05$, d = 1.75). End-T$_c$ pre-post heat tolerance test was significantly reduced in both groups ($p = 0.007$), but no interaction between groups ($p = 0.545$). Both groups revealed a nonsignificant increase (5% and 6% in DEH and EUH) in sweat rate from pre-post heat acclimation ($p = 0.412$), with no difference between groups ($p = 0.773$).

Table 3. Physiological responses during the heat tolerance test following 7 days of heat acclimation (mean ± SD).

Parameter	EUH		DEH	
	Pre	Post	Pre	Post
HTT$_{end}$ HR (b × min^{-1})	163 ± 13	152 ± 14	166 ± 9	143 ± 9 [†]
HTT$_{end}$ T$_c$ (°C)	38.7 ± 0.4	38.4 ± 0.3	38.8 ± 0.4	38.3 ± 0.3
HTT sweat rate (L × h^{-1})	1.38 ± 0.11	1.47 ± 0.22	1.06 ± 0.25	1.11 ± 0.42

EUH, euhydrated; DEH, dehydrated; HTT, heat tolerance test; HR, heart rate; T$_c$, core temperature; [†] indicating a significant interaction, $p < 0.05$. $n = 6$ in the EUH group and $n = 6$ in the DEH group.

3.3. Changes in VO_{2max} and Time-Trial Performance in Response to Heat Acclimation

There was no difference in VO_{2max} in response to heat acclimation ($p = 0.099$) and no significant interaction between groups ($p = 0.491$). However, there was a significant time effect for PPO ($p = 0.001$), yet no differences in maximal HR ($p = 0.068$) or RPE ($p = 0.183$) in either group following heat acclimation (Table). Seven days of heat acclimation led to a 3% improvement in TT performance in both groups ($p < 0.01$; d = 2.45, d = 3.04), but no interaction was revealed ($p = 0.485$). Peak power output during the TT was not different following 7 days of heat acclimation ($p = 0.374$); however, mean power output was significantly increased in both groups ($p < 0.01$, d = 2.64, d = 2.79), with no interaction between groups ($p = 0.865$). End-exercise HR during the TT did not change in response to heat acclimation ($p = 0.766$, $p = 0.147$). However, average RPE during the TT was significantly different in both groups following heat acclimation ($p = 0.004$), but no interaction was revealed ($p = 0.429$; Table).

Table 4. Effect of 7 days of heat acclimation on maximal oxygen consumption and 16-km cycling time-trial performance (mean ± SD).

Parameter	EUH		DEH	
	Pre	Post	Pre	Post
VO_{2max} (mL × kg^{-1} × min^{-1})	52.9 ± 7.1	54.8 ± 6.2	50.3 ± 8.5	51.1 ± 8.2
VO_{2max} (L × min^{-1})	4.2 ± 1.0	4.3 ± 0.9	3.7 ± 0.3	3.7 ± 0.3
HR_{max} (b × min^{-1})	186 ± 9	183 ± 6	184 ± 8	178 ± 8
VO_{2max} PPO (W)	351 ± 24	372 ± 29	332 ± 25	348 ± 36
TT time (s)	1692.9 ± 57.8	1645.4 ± 53.7	1777.3 ± 63.7	1718.3 ± 51.2
TT average PO (W)	217 ± 21	233 ± 20	191 ± 16	208 ± 15
TT end HR (b × min^{-1})	185 ± 9	183 ± 10	180 ± 13	181 ± 9
TT average RPE	15 ± 1	16 ± 1	14 ± 1	15 ± 1

EUH, euhydrated; DEH, dehydrated; VO_{2max}, maximal oxygen consumption; TT, 16-km cycling time-trial; HR, heart rate; PPO, peak power output; PO, power output; RPE, rating of perceived exertion.

3.4. Markers of Dehydration and Kidney Function

One blood sample from the EUH group was missing during data analysis. Urine specific gravity increased from pre-to-post exercise on day 1 and 7 of heat acclimation ($p = 0.011$), but there was no interaction ($p = 0.200$). Plasma osmolality significantly increased from pre-to-post exercise on day 1 and 7 ($p = 0.009$), and there was a significant interaction between groups ($p = 0.044$). Tukey's post-hoc test revealed a greater increase in plasma osmolality in the DEH group ($p < 0.05$, d = 2.23; Table). Compared to pre-exercise, urine NGAL was not significantly increased following day 1 and 7 of heat acclimation ($p = 0.113$) and there was no significant interaction between groups ($p = 0.667$). However, there was a significant increase in urine KIM-1 following day 1 and 7 of heat acclimation ($p = 0.002$), but no interaction occurred ($p = 0.307$; Figure). It should be noted one participant's pre-exercise urine sample from the DEH group was lost during data collection.

Table 5. Urine and kidney markers following 7 days of heat acclimation (mean ± SD).

Parameter	EUH Day 1		EUH Day 7	
	Pre	Post	Pre	Post
USG (g/mL)	1.007 ± 0.003	1.009 ± 0.004	1.005 ± 0.003	1.014 ± 0.007
Plasma osmolality (mOsm/kg)	300 ± 4	299 ± 2	298 ± 6	300 ± 3 [†]

Parameter	DEH Day 1		DEH Day 7	
	Pre	Post	Pre	Post
USG (g/mL)	1.006 ± 0.005	1.012 ± 0.008	1.006 ± 0.005	1.009 ± 0.007
Plasma osmolality (mOsm/kg)	301 ± 5	307 ± 6	301 ± 4	308 ± 3 [†]

EUH, euhydrated; DEH, dehydrated; USG, urine specific gravity; [†] indicating a significant interaction, $p < 0.05$. $n = 6$ for the EUH group was assessed for plasma osmolality.

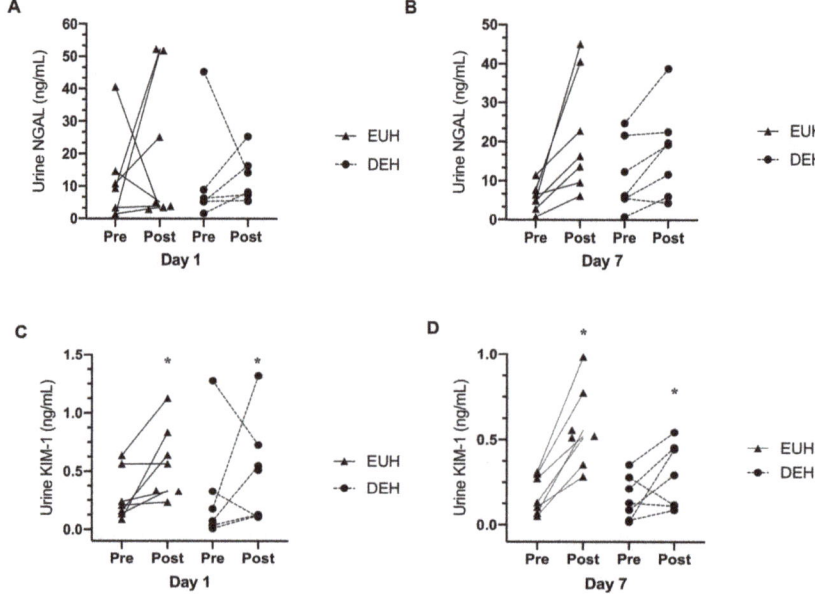

Figure 2. Individual data for kidney injury markers before and after 7 days of heat acclimation. (**A**) urinary neutrophil gelatinase-associated lipocalin (NGAL) response before and after day 1 of heat acclimation; (**B**) NGAL response before and after day 7 of heat acclimation; (**C**) urine kidney injury molecule-1 (KIM-1) response before and after day 1 of heat acclimation; (**D**) KIM-1 response before and after day 7 of heat acclimation; EUH, euhydrated; DEH, dehydrated; * indicating a significant main effect, $p < 0.05$. $n = 6$ for the DEH group was assessed for urine NGAL and KIM-1.

4. Discussion

Heat acclimation has repeatedly been shown to induce thermoregulatory changes which improve tolerance to exercise in a hot environment [7,24,44] However, it is unclear whether undergoing heat acclimation with permissive dehydration is an effective approach to increase endurance performance in a temperate environment more so than with adequate hydration. Further, the impact of heat acclimation with permissive dehydration on markers of AKI is unknown. Our findings suggest that (1) thermoregulatory adaptations from 7 days of heat acclimation occur independent of hydration, (2) this approach of heat acclimation does not lead to increases in VO_{2max}, (3) exercise performance in a temperate environment is increased independent of hydration, and (4) a heat acclimation protocol associated with DEH did not increase markers of AKI.

There has been increased interest in examining the feasibility of short-term heat acclimation protocols [, , , ,]; however, many studies recruited well-trained participants and only two studies employed short-term heat acclimation and permissive dehydration in comparison to euhydration [,]. In the present study, we recruited moderately trained participants who completed a 7-day controlled hyperthermia protocol. Results showed that both groups observed a similar increase in sweat rate from day 1 to day 7 equal to 13% in the EUH group, and 8% in the DEH group. This suggests that our protocol did provide a stimulus for sudomotor adaptation, but hydration does not mediate changes in sweat rate. Resting HR significantly decreased in both groups following heat acclimation, and there was a significant reduction in resting T_c by the 7th day of heat acclimation, with no differences between groups. End-exercise HR and end-exercise T_c during the heat tolerance test were significantly reduced after heat acclimation, which corroborates previous studies [, ,]. Our findings demonstrate that 7 days of exercise in the heat result in cardiovascular and thermoregulatory adaptations, as shown in other studies [, ,]; however, permissive dehydration did not result in greater improvements in comparison to euhydration, supporting previous findings in well-trained participants [ ].

As a result of exercising in the heat, participants in the DEH group lost ~2.4% of body weight on day 1 and day 7 of heat acclimation, which supports prior findings [, ,], and plasma osmolality significantly increased following permissive dehydration. This level of dehydration significantly increases electrolyte and water retention [ ], which may lead to greater thermoregulatory and cardiovascular adaptations following heat acclimation and improved fluid balance in comparison to euhydration [ ]. However, participants were dehydrated for a minimal duration during exercise and this did not induce superior changes in resting and exercise HR or T_c, PV expansion, or improvements in exercise performance. Pethick et al., [ ] reported that a 1.5–2% BW loss for 10 h during 5 days of heat acclimation did not further expand PV or improve TT performance. Additionally, Travers et al., [ ] concluded that maintaining euhydration during heat acclimation reduced skin temperature and enhanced sweat rate and TT performance in the heat when compared to dehydration (~3% BW loss). Thus, dehydration during heat acclimation may not enhance heat adaptations or performance outcomes.

Permissive dehydration during short-term heat acclimation has been shown to accelerate physiological adaptations in trained participants due to increased electrolyte retention, PV expansion, and reducing cardiovascular and thermal strain [,]. However, our findings support data from Neal et al. [ ] who showed that permissive dehydration does not further augment changes in HR, T_c, or sweat rate during heat acclimation or further improve VO_{2max} or exercise performance in a temperate environment. One explanation for this result is that maintaining high cardiorespiratory fitness reduces the physiological strain imposed by mild hypohydration [ ] and it is apparent that trained individuals will require greater fluid regulatory strain than individuals who are less fit [ ]. Our participants had a lower VO_{2max} (~51.6 mL $\times$ kg^{-1} $\times$ min^{-1}) than participants in previous studies (~58.5 mL $\times$ kg^{-1} $\times$ min^{-1}) [,], and permissive dehydration did not induce different responses compared to euhydration. However, PPO during the VO_{2max} test and mean power output during the 16-km TT were significantly higher in both the EUH and DEH group, but the mechanism leading to this improvement is unclear as VO_{2max} did not improve in either group.

Our data show that VO_{2max} did not change after 7 days of heat acclimation despite a significant PV expansion, but PPO was increased on average by 19 W, similar to Neal et al. [ ] in response to heat acclimation and permissive dehydration. This result contrasts with data from Lorenzo et al. [ ] who demonstrated that a 6.5% (200 mL) increase in PV resulted with a 5% increase in VO_{2max} after 10 days of exercising in the heat at 50% of VO_{2max}. Our data corroborate other studies showing no effect of heat acclimation on VO_{2max} in either group even in the presence of PV expansion [, ,]. Karlsen et al. [ ]

reported a PV expansion of 15% (559 mL) following 2 weeks of heat acclimatization and a 12% expansion (503 mL) in the control group; however, there were no changes in VO_{2max} tested in a cool environment. Similarly, Keiser et al. [51] reported a PV expansion equal to 6% (201 mL) in participants who were heat acclimated with no change in the control group. Yet, these authors [51] revealed no change in VO_{2max} or TT performance in a temperate environment in either group. It is evident that any expected benefit from an expanded PV is most likely compensated by hemodilution [52] which we showed in the form of reductions in Hb and Hct that may have led to no change in VO_{2max} following heat acclimation.

Both groups exhibited similar improvements in cycling performance and mean power output in a temperate environment following heat acclimation. A previous study [7] revealed similar improvements in cycling performance in both a hot and cool environment in response to 10 days of heat acclimation. Nevertheless, in trained cyclists undergoing a 5-day heat protocol also instituting dehydration, results showed no improvement in 20-km TT performance in a temperate environment following heat acclimation [20]; however, no control group was used. Improvements in temperate TT performance following heat acclimation are believed to be due to a reduction in exercising HR and T_c at any given intensity throughout exercise [53–55]. In addition, we observed a significant increase in sweat rate during heat acclimation in both groups and this is likely to have contributed to enhanced evaporative cooling, resulting in improved blood flow to skeletal muscle and likely improved exercise performance in a temperate environment [56]. Although this was not measured in our study, another possible reason for the improvement in temperate cycling performance could be a reduction in muscle glycogen utilization during exercise following heat acclimation [57]. In response to heat stress, skeletal muscle cellular adaptations might occur which may increase mitochondrial biogenesis [58] resulting in enhanced oxidative capacity that may induce improvements in cycling performance. In summary, our data suggest that cycling performance in a temperate environment lasting approximately 25–30 min can be increased through 7 days of heat acclimation, and this adaptation is unaffected by hydration state.

Many studies [27,28,32,35,36,59] have consistently demonstrated increases in AKI markers with an acute bout of exercise completed in the heat or with dehydration. In the present study, there was a significant increase in plasma osmolality in the DEH group pre- and post-heat acclimation on day 1 and 7, but no difference in urine NGAL in either group. A significant increase in urine KIM-1 was observed in both groups from pre- to post-exercise on days 1 and 7 of heat acclimation, but no difference between groups. Although the elevations in these AKI biomarkers have been proposed to indicate intrinsic renal damage, it seems that the mild dehydration (~2.4% body weight loss) and heat strain (T_c = 38.5 °C) implemented in the present study were insufficient to consistently increase markers of AKI. A previous study examining firefighters [29] showed that the change in NGAL is mediated by the magnitude of increase in T_c and the degree of dehydration during exercise in the heat. In the present study, the elevation in T_c was similar between the groups, but body water loss was higher in the DEH group compared to EUH. It is plausible that this moderate dehydration (~2.4% body weight loss) did not result in significant renal ischemia and glomerular dysfunction. In addition, levels of KIM-1 increased pre-to post-exercise on day 1 and day 7 and this response occurred regardless of hydration. An increase in KIM-1 indicates proximal tubule injury and perhaps is more sensitive to AKI in the context of exercise than NGAL. Using creatinine and glomerular filtration rate as markers of AKI, Pryor et al. [28] demonstrated that 6 days of heat acclimation in healthy participants led to a reduction in the number of participants classified with AKI, but overall kidney function remained impaired. Although these two markers are frequently used in clinical settings, the observed increase may not always be indicative of kidney injury in healthy individuals exposed to mild dehydration and heat strain.

A limitation of this study is that we did not have a control group and only recruited male participants. Men and women differ in their thermoregulatory responses during exercise in the heat; therefore, the results of this study may not be generalizable to women.

It is possible that because our participants were moderately fit, the 7-day heat acclimation protocol may have resulted in a training effect independent of the heat stimulus; however, we observed no changes in VO_{2max} after heat acclimation and we made sure that the participants documented and maintained their current exercise regimen throughout the study. Also, any change in VO_{2max} in our study was strengthened by using a verification test which confirmed VO_{2max} attainment before and after heat acclimation. It is possible that a learning effect may lead to increased cycling performance following heat acclimation. However, we implemented two familiarization trials prior to heat acclimation, which ensured that any learning effect would have been eliminated. The present study only examined two AKI markers; thus, the study could be strengthened by assessing markers of kidney function such as creatinine and calculated glomerular filtration rate.

5. Conclusions

Our results suggest that 7 days of heat acclimation does not improve VO_{2max} in moderately trained participants, yet endurance performance was significantly increased; thus, heat acclimation with permissive dehydration did not provide an additional stimulus for improving performance in a temperate environment. Moreover, heat acclimation increased KIM-1, but dehydration did not further increase markers of AKI. Maintaining hydration during exercise in the heat is important, but an increased risk of AKI may not be as prevalent for individuals who experience mild dehydration during exercise in the heat. Future research should continue to explore the incidence of kidney injury in larger groups during acute and chronic exercise in the heat with dehydration as well as examine sex differences and other kidney and inflammatory markers such as serum creatinine, glomerular filtration rate, cytokines, and cortisol.

Author Contributions: Conceptualization, A.C.S., A.H., and F.T.A.; methodology, A.C.S., A.H., F.T.A., T.A.A., and N.K.; validation, A.C.S., A.H., F.T.A.; formal analysis, A.C.S., A.H., F.T.A., T.A.A., N.K., Z.F., Z.M., and R.N.; investigation, A.C.S., A.H., K.M.C., A.R.D.M., and M.J.E.; resources, A.C.S., A.H., and F.T.A.; data curation, A.C.S., A.H., F.T.A., T.A.A., N.K.,K.M.C., A.R.D.M., M.J.E., Z.F., Z.M., R.N.; writing—original draft preparation, A.C.S., A.H., F.T.A., T.A.A., N.K.; writing—review and editing, A.C.S., A.H., F.T.A., T.A.A., N.K., K.M.C., A.R.D.M., M.J.E., Z.F., Z.M., and R.N.; visualization, A.C.S., A.H., and F.T.A.; supervision, A.C.S., A.H., and F.T.A.; project administration, A.C.S., A.H., and F.T.A.; funding acquisition, A.C.S. and A.H. All authors have read and agreed to the published version of the manuscript.

Funding: This research was funded by the Research, Scholarship, and Creative Activities grant from California State University, Los Angeles.

Institutional Review Board Statement: The study was conducted according to the guidelines of the Declaration of Helsinki and approved by the Institutional Review Board of California State University, Los Angeles (protocol code 1066319-5; 02/19/2019).

Informed Consent Statement: Informed consent was obtained from all subjects involved in the study.

Data Availability Statement: Data sharing is not applicable to this article. The participants in this study did not consent to access to this information by third parties for uses outside the scope of this project.

Acknowledgments: The authors would like to thank Michael Cardenas and Alex Moreno for their assistance and expertise in data collection. The authors would also like to thank the participants for their dedication in completing the study.

Conflicts of Interest: The authors declare no conflict of interest. The funders had no role in the design of the study; in the collection, analyses, or interpretation of data; in the writing of the manuscript, or in the decision to publish the results.

References

1. Wenger, C.B. Human heat adaptation to hot environments. In *Medical Aspects of Harsh Environments*; Pandolf, K.B., Burr, R.E., Eds.; Office of the Surgeon General, Department of the Army: Washington, DC, USA, 2001; Volume 1, pp. 51–86.
2. Sawka, M.N.; Wenger, C.B.; Pandolf, K.B. Thermoregulatory responses to acute exercise-heat stress and heat acclimation. In *Handbook of Physiology*; Sec. 4, Environmental Physiology; Fregly, M.J., Blatteis, C.M., Eds.; Oxford University Press: New York, NY, USA, 1996; pp. 157–185.
3. Nunneley, S.A.; Reardon, M.J. Prevention of heat illness. In *Medical Aspects of Harsh Environments*; Pandolf, K.B., Burr, R.E., Eds.; Office of the Surgeon General, Department of the Army: Washington, DC, USA, 2001; Volume 1, pp. 209–230.
4. Minson, C.T.; Cotter, J.D. CrossTalk proposal: Heat acclimatization does improve performance in a cool condition. *J. Physiol.* **2015**, *594*, 241. [CrossRef]
5. Nybo, L.; Lundby, C. Rebuttal by Lars Nybo and Carsten Lundby. *J. Physiol.* **2015**, *594*, 251. [CrossRef] [PubMed]
6. Garrett, A.T.; Goosens, N.G.; Rehrer, N.J.; Patterson, M.J.; Harrison, J.; Sammut, I.; Cotter, J.D. Short-term heat acclimation is effective and may be enhanced rather than impaired by dehydration. *Am. J. Hum. Biol.* **2014**, *26*, 311–320. [CrossRef] [PubMed]
7. Lorenzo, S.; Halliwill, J.R.; Sawka, M.N.; Minson, C.T. Heat acclimation improves exercise performance. *J. Appl. Physiol.* **2010**, *109*, 1140–1147. [CrossRef]
8. Moseley, P.L. Heat shock proteins and heat adaptation of the whole organism. *J. Appl. Physiol.* **1997**, *83*, 1314–1417. [CrossRef] [PubMed]
9. Moss, J.N.; Bayne, F.M.; Castelli, F.; Naughton, M.R.; Reeve, T.C.; Trangmar, S.J.; Mackenzie, R.W.A.; Tyler, C.J. Short-term isothermic heat acclimation elicits beneficial adaptations but medium-term elicits a more complete adaptation. *Eur. J. Appl. Physiol.* **2019**, *120*, 243–254. [CrossRef]
10. Garrett, A.T.; Goosens, N.G.; Rehrer, N.J.; Patterson, M.J.; Cotter, J.D. Induction and decay of short-term heat acclimation. *Eur. J. Appl. Physiol.* **2009**, *107*, 659–670. [CrossRef] [PubMed]
11. McClung, J.P.; Hasday, J.D.; He, J.R.; Montain, S.J.; Cheuvront, S.N.; Sawka, M.N.; Singh, I.S. Exercise-heat acclimation in humans alters baseline levels and ex vivo heat inducibility of HSP72 and HSP90 in peripheral blood mononuclear cells. *Am. J. Physiol. Regul. Integr. Comp. Physiol.* **2008**, *294*, 185–191. [CrossRef]
12. Cheung, S.S.; McLellan, T.M. Influence of hydration status and fluid replacement on heat tolerance while wearing NBC protective clothing. *Eur. J. Appl. Occup. Physiol.* **1998**, *77*, 139–148. [CrossRef] [PubMed]
13. Neal, R.A.; Massey, H.C.; Tipton, M.J.; Young, J.S.; Corbett, J. Effect of permissive dehydration on induction and decay of heat acclimation, and temperate exercise performance. *Front. Physiol.* **2016**, *7*, 564. [CrossRef]
14. Pandolf, K.B. Time course of heat acclimation and its decay. *Int. J. Sports Med.* **1998**, *19*, S157–S160. [CrossRef]
15. Sawka, M.N.; Pandolf, K.B. Physical exercise in hot climates: Physiology, performance, and biomedical issues. In *Medical Aspects of Harsh Environments*; Pandolf, K.B., Burr, R.E., Eds.; Office of the Surgeon General, Department of the Army: Washington, DC, USA, 2001; Volume 1, pp. 87–133.
16. Periard, J.D.; Racinais, S.; Sawka, M.N. Adaptations and mechanisms of human heat acclimation: Applications for competitive athletes and sports. *Scand. J. Med. Sci. Sports* **2015**, *25*, 20–38. [CrossRef]
17. Yamada, P.M.; Amorim, F.T.; Moseley, P.; Robergs, R.; Schneider, S.M. Effect of heat acclimation on heat shock protein 72 and interleukin-10 in humans. *J. Appl. Physiol.* **2007**, *103*, 1196–1204. [CrossRef]
18. Poirier, M.P.; Gagnon, D.; Friesen, B.J.; Hardcastle, S.G.; Kenny, G.P. Whole-body heat exchange during heat acclimation and its decay. *Med. Sci. Sports Exerc.* **2015**, *47*, 390–400. [CrossRef]
19. White, A.C.; Salgado, R.M.; Astorino, T.A.; Loeppky, J.A.; Schneider, S.M.; McCormick, J.J.; McLain, T.A.; Kravitz, L.; Mermier, C.M. The effect of ten days of heat acclimation on exercise performance at acute hypobaric hypoxia (4350 m). *Temperature* **2015**, *3*, 1–10. [CrossRef]
20. Neal, R.A.; Corbett, J.; Massey, H.C.; Tipton, M.J. Effect of short-term heat acclimation with permissive dehydration on thermoregulation and temperate exercise performance. *Scand. J. Med. Sci. Sports* **2016**, *26*, 875–884. [CrossRef]
21. Akerman, A.P.; Tipton, M.; Minson, C.T.; Cotter, J.D. Heat stress and dehydration in adapting for performance—Good, bad, both, or neither. *Temperature* **2016**, *3*, 1–25. [CrossRef]
22. Merry, T.L.; Ainslie, P.N.; Cotter, J.D. Effects of aerobic fitness on hypohydration-induced physiological strain and exercise impairment. *Acta. Physiol.* **2010**, *198*, 179–190. [CrossRef]
23. Taylor, N.A.S.; Cotter, J. Heat adaptation: Guidelines for the optimization of human performance. *Int. Sport Med. J.* **2006**, *7*, 33–57.
24. Garrett, A.T.; Creasy, R.; Rehrer, N.J.; Patterson, M.J.; Cotter, J.D. Effectiveness of short-term heat acclimation for highly trained athletes. *Eur. J. Appl. Physiol.* **2012**, *112*, 1827–1837. [CrossRef]
25. Wesseling, C.; Crowe, J.; Hogstedt, C.; Jakobsson, K.; Lucas, R.; Wegman, D.H. Resolving the enigma of the mesoamerican nephropathy: A research workshop summary. First International Research Workshop on the Mesoamerican Nephropathy. *Am. J. Kidney Dis. Mar.* **2014**, *63*, 396–404. [CrossRef]
26. Chapman, C.L.; Johnson, B.D.; Sackett, B.D.; Parker, M.D.; Schlader, Z.J. Soft drink consumption during and following exercise in the heat elevates biomarkers of acute kidney injury. *Am. J. Physiol. Regul. Integr. Comp. Physiol.* **2019**, *316*, 189. [CrossRef] [PubMed]

27. Divine, J.G.; Clark, J.F.; Colosimo, A.J.; Donaworth, M.; Hasselfeld, K.; Himmler, A.; Rauch, J.; Mangine, R. American football players in preseason training at risk of acute kidney injury without signs of rhabdomyolysis. *Clin. J. Sport Med.* **2018**, *30*, 556–561.
28. Pryor, R.R.; Pryor, L.J.; Vandermark, L.W.; Adams, E.L.; Brodeur, R.M.; Schlader, Z.J.; Armstrong, L.E.; Lee, E.C.; Maresh, C.M.; Casa, D.J. Acute kidney injury biomarker responses to short-term heat acclimation. *Int. J. Environ. Res. Public Heath* **2020**, *17*, 1325.
29. Schlader, Z.J.; Chapman, C.L.; Sarker, S.; Russo, L.; Rideout, T.C.; Parker, M.D.; Johnson, B.D.; Hostler, D. Firefighter work duration influences the extent of acute kidney injury. *Med. Sci. Sport Exerc.* **2017**, *49*, 1745–1753.
30. Hvidberg, V.; Jacobsen, C.; Strong, R.K.; Cowland, J.B.; Moestrup, S.K.; Borregaard, N. The endocytic receptor megalin binds the iron transporting neutrophil-gelatinase-associated lipocalin with high affinity and mediates its cellular uptake. *FEBS Lett.* **2005**, *579*, 773–779.
31. Jouffroy, R.; Lebreton, X.; Mansencal, N.; Anglicheau, D. Acute kidney injury during an ultra-endurance race. *PLoS ONE* **2019**, *14*, e222544.
32. Mansour, S.G.; Verma, G.; Pata, R.W.; Martin, T.G.; Perazella, M.A.; Parikh, C.R. Kidney injury and repair biomarkers in marathon runners. *Am. J. Kidney Dis.* **2017**, *70*, 252–261.
33. Lei, L.; Li, L.P.; Zeng, Z.; Mu, J.X.; Yang, X.; Zhou, C.; Wang, Z.L.; Zhang, H. Value of urinary KIM-1 and NGAL combined with serum Cys C for predicting acute kidney injury secondary to decompensated cirrhosis. *Sci. Rep.* **2018**, *8*, 7962.
34. Schlader, Z.; Hostler, D.; Parker, M.D.; Pryor, R.R.; Lohr, J.W.; Johnson, B.D.; Chapman, C.L. The potential for renal injury elicited by physical work in the heat. *Nutrients* **2019**, *11*, 2087.
35. Schrier, R.W.; Hano, J.; Keller, H.I.; Finkel, R.M.; Gilliland, P.F.; Cirksena, W.J.; Teschan, P.E. Renal, metabolic, and circulatory responses to heat and exercise: Studies in military recruits during summer training, with implications for acute renal failure. *Ann. Int. Med.* **1970**, *73*, 213–223.
36. Omassoli, J.; Hill, N.E.; Woods, D.R.; Delves, S.K.; Fallowfield, J.L.; Brett, S.J.; Wilson, D.; Corbett, R.W.; Allsopp, A.J.; Stacey, M.J. Variation in renal responses to exercise in the heat with progressive acclimatisation. *J. Sci. Med. Sport* **2019**, *22*, 1004–1009.
37. Borg, G. Psychophysical bases of perceived exertion. *Med. Sci. Sport Exerc.* **1982**, *14*, 377–381.
38. Astorino, T.A.; White, A.C.; Dalleck, L.C. Supramaximal testing to confirm attainment of VO_{2max} in sedentary men and women. *Int. J. Sports Med.* **2009**, *30*, 279–284.
39. Dalleck, L.C.; Astorino, T.A.; Erickson, R.M.; McCarthy, C.M.; Beadell, A.A.; Botten, B.H. Suitability of verification testing to confirm attainment of VO_{2max} in middle-aged and older adults. *Res. Sports Med.* **2012**, *20*, 118–128.
40. Scharhag-Rosenberger, F.; Carlsohn, A.; Cassel, M.; Mayer, F.; Scharhag, J. How to test maximal oxygen uptake: A study on timing and testing procedure of a supramaximal verification test. *Appl. Physiol. Nutr. Metab.* **2011**, *36*, 153–160.
41. Westgarth-Taylor, C.; Hawley, J.A.; Rickard, S.; Myburgh, K.H.; Noakes, T.D.; Dennis, S.C. Metabolic and performance adaptations to interval training in endurance-trained cyclists. *Eur. J. Appl. Physiol. Occup. Physiol.* **1997**, *75*, 298–304.
42. Astorino, T.A.; Cottrell, T.; Talhami Lozano, A.; Aburto-Pratt, K.; Duhon, J. Ergogenic effects of caffeine on simulated time-trial performance are independent of fitness level. *J. Caffeine Res.* **2011**, *1*, 179–185.
43. Dill, D.B.; Costill, D.L. Calculation of percentage changes in volumes of blood, plasma, and red cells in dehydration. *J. Appl. Physiol.* **1974**, *37*, 247–248.
44. Racinais, S.; Periard, J.D.; Karlsen, A.; Nybo, L. Effect of heat acclimatization on cycling time trial performance and pacing. *Med. Sci. Sports Exerc.* **2015**, *47*, 601–606.
45. Costello, J.T.; Rendell, R.A.; Furber, M.; Massey, H.C.; Tipton, M.J.; Young, J.S.; Corbett, J. Effects of acute or chronic heat exposure, exercise and dehydration on plasma cortisol, IL-6 and CRP levels in trained males. *Cytokine* **2018**, *110*, 277–283.
46. McConell, G.K.; Burge, C.M.; Skinner, S.L.; Hargreaves, M. Influence of ingested fluid volume on physiological responses during prolonged exercise. *Acta Physiol. Scand.* **1997**, *160*, 149–156.
47. Pethick, W.A.; Murray, H.J.; McFadyen, P.; Brodie, R.; Gaul, C.A.; Stellingwerff, T. Effects of hydration status during heat acclimation on plasma volume and performance. *Scand. J. Med. Sci. Sports* **2019**, *29*, 189–199.
48. Travers, G.; Nichols, D.; Riding, N.; Gonzalez-Alonso, J.; Periard, J.D. Heat acclimation with controlled heart rate: Influence of hydration status. *Med. Sci. Sports Exerc.* **2020**, *52*, 1815–1824.
49. Merry, T.L.; Ainslie, P.N.; Walker, R.; Cotter, J.D. Fitness alters regulatory but not behavioural responses to hypohydrated exercise. *Physiol. Behav.* **2008**, *95*, 348–352.
50. Karlsen, A.; Nybo, L.; Norgaard, S.J.; Jensen, M.V.; Bonne, T.; Racinais, S. Time course of natural heat acclimatization in well-trained cyclists during a 2-week training camp in the heat. *Scand. J. Med. Sci. Sports* **2015**, *25*, 240–249.
51. Keiser, S.; Fluck, D.; Huppin, F.; Stravs, A.; Hilty, M.P.; Lundby, C. Heat training increases exercise capacity in hot but not in temperate conditions: A mechanistic counter-balanced cross-over study. *Am. J. Physiol. Heart Circ. Physiol.* **2015**, *309*, 750–761.
52. Armstrong, L.E.; Costill, D.L.; Fink, W.J. Changes in body water and electrolytes during heat acclimation: Effects of dietary sodium. *Aviat. Space Environ. Med.* **1987**, *58*, 143–148.
53. Nielsen, B.; Strange, S.; Christensen, N.J.; Warberg, J.; Saltin, B. Acute and adaptive responses in humans to exercise in a warm, humid environment. *Pflug. Arch.* **1997**, *434*, 49–56.

54. Senay, L.C.; Mitchell, D.; Wyndham, C.H. Acclimatization in a hot, humid environment: Body fluid adjustments. *J. Appl. Physiol.* **1976**, *40*, 786–796. [CrossRef]
55. Wyndham, C.H.; Benade, A.J.; Williams, C.G.; Strydom, N.B.; Goldin, A.; Heyns, A.J. Changes in central circulation and body fluid spaces during acclimatization to heat. *J. Appl. Physiol.* **1968**, *25*, 586–593. [CrossRef] [PubMed]
56. Lorenzo, S.; Minson, C.T. Heat acclimation improves cutaneous vascular function and sweating in trained cyclists. *J. Appl. Physiol.* **2010**, *109*, 1736–1743. [CrossRef] [PubMed]
57. Young, A.J.; Sawka, M.N.; Levine, L.; Cadarette, B.S.; Pandolf, K.B. Skeletal muscle metabolism during exercise is influenced by heat acclimation. *J. Appl. Physiol.* **1985**, *59*, 1929–1935. [CrossRef] [PubMed]
58. Liu, C.T.; Brooks, G.A. Mild heat stress induces mitochondrial biogenesis in C2C12 myotubes. *J. Appl. Physiol.* **2012**, *112*, 354–361. [CrossRef]
59. McCullough, P.A.; Chinnaiyan, K.M.; Gallagher, M.J.; Colar, J.M.; Geddes, T.; Gold, J.M.; Trivax, J.E. Changes in renal markers and acute kidney injury after marathon running. *Nephrology* **2011**, *16*, 194–199. [CrossRef]

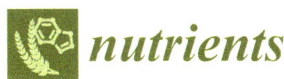

Article

Awareness of Fluid Losses Does Not Impact Thirst during Exercise in the Heat: A Double-Blind, Cross-Over Study

Catalina Capitán-Jiménez [1,2,*] and Luis F. Aragón-Vargas [1]

[1] Human Movement Science Research Center, University of Costa Rica, Montes de Oca, San José 11-501-2060, Costa Rica; luis.aragon@ucr.ac.cr
[2] Department of Nutrition, Hispanoamerican University, El Carmen, San José 10101, Costa Rica
* Correspondence: ccapitan@uh.ac.cr

Abstract: Background: Thirst has been used as an indicator of dehydration; however, as a perception, we hypothesized that it could be affected by received information related to fluid losses. The purpose of this study was to identify whether awareness of water loss can impact thirst perception during exercise in the heat. Methods: Eleven males participated in two sessions in random order, receiving true or false information about their fluid losses every 30 min. Thirst perception (TP), actual dehydration, stomach fullness, and heat perception were measured every 30 min during intermittent exercise until dehydrated by ~4% body mass (BM). Post exercise, they ingested water ad libitum for 30 min. Results: Pre-exercise BM, TP, and hydration status were not different between sessions ($p > 0.05$). As dehydration progressed during exercise, TP increased significantly ($p = 0.001$), but it was the same for both sessions ($p = 0.447$). Post-exercise water ingestion was almost identical ($p = 0.949$) in the two sessions. Conclusion: In this study, thirst was a good indicator of fluid needs during exercise in the heat when no fluid was ingested, regardless of receiving true or false water loss information.

Keywords: voluntary fluid intake; dehydration; thirst perception

1. Introduction

Hydration is a factor to take into consideration for health and performance during prolonged exercise, especially in the heat, when fluid replacement of sweat losses is relevant. Thirst has been widely studied as a mechanism of hydration control during exercise, but whether it is good enough to maintain euhydration is still controversial [1–4].

Previous studies have shown that thirst perception is strongly associated with actual fluid deficits during exercise, provided no fluid ingestion is allowed [5]. Manipulation of thirst perception has been studied to see how it can affect performance [6,7], using protocols to control thirst through saline infusions and mouth rinsing. Other behaviors and perceptions may be modified by external variables, such as publicity, noise, and vibrations. The so-called Hawthorne effect [8], as an example, is normally understood to describe how the behavior of workers—or patients—is modified when they become aware of being observed. Thirst may be easily affected by environmental conditions, fatigue, and especially by drinking [9]. Studies have clearly shown that the major issue with thirst-driven intake is a rapid decrease of the desire to drink after fluid ingestion, even when people replace less than 60% of what they lose [9,10]. We do not know, however, whether thirst perception can be intentionally modified by providing information or whether humans will change their perceptions of thirst just because they know how much their fluid losses are. Thirst perception, and its corresponding behavior, drinking, may be susceptible to change depending on awareness of fluid losses.

Therefore, the aim of the study was to identify whether thirst perception (TP) can be affected by awareness of fluid losses incurred during exercise in the heat.

2. Materials and Methods

The current investigation used a double-blind, cross-over design to determine whether thirst perception (TP) can be affected by receiving information about fluid losses during exercise in the heat. Subjects completed two randomly assigned sessions. Experimental testing procedures required subjects to exercise in the heat until they dehydrated by ~4% BM. Subjects were asked to report using the thirst perception scale every 30 min from the onset of exercise until they reached the target level of dehydration, and then to drink as much as they wanted for 30 min.

2.1. Subjects

Eleven apparently healthy, physically active males participated in the study. The sample size of the study was determined from previous studies that were similar in design [10,11]. Informed consent was obtained from all subjects involved in the study. The protocol was approved by the Institutional Ethics Committee.

2.2. Procedures

In one session, subjects received real information (RI) about their fluid losses, and in the other session they received information corresponding to 60% of their real fluid losses (false information, FI), which is close to the average voluntary drinking reported in other studies [10,11]; sessions were randomly assigned. Each participant arrived in the laboratory after overnight fasting, performed the baseline procedures, exercised in the heat, and rehydrated ad libitum. At different points during the protocol, self-reported measures were obtained for thirst, fullness, and heat perception.

On testing days, participants reported to the laboratory and voided their bladders completely. Urine was collected and analyzed with a refractometer for urine-specific gravity (manual refractometer ATAGO® model URC-Ne, Minato-ku, Tokyo, Japan, with a spectrum of 1.000 to 1.050). Urine osmolality (U_{osm}) was also measured via freezing point depression (Advanced Instruments 3250 osmometer; Norwood, MA, USA). Nude baseline body weight was measured to the nearest 10 g (e-Accura® scale, model DSB921, Qingpu, Shanghai, China).

Self-reported thirst was recorded with a visual analog scale. The scale consisted of a continuous 100 mm line with a mark on the left end indicating "not at all," and on the right "extremely," corresponding to the question, "How thirsty do you feel?" Perceived heat sensation was measured with an analog scale from "1: incredibly cold" to "8: incredibly hot." Finally, for the feeling of fullness, the question was: "How full do you feel?" Scoring between 1 (not at all) and 5 (very, very) was used. This group of scales had been used in previous studies [10,11].

Baseline measurements were taken for both sessions upon arrival to the laboratory. These consisted in nude body weight, urine-specific gravity, urine osmolality, and perceptions of thirst, heat, and fullness. Participants were asked to use the same clothing for both sessions.

Each participant ingested a standardized breakfast after baseline measurements (750 kilocalories: 24.6% fat, 20.7% protein, and 54.7% carbohydrates; 250 mL of fluid; 1500 mg sodium). After resting for thirty minutes, baseline measurements were taken, and the exercise session started.

In both sessions, each participant exercised intermittently (30 min bicycle/30 min treadmill, at 70–80% HRmax) in the heat (WBGT = 28.8 ± 0.1 °C and 28.9 ± 0.3 °C, for RI and FI, respectively; T = 32.5 ± 0.7 and H = 73 ± 3 for RI, and T = 32.2 ± 1.1 and H = 70 ± 3 for FI), to a target dehydration equivalent to 4% body mass (BM). Subjects were weighed every 30 min to monitor their fluid losses; after every weighing, subjects received information according to the session. Thirst perception was measured every 15 min after they received information. Water ingestion during exercise was not allowed. Heat stress was monitored with a Questemp36® monitor (3M, Oconomowoc, WI, USA).

To achieve the double-blind design of the study, an assistant was responsible for monitoring body weight and providing the information about weight losses to the participants; he did not know the objective of the study. This assistant measured body weights and passed the information on to the researchers outside the chamber, who performed the calculations of weight loss that had to be communicated to the participants. The participants were weighed naked behind a curtain; therefore, the scale display was not visible to them. This ensured that they could only obtain information from the assistant. Both the participant and the assistant in the chamber were informed of the real aim of the study upon completion.

Upon exercise termination, participants were instructed to drink as much as they needed from previously weighed bottles for 30 min. Water intake was measured with an OHAUS® Compact Scales, model CS2000 (Parsippany, NJ, USA) food scale. Urine-specific gravity (USG) and osmolality (U_{osm}), fullness, heat sensation, and thirst perception (TP) were measured pre- and post-exercise, and post-rehydration.

2.3. Statistical Analysis

Mean and standard deviation were used for descriptive statistics. Normality was checked for all variables. A t-test was performed to identify differences between sessions for each variable (body mass, USG, Uosm, thirst, WBGT, fullness, and heat sensation). One-way analyses of variance were performed to see differences over time for each variable (urine osmolality, thirst, heat sensation, and fullness). Where ANOVA showed a statistically significant main effect, Tukey's post hoc tests were performed to compare time differences.

3. Results

Participants were 23.0 ± 3.0 years old, 1.75 ± 0.07 m tall, and weighed (upon arrival) 76.7 ± 4.9 kg. Pre-exercise conditions were the same for both sessions; see Table 1.

Table 1. Pre-exercise conditions for each session.

Variable	Real Information (RI)	False Information (FI)	t	p
Body Mass (kg)	77.1 ± 4.9	77.1 ± 5.0	-0.389	0.706
USG (a.u)	1.017 ± 0.007	1.017 ± 0.007	0.135	0.895
Uosm (mmol·kg^{-1})	654.3 ± 296.4	663.2 ± 297.4	0.279	0.786
Thirst perception (mm)	12.8 ± 10.8	14.1 ± 7.5	-1.38	0.199
WBGT (°C)	28.8 ± 0.1	28.9 ± 0.3	-0.814	0.461
Fullness	2.9 ± 1.0	2.9 ± 0.5	-1.27	0.232
Heat sensation	3.8 ± 1.0	3.7 ± 1.0	1.02	0.860

Participants exercised for 110.0 ± 24.8 or 115.0 ± 22.3 min (t = -1.27; p = 0.232) during the RI and FI sessions, respectively, and achieved body mass losses of 2.98 ± 0.37 kg and 2.93 ± 0.33 kg, respectively, representing actual dehydration of $3.88 \pm 0.43\%$ and $3.81 \pm 0.38\%$ (t = -0.30; p = 0.756), respectively. Subjects ingested the same amounts of water at the ends of the sessions (1220 ± 249 mL and 1228 ± 422 mL; t = -0.66, p = 0.949). At the end of the rehydration period, hypohydration was still equivalent to $2.50 \pm 0.48\%$ or $2.48 \pm 0.68\%$ of pre-exercise body mass, respectively.

Figure 1 shows urine osmolality between conditions over time, pre-exercise (RI: 654.3 ± 296.4 and FI: 663.2 ± 297.4), post-exercise (RI: 630.1 ± 295.5 and FI: 579.1 ± 279.3), and after rehydration (RI: 695.2 ± 259.5 and FI: 665.9 ± 288.5). Uosm was not different between sessions (f = 0.134; p = 0.722), and there was no difference over time (f = 0.65; p = 0.804) and no interaction (f = 0.243; p = 0.633) either.

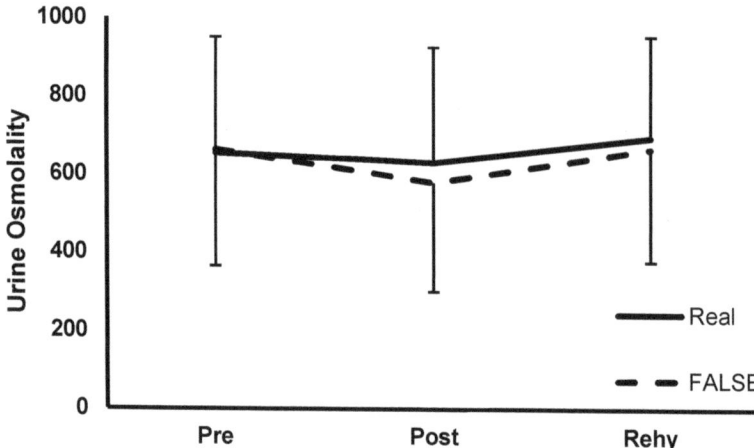

Figure 1. Urine osmolatity values (mean ± s.d): no difference between sessions ($p = 0.722$) or over time ($p = 0.804$). PRE = pre-exercise. POST = post-exercise. REHY = upon completion of rehydration.

A strong and significant association was found between the perception of thirst and the percentage of dehydration in both sessions ($r = 0.992$ and $r = 0.979$, $p < 0.05$, for RI and FI, respectively)

Thirst perception showed no difference between sessions (F = 0.661; $p = 0.447$). There was a difference over time (F = 44.6; $p = 0.001$) pre-exercise, but no interaction (F = 0.382; $p = 0.559$). Percentages of dehydration did not differ between sessions (t = −0.30; $p = 0.756$). Fullness showed no differences between sessions (F = 3.74; $p = 0.205$), nor over time (F = 3.74; $p = 0.304$). Meanwhile, sensation of heat did not differ between sessions (F = 0.982; $p = 0.360$) or over time (F = 2.88; $p = 0.140$). See Figure 2A–D.

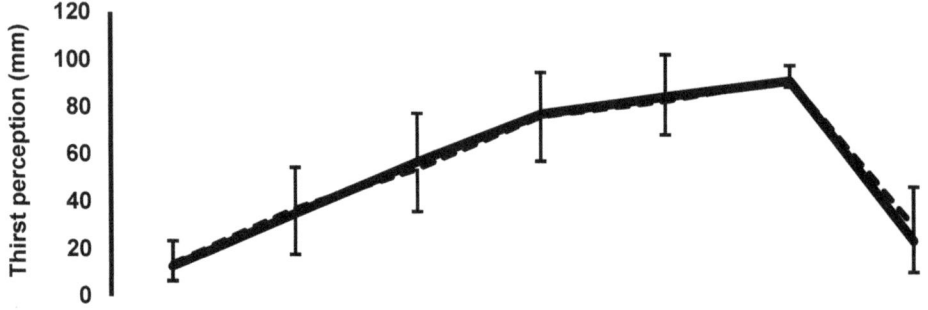

(A)

Figure 2. Cont.

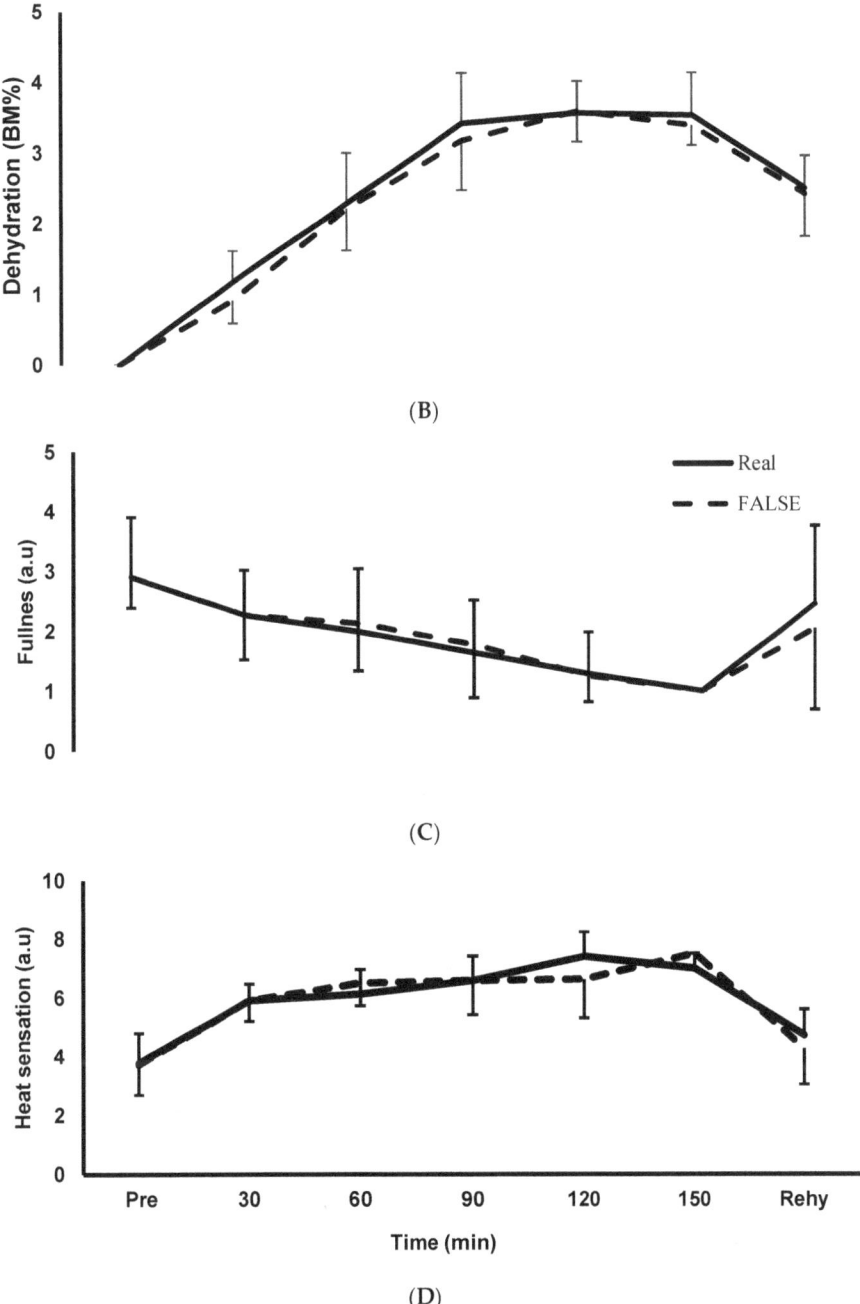

Figure 2. Values shown are mean ± s.d. (**A**) Thirst perception shows no difference between sessions ($p = 0.447$). There is a difference over time ($p = 0.001$) for pre-exercise, but no interaction ($p = 0.559$). (**B**) Percentage of dehydration did not differ between sessions (t = −0.30; $p = 0.756$). (**C**) Fullness: no differences between sessions ($p = 0.205$), nor over time ($p = 0.304$). (**D**) Heat sensation did not differ between sessions ($p = 0.360$) or over time ($p = 0.140$). By design, not all subjects finished at the same time: at 120 min, $n = 9$; at 150 min, $n = 2$; at REHY $n = 11$. Real: real information trial. False: false information trial, equivalent to 60% of actual water loss.

4. Discussion

The aim of the study was to identify whether thirst perception (TP) can be affected by awareness of fluid losses during exercise in the heat. The main finding of this study was that thirst perception during exercise in the heat was not influenced by true or false information about fluid losses. After exercise, subjects drank one-third of their losses ($\approx$1.2 L), a large volume for 30 min of rehydration, independently of the information they received. Thirst perception was markedly reduced at this point.

This study design differs from others because we manipulated thirst through the information of fluid losses of the subjects, contrary to others that manipulated thirst with saline infusions, mouth rinsing, or small quantities of water [7]. We also focused only on thirst perception during exercise and not on performance, which was done by other studies [5,12–14]. This could be relevant because an important proportion of the physically active population may be relying on thirst to drive their hydration, while not caring much about performance. Athletes, who care about performance, represent a small percentage of the population. This study confirms that thirst perception can detect dehydration and it will go higher as the level of dehydration increases during exercise in the heat (Figure 2A,B). However, as has been shown in other studies, this association between thirst perception and hydration needs quickly deteriorates as soon as subjects drink some fluid [5,6,10,12,15]. In our case, after 30 min of ad libitum rehydration, TP was markedly reduced, but the fluid deficit remained high. This behavior of thirst perception has been reported in previous studies [7,10,11]. Others have shown that thirst decreases rapidly as soon as liquid is ingested, long before the fluid lost during exercise has been replenished [2,7,8]. In the present study, thirst perception was evaluated at the end of the protocol, 30 min after finishing exercise. Unfortunately, the protocol used in the present study was focused on thirst responses during exercise, and post-exercise fluid intake and TP were only recorded once over those 30 min. We acknowledge that it would have been interesting to follow TP for a longer period, to complement the information on reduced ad libitum water intake reported by others [2,5,7].

Even when WBGT and exercise intensity were high, thirst perception between sessions was the same and had the same behavior over time, regardless of receiving true or false information about fluid loss, reflecting the percentage of dehydration [10] (see Figure 2A,B). It should be noticed that in this study, drinking during exercise was not allowed. We expect that this behavior will change when drinking or mouth rinsing is allowed, as others have shown [10,16]. Possibly, knowing that drinking would not be possible until the end of exercise could alter thirst perception, but this was a necessary element in the study design.

Thirst perception is widely used as a reference for hydration needs, especially in physically active persons (not necessarily athletes). Moreover, thirst could be used as a parameter as long as no liquid is ingested during exercise [7,10]. From this particular study, it may be added that internal signals such as increases in plasma osmolality or decreases in plasma volume [13,17] seem to be adequate to reflect dehydration in the absence of drinking, despite inaccurate external information that a person may receive about his hydration status. However, this does not mean that thirst perception should be recommended as a hydration strategy during exercise, due to its limitations whenever fluid is ingested [7,10]. As a hydration strategy during exercise, a pre-established protocol seems to be a better alternative.

5. Conclusions

In conclusion, thirst perception (TP) was not affected by receiving information about fluid losses during exercise in the heat in the absence of drinking. This might suggest that awareness of fluid losses during exercise cannot override the dehydration-induced hypothalamic signal for thirst.

Author Contributions: Conceptualization, C.C.-J. and L.F.A.-V.; Methodology, C.C.-J. and L.F.A.-V.; Software, C.C.-J. and L.F.A.-V.; Validation, C.C.-J. and L.F.A.-V.; Formal Analysis, C.C.-J. and L.F.A.-V.;

Investigation, C.C.-J. and L.F.A.-V. Resources, L.F.A.-V. Data Curation, C.C.-J. and L.F.A.-V. Writing—Original Draft Preparation, C.C.-J.; Writing—Review and Editing, C.C.-J. and L.F.A.-V.; Visualization, C.C.-J. and L.F.A.-V.; Supervision, L.F.A.-V. Project Administration, L.F.A.-V. Funding Acquisition, L.F.A.-V. All authors have read and agreed to the published version of the manuscript.

Funding: This research was funded by Gatorade Sports Science Institute® and University of Costa Rica project VI-838-B4-309.

Institutional Review Board Statement: The study was conducted according to the guidelines of the Declaration of Helsinki, and approved by the Institutional Ethics Committee of University of Costa Rica (protocol code VI-838-B4-309 and date of approval 14 August 2013).

Data Availability Statement: Raw data for this research is available in the institutional repository: http://hdl.handle.net/10669/83765 (accessed 18 August 2021).

Conflicts of Interest: The authors declare no conflict of interest.

References

1. Cotter, D.J.; Thornton, N.S.; Lee, K.J.; Laursen, B.P. Are we being drowned in hydration advice? Thirsty for more? *Extrem. Physiol. Med.* **2014**, *3*, 18. [CrossRef] [PubMed]
2. Mears, S.A.; Watson, P.; Shirreffs, S.M. Thirst responses following high intensity intermittent exercise when access to ad libitum water intake was permitted, not permitted or delayed. *Physiol. Behav.* **2016**, *157*, 47–54. [CrossRef] [PubMed]
3. Noakes, T.D. Drinking guidelines for exercise: What evidence is there that athletes should drink "as much as tolerable", "to replace the weight lost during exercise" or "ad libitum"? *J. Sports Sci.* **2007**, *25*, 781–796. [CrossRef] [PubMed]
4. Noakes, T.D. Is Drinking to Thirst Optimum? *Ann. Nutr. Metab.* **2010**, *57*, 9–17. [CrossRef] [PubMed]
5. Armstrong, L.E.; Johnson, E.C.; Kunces, L.J.; Ganio, M.S.; Judelson, D.A.; Kupchak, B.R.; Vingren, J.L.; Munoz, C.X.; Huggins, R.A.; Hydren, J.R.; et al. Drinking to Thirst Versus Drinking Ad Libitum During Road Cycling. *J. Athl. Train.* **2014**, *49*, 624–631. [CrossRef] [PubMed]
6. Kenefick, R.W. Drinking Strategies: Planned Drinking Versus Drinking to Thirst. *Sports Med.* **2018**, *48*, 31–37. [CrossRef] [PubMed]
7. Adams, J.D.; Sekiguchi, Y.; Suh, H.G.; Seal, A.D.; Sprong, C.A.; Kirkland, T.W.; Kavouras, S.A. Dehydration Impairs Cycling Performance, Independently of Thirst: A Blinded Study. *Med. Sci. Sports Exerc.* **2018**, *50*, 1697–1703. [CrossRef] [PubMed]
8. James, L.J.; Moss, J.; Henry, J.; Papadopoulou, C.; Mears, S.A. Hypohydration impairs endurance performance: A blinded study. *Physiol. Rep.* **2017**, *5*, e13315. [CrossRef] [PubMed]
9. McCarney, R.; Warner, J.; Iliffe, S.; van Haselen, R.; Griffin, M.; Fisher, P. The Hawthorne Effect: A randomised, controlled trial. *BMC Med. Res. Methodol.* **2007**, *7*, 30. [CrossRef] [PubMed]
10. Capitán-Jiménez, C.; Aragón-Vargas, L.F. Percepción de la sed durante el ejercicio y en la rehidratación ad libitum post ejercicio en calor húmedo y seco. *Pensar Mov. Rev. Cienc. Ejerc. Salud* **2018**, *16*, e31479. [CrossRef]
11. Capitán-Jiménez, C.; Aragón-Vargas, Y.L. Thirst response to post-exercise fluid replacement needs and controlled drinking. *Pensar Mov. Rev. Cienc. Ejerc. Salud* **2016**, *14*, 1–16. [CrossRef]
12. Berkulo, M.A.R.; Bol, S.; Levels, K.; Lamberts, R.P.; Daanen, H.A.M.; Noakes, T.D. Ad-libitum drinking and performance during a 40-km cycling time trial in the heat. *Eur. J. Sport Sci.* **2016**, *16*, 213–220. [CrossRef] [PubMed]
13. Hew-Butler, T.; Hummel, J.; Rider, B.C.; Verbalis, J.G. Characterization of the effects of the vasopressin V2 receptor on sweating, fluid balance, and performance during exercise. *Am. J. Physiol. Regul. Integr. Comp. Physiol.* **2014**, *307*, R366–R375. [CrossRef] [PubMed]
14. Wall, B.A.; Watson, G.; Peiffer, J.J.; Abbiss, C.R.; Siegel, R.; Laursen, P.B. Current hydration guidelines are erroneous: Dehydration does not impair exercise performance in the heat. *Br. J. Sports Med.* **2015**, *49*, 1077–1083. [CrossRef] [PubMed]
15. Armstrong, L.E.; Johnson, E.C.; McKenzie, A.L.; Ellis, L.A.; Williamson, K.H. Endurance Cyclist Fluid Intake, Hydration Status, Thirst, and Thermal Sensations: Gender Differences. *Int. J. Sport Nutr. Exerc. Metab.* **2016**, *26*, 161–167. [CrossRef] [PubMed]
16. Cheung, S.S.; McGarr, G.W.; Mallette, M.M.; Wallace, P.J.; Watson, C.L.; Kim, I.M.; Greenway, M.J. Separate and combined effects of dehydration and thirst sensation on exercise performance in the heat. *Scand. J. Med. Sci. Sports* **2015**, *25*, 104–111. [CrossRef] [PubMed]
17. Peyrot des Gachons, C.; Avrillier, J.; Gleason, M.; Algarra, L.; Zhang, S.; Mura, E.; Breslin, P.A.S. Oral Cooling and Carbonation Increase the Perception of Drinking and Thirst Quenching in Thirsty Adults. *PLoS ONE* **2016**, *11*, e0162261. [CrossRef] [PubMed]

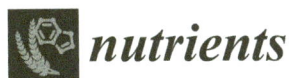

Article

Fluid Balance, Sweat Na+ Losses, and Carbohydrate Intake of Elite Male Soccer Players in Response to Low and High Training Intensities in Cool and Hot Environments

Ian Rollo [1,2,*,†], Rebecca K. Randell [1,2], Lindsay Baker [1], Javier Yanguas Leyes [3], Daniel Medina Leal [3], Antonia Lizarraga [3], Jordi Mesalles [3], Asker E. Jeukendrup [2], Lewis J. James [2] and James M. Carter [1]

1. Gatorade Sports Science Institute, PepsiCo Life Sciences, Global R&D, Leicestershire LE4 1ET, UK; rebecca.randell@pepsico.com (R.K.R.); lindsay.baker@pepsico.com (L.B.); james.carter@pepsico.com (J.M.C.)
2. School of Sports Exercise and Health Sciences, Loughborough University, Leicestershire LE11 3TU, UK; a.e.jeukendrup@lboro.ac.uk (A.E.J.); L.James@lboro.ac.uk (L.J.J.)
3. FC Barcelona Medical Department, FC, 08014 Barcelona, Spain; xavier.yanguas@fcbarcelona.cat (J.Y.L.); damele@me.com (D.M.L.); mlizarraga@ub.edu (A.L.); j.Mesalles@fcbarcelona.cat (J.M.)
* Correspondence: ian.rollo@pepsico.com; Tel.: +116-2348846
† Current address: Gatorade Sports Science Institute, PepsiCo Global Nutrition R&D, Leicestershire LE65 3TU, UK.

Abstract: Hypohydration increases physiological strain and reduces physical and technical soccer performance, but there are limited data on how fluid balance responses change between different types of sessions in professional players. This study investigated sweat and fluid/carbohydrate intake responses in elite male professional soccer players training at low and high intensities in cool and hot environments. Fluid/sodium (Na^+) losses and ad-libitum carbohydrate/fluid intake of fourteen elite male soccer players were measured on four occasions: cool (wet bulb globe temperature (WBGT): 15 ± 7 °C, $66 \pm 6\%$ relative humidity (RH)) low intensity (rating of perceived exertion (RPE) 2–4, m·min^{-1} 40–46) (CL); cool high intensity (RPE 6–8, m·min^{-1} 82–86) (CH); hot (29 ± 1 °C, $52 \pm 7\%$ RH) low intensity (HL); hot high intensity (HH). Exercise involved 65 ± 5 min of soccer-specific training. Before and after exercise, players were weighed in minimal clothing. During training, players had ad libitum access to carbohydrate beverages and water. Sweat [Na^+] (mmol·L^{-1}), which was measured by absorbent patches positioned on the thigh, was no different between conditions, CL: 35 ± 9, CH: 38 ± 8, HL: 34 ± 70.17, HH: 38 ± 8 ($p = 0.475$). Exercise intensity and environmental condition significantly influenced sweat rates (L·h^{-1}), CL: 0.55 ± 0.20, CH: 0.98 ± 0.21, HL: 0.81 ± 0.17, HH: 1.43 ± 0.23 ($p = 0.001$), and percentage dehydration ($p < 0.001$). Fluid intake was significantly associated with sweat rate ($p = 0.019$), with no players experiencing hypohydration > 2% of pre-exercise body mass. Carbohydrate intake varied between players (range 0–38 g·h^{-1}), with no difference between conditions. These descriptive data gathered on elite professional players highlight the variation in the hydration status, sweat rate, sweat Na$^+$ losses, and carbohydrate intake in response to training in cool and hot environments and at low and high exercise intensities.

Keywords: hydration; fluid; carbohydrate; professional; soccer

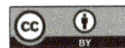

1. Introduction

The consequences of high-intensity intermittent running include an elevation in core temperature (39–40 °C) [1] and a gradual depletion of endogenous carbohydrates [2]. The subsequent thermoregulatory responses include an increased skin blood flow and the onset of sweating to allow evaporative heat loss [3]. A depletion of muscle glycogen and elevations in core temperature during exercise can be associated with fatigue, which, in soccer, may manifest as a reduction in overall distance covered and reduction in high-intensity running [4,5].

Despite fluid availability, soccer players have been reported to experience net fluid deficits during exercise because of fluid lost through sweat. Hypohydration has been reported to increase physiological strain [3] and is associated with reduced physical [6] and technical soccer performance [7], although not all studies report this [8]. Fluid losses vary greatly among elite soccer players, even in response to the same exercise conditions [9]. Furthermore, fluid losses are highly influenced by the environment [10,11] and exercise intensity [12]. Elite players' sweat rates have been reported to be lower (1.13 ± 0.30 L·h^{-1}, 0.71–1.77 L·h^{-1}) when training in cool temperatures (5 ± 1 °C), in comparison with hot conditions (37 ± 3 °C) (1.46 ± 0.24 L·h^{-1}, 1.12–2.09 L·h^{-1}) [11]. Nevertheless, levels of hypohydration are still evident when training in cool environments (1.62 ± 0.55%, range 0.87%–2.55%) [10]. This is because training intensity will continue to help determine the level of metabolic heat production and corresponding sweat response [13].

Studies investigating fluid balance in professional soccer players have reported voluntary fluid intake to be highly varied among players on the same team and influenced by the environmental conditions. Maughan et al. (2005) tabulated results from five studies that investigated fluid loss and intake of elite male soccer players at temperatures ranging from 5 to 32 °C. Ad-libitum fluid intake ranged from 0.42 to 1.40 L [10].

Less information is available on carbohydrate intake during soccer training and matches. This is of interest because the routine ingestion of carbohydrates provided in combination with fluid, typically via carbohydrate–electrolyte beverages, has been reported to delay fatigue and positively influence various aspects of soccer-specific performance [14]. In addition, practicing carbohydrate intake during exercise of similar "match" intensities may help the player better tolerate carbohydrate ingestion during competition [15]. In a study assessing the overall energy intake and energy expenditure of professional soccer players, carbohydrate intake during training was reported to be significantly lower (3.1 ± 4.4 g·h^{-1}) in comparison with a competitive match (32.3 ± 21.9 g·h^{-1}) [16]. Although carbohydrate intake during training was collected on multiple days, the training intensity was consistently low (< 48 m·min^{-1}). Therefore, to date, it has not been reported if professional players adjust their carbohydrate intake to an increase in training intensity.

Finally, post exercise, the ingestion of fluid and replenishment of electrolytes is required for rapid rehydration [17]. Sweat [Na$^+$] has been reported in separate groups of professional players in both cool [10] and hot conditions [11] and at different intensities [12]. However, since these earlier studies, performance parameters in professional soccer have become more intense [18] and technologies have been developed to rapidly quantify sweat [Na$^+$] [19].

Thus, the aim of the present study was to investigate the sweat response, ab-libitum fluid, and carbohydrate intake of the same group of elite male professional soccer players during training at low and high exercise intensities performed in cool and hot environments.

2. Materials and Methods

2.1. Study Participants

Thirty elite professional soccer players participated in the present study. Five players did not return to the club following the first test and 11 players were unavailable on two of the four test days. Therefore, 14 male first-team players of Futbol Club (FC) Barcelona (Spanish first division; La Liga) completed this study. All players completed a health screening questionnaire and provided written informed consent to participate after the details of the study had been explained. The study was approved by the Research Ethics Committee of Loughborough University, U.K. (R16-P133). All players were professional, accustomed to training and/or match durations of between 60 and 120 min 3–6 times per week. The physical characteristics of the players were age: 24 ± 4 years; body mass: 75.2 ± 6.2 kg; stature 180.9 ± 7.1 cm; $\dot{V}O_{2max}$: 57.9 ± 3.8 mL·kg BM·min^{-1} ($\dot{V}O_{2max}$ assessments were performed in July).

2.2. Experimental Design

The measurements were made on four separate training days during the competitive season. The study design was observational and thus the results are descriptive only of those training days on which the tests were completed. Training began at approximately 11.00 a.m. and lasted 65 ± 5 min. Each training session was completed outside on a grass pitch in dry conditions. Environmental temperature and relative humidity were recorded (Kesteral 4500, Nielsen-Kellerman, Pennsylvania, USA) at the beginning and at 15-min intervals during training. The training was that which was normally conducted by the players at that time of the season, with no interference from the research team. Furthermore, players were free-living with no research-requested dietary controls.

All players participated in the same training sessions. The training intensity was classified by a global positioning satellite system (STATSport, 10 Hz Viper [20]). In addition, at the cessation of training, players were asked to rate "how hard" the training session was on a 1–10 rating of perceived exertion (RPE) scale [21]. For the purpose of the present study, ratings of 1–5 were indicative of low intensity and ratings of 6–10 were indicative of high intensity (Table 1).

Table 1. Global positioning satellite parameters and player rating of perceived exertion (RPE) for training intensity classification. High speed running defined as > 14 km·h^{-1} < 20 km·h^{-1}. Sprint defined as > 20 km·h^{-1}.

Parameter	Intensity	
	Low	High
Rating of Perceived Exertion	2–4	6–8
Total distance (m)	2509–2593	4889–4949
m·min^{-1}	40–46	82–86
High Speed Running (m)	33–35	191–232
Number of Sprints	2–3	10–12

Data were collected under the following conditions classified by wet bulb globe temperature (WBGT): cool (14 ± 7 °C, 67 ± 7% relative humidity (RH)) low intensity (CL); cool (14 ± 8 °C, 69 ± 7 RH) high intensity (CH); hot (28 ± 1 °C, 55 ± 9 RH) low intensity (HL); hot (28 ± 2 °C, 55 ± 10 RH) high intensity (HH) [22]. Testing in the two hot conditions was completed in Barcelona, Spain (July). Testing in the cool high intensity condition was completed in the United Kingdom (July) and the cool low intensity condition was completed in Barcelona, Spain (January) of the same competitive season. The testing schedule was dictated by players' availability during the pre-season and winter break schedule. Players self-selected the clothing worn on each testing occasion. Outfield players wore a training shirt, shorts, soccer socks, and soccer boots in hot conditions. In the cool conditions, players also wore base layers that covered limbs and torso, and neck scarves. During the training sessions, all players had free access to water and a 6% carbohydrate–electrolyte beverage (Gatorade Thirst Quencher, PepsiCo Ltd.) in individually labelled drinks bottles, but drinking was limited to during coach-allocated "drinks breaks".

2.3. Assessment of Fluid Balance

A pre-exercise urine sample was collected from all players 30–60 min prior to exercise. These samples were analysed for urine specific gravity (USG) (Atago 3730 Pen-Pro Dip-Style Digital Refractometer, Washington, USA) to provide an indication of pre-training hydration status. Hydration status was classified as follows: < 1.020 euhydrated, 1.021–1.024 minimally hypohydrated, > 1.024 hypohydrated [23]. Containers were allocated to each player to collect any urine passed during practice. In the hour before training, players were encouraged to void their bladder before body mass (kg) was recorded in minimal clothing. Sweat loss was calculated from the change in body mass collected after exercise, following the correction for fluid intake and any urine/stool loss [24]. Relatively small changes in mass due to substrate oxidation and other sources of water loss were ignored [25].

2.4. Assessment of Sweat [Na^+]

Full details of the sweat collection protocol have been described in detail by Baker and colleagues (2014). In summary, sweat patches (Tegaderm + Pad, 3M, Loughborough, UK) were applied to specific landmarks on the surface of the thigh and back (in case no sample was available from the thigh). In all 14 players across all four conditions, the thigh patch was used with no exceptions. The sweat samples were analysed with a compact wireless analyser that uses ion-selective electrode technology to derive measures of [Na^+] (Horiba B-722) [19]. Regional sweat [Na^+] was normalised to whole-body concentrations [26]. Sodium chloride losses per hour of exercise were calculated from the sweat [Na^+] and individual sweat rate [24].

2.5. Statistical Analysis

Data are reported as mean and standard deviation (mean, s), with the range of data given in parentheses. All data were analysed using Minitab software package (version 17; Minitab Inc, State College, PA, USA). A Shapiro–Wilk test was used to determine normality of distribution. All variables (sweat rate, percentage dehydration, sweat [Na^+], sodium chloride loss, fluid intake, and carbohydrate intake) were checked for homoscedasticity using the Levene test, and analysed using a one-way repeated measures analysis of variance (ANOVA), and with Tukey's Honestly Significant Difference (HSD) pairwise comparison when a significant main effect was identified. A Pearson Correlation Coefficient was used to determine the strength of the relationship between USG and sweat rate, and sweat rate and fluid intake. Statistical significance was declared when $p < 0.05$.

3. Results

The players' physical performance during the training sessions was classified as low or high-intensity exercise by the parameters listed in Table 1. Pre-exercise body mass was not different between trials 75.2 ± 6.2 kg (67.1–86.0 kg) ($p > 0.05$). Three of the 14 players (21%) (four players (29%) in the HL trial) had urine specific gravity indicative of "euhydration" prior to each trial. The majority of players, 57%, 64%, 57%, and 50%, had urine specific gravity indicative of "hypohydration" prior to the CL, CH, HL, and HH trials, respectively.

The fluid balance variables for the four exercise conditions were normally distributed (Shapiro–Wilk test, $p = 0.328$) and are reported in Table 2. Levene tests were run on each dataset, comparing all four levels to check for equality of variance. As $p > 0.05$ for every test, we can assume that variances are equal across groups. No urine was produced by players during the training sessions. For each trial, there were three drinks breaks per hour of exercise. The duration of each drinks break was 90 ± 30 s. The mean and range of carbohydrate intake are reported in Table 2. The frequency of players ingesting 0 g of carbohydrate was $n = 2$ for the CL trial, $n = 4$ in the CH trial, $n = 1$ for the HL trial, and $n = 2$ in the HH trial. Three of the 14 players showed consistency in their choice of beverage, opting for no carbohydrate in two to three of the four trials. Nine of the 14 players ingested carbohydrates during all exercise conditions.

Table 2. The mean ± s and (range) of variables recorded before and during each training session in response to exercise at low and high exercise intensities in cool and hot conditions. Predicted whole-body sweat [Na⁺], predicted whole-body sweat Na⁺ losses, and assumed sodium chloride losses during exercise. The loss of sodium chloride is calculated on the assumption that all Na⁺ loss is sodium chloride [27]. a = significantly different from Cool Low, b = significantly different from Cool High, c = significantly different from Hot Low.

	Condition					
	Cool		Hot			
Intensity	Low	High	Low	High	F	p
Urine Specific Gravity	1.024 ± 0.005	1.023 ± 0.004	1.023 ± 0.006	1.025 ± 0.005	(3,52) = 0.35	0.786
	(1.016–1.032)	(1.014–1.028)	(1.011–1.033)	(1.017–1.034)		
Sweat rate (L·h^{-1})	0.55 ± 0.20	0.98 ± 0.21 [a]	0.81 ± 0.17 [a]	1.43 ± 0.23 [abc]	(3,52) = 46.37	0.001
	(0.20–0.85)	(0.67–1.50)	(0.50–1.20)	(1.10–1.81)		
Fluid intake (mL·h^{-1})	394 ±160	505 ± 265	572 ± 214	663 ± 229 [a]	(3,52) = 3.68	0.018
	(184–719)	(220–1058)	(308–898)	(266–933)		
Carbohydrate intake (g·h^{-1})	12 ± 9	11 ± 11	15 ± 12	15 ± 14	(3,52) = 0.57	0.637
	(0–37)	(0–32)	(0–36)	(0–50)		
Sweat [Na⁺] (mmol·L^{-1})	35 ± 9	38 ± 8	34 ± 7	38 ± 8	(3,52) = 0.85	0.475
	(21–54)	(26–48)	(24–45)	(22–53)		
Sweat Na⁺ loss (mmol·h^{-1})	19 ± 9	38 ± 13 [a]	28 ± 9 [a]	54 ± 15 [abc]	(3,52) = 22.98	0.001
	(7–36)	(19–68)	(13–52)	(33–81)		
NaCl loss (g·h^{-1})	1.1 ± 0.5	2.2 ± 0.8 [a]	1.6 ± 0.5 [a]	3.2 ± 0.9 [abc]	(3,52) = 22.98	0.001
	(0.4–2.1)	(1.1–3.9)	(0.8–3.0)	(1.9–4.8)		

There was no association between pre-exercise urine specific gravity and sweat rate ($r = 0.065$, $r^2 = 0.004$, $p > 0.05$). The relationship between sweat rate (L·h^{-1}) and the volume of drink consumed (mL·h^{-1}) during all training sessions was significant ($p = 0.019$) (Figure 1). The respective sodium chloride losses during exercise and carbohydrate intake are reported in Table 2. The distribution and central tendency of player percentage dehydration are displayed in Figure 2 and player sweat [Na⁺] is displayed in Figure 3. Mean sweat [Na⁺] did not change significantly over the four testing occasions. The individual change in sweat [Na⁺] over the four trials was 10 ± 10 mmol·L^{-1} (3.6–16.7 mmol·L^{-1}).

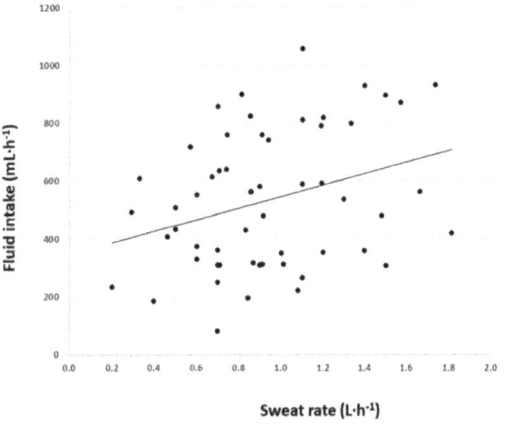

Figure 1. The relationship between sweat rate (L·h^{-1}) and the volume of drink consumed (mL·h^{-1}) during all training sessions was significant (p= 0.019, r = 0.31, r^2 = 0.098).

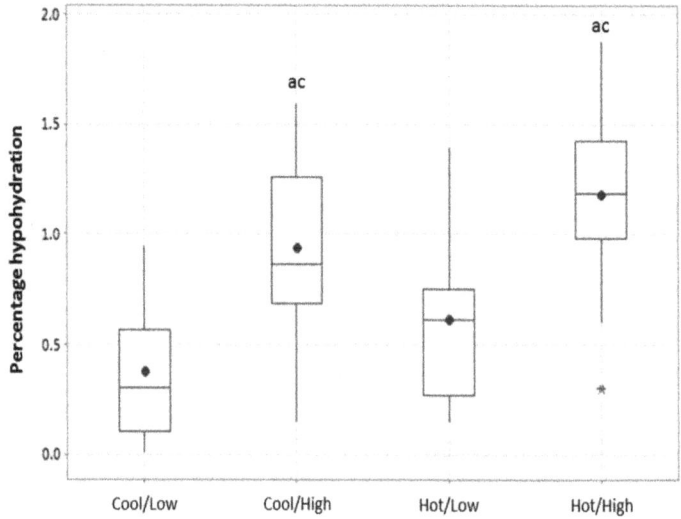

Figure 2. The percentage of hypohydration experienced by players in response to exercise at low and high exercise intensities in cool and hot conditions. The mean (•), median (-), interquartile range box (middle 50% of the data), and upper and lower error bars representing the upper and lower 25% of the distribution, respectively, are displayed. a = significantly different from Cool Low, c = significantly different from Hot Low. * indicates outlier in results.

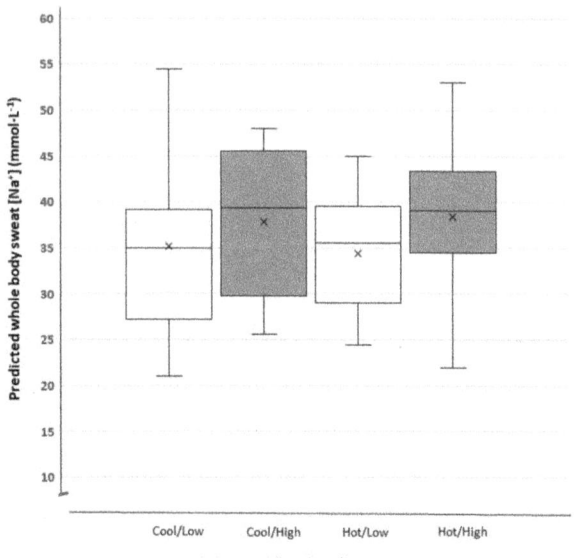

Figure 3. Predicted whole-body sweat sodium concentration (mmol·L^{-1}; from thigh sweat [Na$^+$]) during exercise at low and high exercise intensities in cool and hot conditions. The mean (x), median (-), interquartile range box (middle 50% of the data), and upper and lower error bars representing the range. No significant difference between trials ($p > 0.05$).

4. Discussion

The aim of the present study was to investigate the fluid balance and carbohydrate intake of elite professional male soccer players in response to exercise at different intensities and in different environmental conditions. Consistent with the literature in this population, all players experienced a reduction in body mass over the duration of the training sessions. However, the novel findings of the present study were: (1) players adequately adjusted ad-libitum fluid intake to prevent hypohydration greater than 2% of pre-exercise body mass; (2) carbohydrate ingestion was no different between conditions, with a large range in the rate of ingestion between individual players; and (3) thigh sweat [Na$^+$] was not different across conditions.

In the present study, sweat rates were similar to those reported in the soccer literature (1.0–2.2 L·h^{-1}) [9,28]. Furthermore, the change in sweat rate across conditions was similar to those previously reported in hot (~35 °C) (1.48 ± 0.36 L·h^{-1}) [11] and cool environments (5 °C) (1.13 ± 0.30 L·h^{-1}) [10] and in response to an increase in exercise intensity [12]. However, the present study is the first to show this pattern of responses in the same group of elite professional players in the same competitive season. Interestingly, a player's level of hypohydration during the cool high intensity condition was not significantly different from high intensity exercise in the heat. Our observations would suggest that, beyond exercise intensity, this may be a consequence of players wearing more clothing in response to the cold environment. Hypohydration ensues when multiple layers of clothing increase sweat rates [29], combined with reduced fluid intake when exercising in cool environments [10].

In contrast to previous studies, no player experienced hypohydration > 2% of pre-exercise body mass values [9,12]. This observation may be due to the shorter duration of exercise in the present study (~60 min), to that reported previously (100 min) [9]. Fluid loss is of interest in professional soccer because acute hypohydration has been reported to lead to decrements in both physical and technical performance [7]. The typical threshold for hypohydration to impact exercise performance is reported as 2% of pre-exercise values [30]. However, this assumes a pre-exercise hydration status of "euhydration". The urine specific gravity data suggest that this was not always the case. In professional soccer, pre-exercise hypohydration as indicated by urine concentration is common [25,31]. Consequently, it is likely that the resulting fluid balance data underestimate the extent of subsequent hypohydration that occurs during exercise. Interestingly, recent evidence suggests that routine exposure to hypohydration, potentially such as that resulting from day-to-day training in soccer, may alleviate some performance detriments [32]. Whilst the limitations of urine specific gravity as a "hydration assessment" are recognised, more invasive measures, such as measuring plasma osmolality, were not possible in the present study [33]. Despite potential "familiarisation" to hypohydration, it is important to note that performance remains "optimised" by commencing exercise euhydrated [32]. Thus, care should be taken that players are not simply accustomed to hypohydration. To achieve this, appropriate rehydration strategies are recommended between exercise sessions [17]. In addition, daily changes in body mass, thirst, and urine USG may be collected to track changes in players' hydration status [34].

The mean carbohydrate intake was approximately 15 g·h^{-1} and remained unchanged between exercise occasions (Table 2). The guidelines for carbohydrate intake for exercise durations of 60–70 min, especially during training as in the present study, are a "grey area" in sports nutrition. Specifically, the most recent The American College of Sports Medicine(ACSM) position recommends "small amounts of carbohydrate including mouth rinse" for exercise durations of 45–75 min, and 30–60 g of carbohydrate per hour for durations of 1–2.5 h, "including stop and start" sports [23]. Therefore, it is reasonable to suggest that most players met the minimum recommendation (i.e., small amounts), especially as the players were fed, and that exercise durations were closer to 1 h than to 2.5 h. The requirement for carbohydrate ingestion during exercise depends upon the demands and duration of the exercise and the goal of the individual player [35]. Thus, during low-intensity sessions, in cool environments, there may be little benefit of carbohydrate ingestion. Furthermore, some aerobic adaptation may be augmented by abstaining from carbohydrate ingestion before and during exercise [36]. Conversely, carbohydrate ingestion is associated with improved physical and technical performance in soccer [37]. Thus, it is advised that players practice ingesting those volumes and quantities associated with improved performance [15]. Glycogen stores will be depleted during 60 min of soccer activity [5] and the rate of glycogen use is elevated when playing in hot environments [38]. Nevertheless, there is no evidence that increasing the quantity of carbohydrate ingested (to quantities recommended for exercise durations > 3 h, 90 g carbohydrate h^{-1}) would result in further physical and technical performance benefits [23,39].

Previous studies have reported sweat [Na$^+$] and subsequent sodium chloride losses in different squads of professional male players in response to single training sessions [10,11]. Duffield et al. (2012) reported that sweat [Na$^+$] of the same squad of professional players increased in response to higher exercise intensities. This finding was consistent with laboratory-based investigations that report a proportional increase in forearm sweat [Na$^+$] as sweat rate is increased [40]. This is because at higher sweat rates Na$^+$ secretion increases proportionally faster than the rate at which Na$^+$ can be reabsorbed along the distal duct of the sweat gland [35]. In the present study, only four of the 16 players' sweat [Na$^+$] changed sufficiently to re-classify their values from low (< 36 mmol·L^{-1}) to moderate (36–58 mmol·L^{-1}) [41]. One possible reason for the discrepancy between our results and previous studies could be differences in the site of sweat collection. The study by Duffield and colleagues collected sweat from the scapula, whereas in the present study it was collected from the thigh. In a recent laboratory study, sweat rate and sweat [Na$^+$] significantly increased on several upper body regions (including the scapula and forearm) in response to increased exercise intensity, but there were no changes on the lower body (thigh and calf) [42]. Of course, this is difficult to confirm in the present study without concomitant local sweat rates on the thigh or data from additional anatomical regions. Future field research measuring sweat [Na$^+$] from several upper and lower body sites is needed. Nevertheless, sodium chloride loss significantly increased in the heat and at higher intensities because of the increased sweat rate. Thus, the results of the present study support previous recommendations that re-hydration strategies be modified to the exercise intensity, environmental condition, and individual player [12,28].

4.1. Limitations, Strengths, and Future Research

The present study was descriptive and thus several limitations are acknowledged. First, the final assessment was completed 5 months after the first tests completed in July. It is unknown if the players' acclimation and/or physical status changed over this duration, which may have influenced both the sweat rate and sweat [Na$^+$] response to exercise. Second, the analysis of sweat did not include potassium concentration, which would have been preferential as a quality control for sweat samples [43]. Despite this, best practices of sweat collection (clean skin, avoided patch saturation, gloves, etc.) described by Baker [43] were followed, so that we have confidence in our analysis. Other factors reported to influence sweat [Na$^+$] such as hormones [44] and diet [45] were not recorded or controlled for prior to testing, due to the nature of field/descriptive studies. Another limitation of the present study was that fluid intake was only assessed during exercise. The pre-training spot USG measure did not allow for the complete understanding of the players' hydration status before training. Assessing first morning USG, 24-h urine volumes, and/or 24-h fluid intake prior to training would provide insight into the influence of baseline hydration on sweat rates and sweat [Na$^+$]. Finally, as some (n = 3) players ingested no carbohydrate during exercise, future studies could investigate how alternative sources of carbohydrate (i.e., gels, bars, chews) may influence the ad-libitum carbohydrate intake of players. This would be relevant during high-intensity training sessions and prolonged pre-season training, and to encourage practicing match day nutrition.

4.2. Practical Applications

This study shows that observations such as the variability in sweat rate and sweat [Na^+] made in sub-elite soccer populations also apply to professional players. This study is evidence that it is possible to gather hydration-related data on elite players without disruption to normal training or competitive schedules. Furthermore, the results of the present study suggest that sweat [Na^+] does not change over time or between different sessions. Therefore, this kind of sweat [Na^+] analysis, often the expensive and technically time-consuming part of the process, may be completed on a single occasion. The sweat [Na^+] can then be applied to sweat rates, which are more easily measured on multiple occasions. However, further studies are required to confirm this applies over the entirety of the season.

5. Conclusions

These descriptive data gathered on elite professional players highlight the variation in the hydration status, sweat rate, sweat Na^+ loss, and carbohydrate intake in response to training in cool and hot environments and at low and high exercise intensities. Thus, these data support recommendations that fluid and carbohydrate intake strategies should be specific to the individual and exercise occasion.

Author Contributions: Study conceptualisation, I.R., J.M.C., A.E.J., and D.M.L.; methodology, I.R., J.M.C., A.E.J., J.M., A.L., and R.K.R., formal analysis, L.J.J., I.R., and J.Y.L., writing—original draft preparation, I.R. and R.K.R.; writing—review and editing, I.R., L.B., A.E.J., D.M.L., J.M.C., J.Y.L., J.M., A.L., and R.K.R. All authors have read and agreed to the published version of the manuscript.

Funding: Financial support for this study was provided by the Gatorade Sports Science Institute, a division of PepsiCo, Inc.

Institutional Review Board Statement: The study was conducted according to the guidelines of the Declaration of Helsinki, and approved by the Research Ethics Committee of Loughborough University, U.K. (R16-P133).

Informed Consent Statement: Informed consent was obtained from all subjects involved in the study.

Data Availability Statement: The data presented in this study are available on request from the corresponding author and the permission of all parties involved in the study. The data are not publicly available due to privacy.

Acknowledgments: The authors thank all the players and staff at FC Barcelona for their time and effort in the completion of this study. A special thank you to Eduard Pons for his assistance and expertise in the GPS analysis.

Conflicts of Interest: Authors I.R., R.K.R., L.B., and J.M.C. are employees of the Gatorade Sports Science Institute, a division of PepsiCo, Inc. The views expressed in this article are those of the authors and do not necessarily reflect the position or policy of PepsiCo Inc.

References

1. Ekblom, B. Applied physiology of soccer. *Sports Med.* **1986**, *3*, 50–60. [CrossRef] [PubMed]
2. Saltin, B. Metabolic fundamentals in exercise. *Med. Sci. Sports Excerc.* **1973**, *5*, 137–146. [CrossRef]
3. Armstrong, L.E.; Maresh, C.M.; Gabaree, C.V.; Hoffman, J.R.; Kavouras, S.A.; Kenefick, R.W.; Castellani, J.W.; Ahlquist, L.E. Thermal and circulatory responses during exercise: Effects of hypohydration, dehydration, and water intake. *J. Appl. Physiol.* **1997**, *82*, 2028–2035. [CrossRef] [PubMed]
4. Bangsbo, J. Energy demands in competitive soccer. *J. Sports Sci.* **1994**, *12*, S5–S12. [CrossRef]
5. Bendiksen, M.; Bischoff, R.; Randers, M.B.; Mohr, M.; Rollo, I.; Suetta, C.; Bangsbo, J.; Krustrup, P. The Copenhagen Soccer Test: Physiological response and fatigue development. *Med. Sci. Sports Excerc.* **2012**, *44*, 1595–1603. [CrossRef]
6. Mohr, M.; Krustrup, P. Heat stress impairs repeated jump ability after competitive elite soccer games. *J. Strength Cond. Res.* **2013**, *27*, 683–689. [CrossRef]
7. McGregor, S.J.; Nicholas, W.C.; Lakomy, H.W.; Williams, C. The influence of intermittent high-intensity shuttle running and fluid ingestion on the performance of a football skill. *J. Sports Sci.* **1999**, *17*, 895–903. [CrossRef]
8. Owen, J.A.; Kehoe, S.J.; Oliver, S.J. Influence of fluid intake on soccer performance in a temperate environment. *J. Sports Sci.* **2013**, *31*, 1–10. [CrossRef]

9. Da Silva, R.P.; Mundel, T.; Natali, A.J.; Filho, M.G.B.; Alfenas, R.C.; Lima, J.R.; Belfort, F.G.; Lopes, P.R.; Marins, J.C. Pre-game hydration status, sweat loss, and fluid intake in elite Brazilian young male soccer players during competition. *J. Sports Sci.* **2012**, *30*, 37–42. [CrossRef]
10. Maughan, R.J.; Shirreffs, S.M.; Merson, S.J.; Horswill, C.A. Fluid and electrolyte balance in elite male football (soccer) players training in a cool environment. *J. Sports Sci.* **2005**, *23*, 73–79. [CrossRef]
11. Shirreffs, S.M.; Aragon-Vargas, L.F.; Chamorro, M.; Maughan, R.J.; Serratosa, L.; Zachwieja, J.J. The sweating response of elite professional soccer players to training in the heat. *Int. J. Sports Med.* **2005**, *26*, 90–95. [CrossRef] [PubMed]
12. Duffield, R.; McCall, A.; Coutts, A.J.; Peiffer, J.J. Hydration, sweat and thermoregulatory responses to professional football training in the heat. *J. Sports Sci.* **2012**, *30*, 957–965. [CrossRef] [PubMed]
13. Gleeson, M. Temperature regulation during exercise. *Int. J. Sports Med.* **1998**, *19* (Suppl. 2), S96–S99. [CrossRef] [PubMed]
14. Williams, C.; Rollo, I. Carbohydrate Nutrition and Team Sport Performance. *Sports Med.* **2015**, *45* (Suppl. 1), S13–S22. [CrossRef] [PubMed]
15. Costa, R.J.S.; Miall, A.; Khoo, A.; Rauch, C.; Snipe, R.; Camoes-Costa, V.; Gibson, P. Gut-training: The impact of two weeks repetitive gut-challenge during exercise on gastrointestinal status, glucose availability, fuel kinetics, and running performance. *Appl. Physiol. Nutr. Metab.* **2017**, *42*, 547–557. [CrossRef]
16. Anderson, L.; Orme, P.; Naughton, R.J.; Close, G.L.; Milsom, J.; Rydings, D.; O'Boyle, A.; di Michele, R.; Louis, J.; Hambley, C.; et al. Energy Intake and Expenditure of Professional Soccer Players of the English Premier League: Evidence of Carbohydrate Periodization. *Int. J. Sport Nutr. Exerc. Metab.* **2017**, *27*, 228–238. [CrossRef]
17. Shirreffs, S.M.; Taylor, A.J.; Leiper, J.B.; Maughan, R.J. Post-exercise rehydration in man: Effects of volume consumed and drink sodium content. *Med. Sci. Sports Excerc.* **1996**, *28*, 1260–1271. [CrossRef]
18. Bush, M.; Barnes, C.; Archer, D.T.; Hogg, B.; Bradley, P.S. Evolution of match performance parameters for various playing positions in the English Premier League. *Hum. Mov. Sci.* **2015**, *39*, 1–11. [CrossRef]
19. Baker, L.B.; Ungaro, C.T.; Barnes, K.A.; Nuccio, R.P.; Reimel, A.J.; Stofan, J.R. Validity and reliability of a field technique for sweat Na+ and K+ analysis during exercise in a hot-humid environment. *Physiol. Rep.* **2014**, *2*, e12007. [CrossRef]
20. Bataller-Cervero, A.V.; Gutierrez, H.; DeRenteria, J.; Piedrafita, E.; Marcen, N.; Valero-Campo, C.; Lapuente, M.; Berzosa, C. Validity and Reliability of a 10 Hz GPS for Assessing Variable and Mean Running Speed. *J. Hum. Kinet.* **2019**, *67*, 17–24. [CrossRef]
21. Borg, G. Ratings of perceived exertion and heart rates during short-term cycle exercise and their use in a new cycling strength test. *Int. J. Sports Med.* **1982**, *3*, 153–158. [CrossRef] [PubMed]
22. Armstrong, L.E.; Casa, D.J.; Millard-Stafford, M.; Moran, D.S.; Pyne, S.W.; Roberts, W.O. American College of Sports Medicine position stand. Exertional heat illness during training and competition. *Med. Sci. Sports Excerc.* **2007**, *39*, 556–572. [CrossRef] [PubMed]
23. Thomas, D.T.; Erdman, K.A.; Burke, L.M. American College of Sports Medicine Joint Position Statement. Nutrition and Athletic Performance. *Med. Sci. Sports Excerc.* **2016**, *48*, 543–568.
24. Barnes, K.A.; Anderson, M.L.; Stofan, J.R.; Dalrymple, K.J.; Reimel, A.J.; Roberts, T.J.; Randell, R.K.; Ungaro, C.T.; Baker, L.B. Normative data for sweating rate, sweat sodium concentration, and sweat sodium loss in athletes: An update and analysis by sport. *J. Sports Sci.* **2019**, *37*, 2356–2366. [CrossRef] [PubMed]
25. Maughan, R.J.; Watson, P.; Evans, G.H.; Broad, N.; Shirreffs, S.M. Water balance and salt losses in competitive football. *IJSNEM* **2007**, *17*, 583–594. [CrossRef]
26. Baker, L.B.; Stofan, J.R.; Hamilton, A.A.; Horswill, C.A. Comparison of regional patch collection vs. whole body washdown for measuring sweat sodium and potassium loss during exercise. *J. Appl. Physiol.* **2009**, *107*, 887–895. [CrossRef]
27. Baker, L.B.; Ungaro, C.T.; Sopena, B.C.; Nuccio, R.P.; Reimel, A.J.; Carter, J.M.; Stofan, J.R.; Barnes, K.A. Body map of regional vs. whole body sweating rate and sweat electrolyte concentrations in men and women during moderate exercise-heat stress. *J. Appl. Physiol.* **2018**, *124*, 1304–1318. [CrossRef]
28. Maughan, R.J.; Shirreffs, S.M. Nutrition for soccer players. *Curr. Sports Med. Rep.* **2007**, *6*, 279–280.
29. Dawson, B.; Pyke, F.S.; Morton, A.R. Improvements in heat tolerance induced by interval running training in the heat and in sweat clothing in cool conditions. *J. Sports Sci.* **1989**, *7*, 189–203. [CrossRef]
30. McDermott, B.P.; Anderson, S.A.; Armstrong, L.E.; Casa, D.J.; Cheuvront, S.N.; Cooper, L.; Kenney, W.L.; O'Connor, F.G.; Roberts, W.O. National Athletic Trainers' Association Position Statement: Fluid Replacement for the Physically Active. *J. Athl. Train.* **2017**, *52*, 877–895. [CrossRef]
31. Aragón-Vargas, L.F.; Moncada-Jiménez, J.; Hernández-Elizondo, J.; Barrenechea, A.C.; Monge-Alvarado, A. Evaluation of pre-game hydration status, heat stress, and fluid balance during professional soccer competition in the heat. *Eur. J. Sports Sci.* **2009**, *9*, 269–276. [CrossRef]
32. Fleming, J.; James, L.J. Repeated familiarisation with hypohydration attenuates the performance decrement caused by hypohydration during treadmill running. *Appl. Physiol. Nutr. Metab.* **2014**, *39*, 124–129. [CrossRef] [PubMed]
33. Cheuvront, S.N.; Ely, B.R.; Kenefick, R.W.; Sawka, M.N. Biological variation and diagnostic accuracy of dehydration assessment markers. *Am. J. Clin. Nutr.* **2010**, *92*, 565–573. [CrossRef] [PubMed]
34. Armstrong, L.E.; Ganio, M.S.; Klau, J.F.; Johnson, E.C.; Casa, D.J.; Maresh, C.M. Novel hydration assessment techniques employing thirst and a water intake challenge in healthy men. *Appl. Physiol. Nutr. Metab.* **2014**, *39*, 138–144. [CrossRef] [PubMed]

35. Impey, S.G.; Hammond, K.M.; Shepherd, S.O.; Sharples, A.P.; Stewart, C.; Limb, M.; Smith, K.; Philp, A.; Jeromson, S.; Hamilton, D.L.; et al. Fuel for the work required: A practical approach to amalgamating train-low paradigms for endurance athletes. *Physiol. Rep.* **2016**, *4*, e12803. [CrossRef]
36. Bartlett, J.D.; Louhelainen, J.; Iqbal, Z.; Cochran, A.J.; Gibala, M.J.; Gregson, W.; Close, G.L.; Drust, B.; Morton, J.P. Reduced carbohydrate availability enhances exercise-induced p53 signaling in human skeletal muscle: Implications for mitochondrial biogenesis. *Am. J. Physiol. Regul. Integr. Comp.* **2013**, *304*, R450–R458. [CrossRef]
37. Rodriguez-Giustiniani, P.; Rollo, I.; Witard, O.C.; Galloway, S.D.R. Ingesting a 12% Carbohydrate-Electrolyte Beverage Before Each Half of a Soccer-Match Simulation Facilitates Retention of Passing Performance and Improves High-Intensity Running Capacity in Academy Players. *Int. J. Sport Nutr. Exerc. Metab.* **2018**, *29*, 397–405. [CrossRef]
38. Hargreaves, M.; Angus, D.; Howlett, K.; Conus, N.M.; Febbraio, M. Effect of heat stress on glucose kinetics during exercise. *J. Appl. Physiol.* **1996**, *81*, 1594–1597. [CrossRef]
39. Newell, M.L.; Wallis, G.A.; Hunter, A.M.; Tipton, K.D.; Galloway, S.D.R. Metabolic Responses to Carbohydrate Ingestion during Exercise: Associations between Carbohydrate Dose and Endurance Performance. *Nutrients* **2018**, *10*, 37. [CrossRef]
40. Buono, M.J.; Ball, K.D.; Kolkhorst, F.W. Sodium ion concentration vs. sweat rate relationship in humans. *J. Appl. Physiol.* **2007**, *103*, 990–994. [CrossRef]
41. Baker, L.B.; Barnes, K.A.; Anderson, M.L.; Passe, D.H.; Stofan, J.R. Normative data for regional sweat sodium concentration and whole-body sweating rate in athletes. *J. Sports Sci.* **2016**, *34*, 358–368. [CrossRef] [PubMed]
42. Baker, L.B.; Pde Chavez, J.D.; Ungaro, C.T.; Sopena, B.C.; Nuccio, R.P.; Reimel, A.J.; Barnes, K.A. Exercise intensity effects on total sweat electrolyte losses and regional vs. whole-body sweat [Na(+)], [Cl(-)], and [K(+)]. *EJAP* **2019**, *119*, 361–375. [CrossRef] [PubMed]
43. Baker, L.B. Sweating Rate and Sweat Sodium Concentration in Athletes: A Review of Methodology and Intra/Interindividual Variability. *Sports Med.* **2017**, *47* (Suppl. S1), 111–128. [CrossRef] [PubMed]
44. Castro-Sepulveda, M.; Cancino, J.; Fernandez-Verdejo, R.; Perez-Luco, C.; Jannas-Vela, S.; Ramirez-Campillo, R.; del Coso, J.; Zbinden-Foncea, H. Basal Serum Cortisol and Testosterone/Cortisol Ratio Are Related to Rate of Na+ Lost During Exercise in Elite Soccer Players. *IJSNEM* **2019**, *29*, 658–663. [CrossRef] [PubMed]
45. McCubbin, A.J.; Lopez, M.B.; Cox, G.R.; Odgers, J.N.C.; Costa, R.J.S. Impact of 3-day high and low dietary sodium intake on sodium status in response to exertional-heat stress: A double-blind randomized control trial. *EJAP* **2019**, *119*, 2105–2118. [CrossRef]

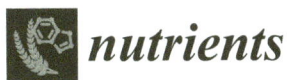

Article

Hydration Status, Fluid Intake, Sweat Rate, and Sweat Sodium Concentration in Recreational Tropical Native Runners

Juthamard Surapongchai [1,*], Vitoon Saengsirisuwan [2], Ian Rollo [3,4], Rebecca K. Randell [3,4], Kanpiraya Nithitsuttibuta [2], Patarawadee Sainiyom [2], Clarence Hong Wei Leow [5] and Jason Kai Wei Lee [5,6,7,8,9,10]

[1] Faculty of Physical Therapy, Mahidol University, Nakhon Pathom 73170, Thailand
[2] Department of Physiology, Faculty of Science, Mahidol University, Bangkok 10400, Thailand; vitoon.sae@mahidol.ac.th (V.S.); kanpiraya.sutt@gmail.com (K.N.); psonepp@gmail.com (P.S.)
[3] Gatorade Sports Science Institute, PepsiCo Life Sciences, Global R&D, Leicestershire LE4 1ET, UK; ian.rollo@pepsico.com (I.R.); rebecca.randell@pepsico.com (R.K.R.)
[4] School of Sport, Exercise and Health Sciences, Loughborough University, Leicestershire LE11 3TU, UK
[5] Human Potential Translational Research Programme, Yong Loo Lin School of Medicine, National University of Singapore, Singapore 119283, Singapore; medhwcl@nus.edu.sg (C.H.W.L.); phsjlkw@nus.edu.sg (J.K.W.L.)
[6] Department of Physiology, Yong Loo Lin School of Medicine, National University of Singapore, Singapore 117593, Singapore
[7] N.1 Institute for Health, National University of Singapore, Singapore 117456, Singapore
[8] Global Asia Institute, National University of Singapore, Singapore 119076, Singapore
[9] Institute for Digital Medicine, Yong Loo Lin School of Medicine, National University of Singapore, Singapore 117456, Singapore
[10] Singapore Institute for Clinical Sciences, Agency for Science, Technology and Research (A*STAR), Singapore 117609, Singapore
* Correspondence: juthamard.sur@mahidol.edu

Abstract: Aim: The purpose of this study was to evaluate hydration status, fluid intake, sweat rate, and sweat sodium concentration in recreational tropical native runners. Methods: A total of 102 males and 64 females participated in this study. Participants ran at their self-selected pace for 30–100 min. Age, environmental conditions, running profiles, sweat rates, and sweat sodium data were recorded. Differences in age, running duration, distance and pace, and physiological changes between sexes were analysed. A p-value cut-off of 0.05 depicted statistical significance. Results: Males had lower relative fluid intake (6 ± 6 vs. 8 ± 7 mL·kg^{-1}·h^{-1}, $p < 0.05$) and greater relative fluid balance deficit (−13 ± 8 mL·kg^{-1}·h^{-1} vs. −8 ± 7 mL·kg^{-1}·h^{-1}, $p < 0.05$) than females. Males had higher whole-body sweat rates (1.3 ± 0.5 L·h^{-1} vs. 0.9 ± 0.3 L·h^{-1}, $p < 0.05$) than females. Mean rates of sweat sodium loss (54 ± 27 vs. 39 ± 22 mmol·h^{-1}) were higher in males than females ($p < 0.05$). Conclusions: The sweat profile and composition in tropical native runners are similar to reported values in the literature. The current fluid replacement guidelines pertaining to volume and electrolyte replacement are applicable to tropical native runners.

Keywords: recreational running; tropical climate; sweat electrolyte; fluid replacement; hydration plan

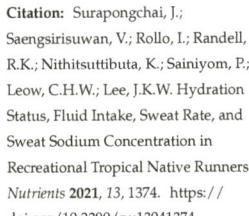

Citation: Surapongchai, J.; Saengsirisuwan, V.; Rollo, I.; Randell, R.K.; Nithitsuttibuta, K.; Sainiyom, P.; Leow, C.H.W.; Lee, J.K.W. Hydration Status, Fluid Intake, Sweat Rate, and Sweat Sodium Concentration in Recreational Tropical Native Runners. Nutrients 2021, 13, 1374. https://doi.org/10.3390/nu13041374

Academic Editors: Douglas J. Casa, Stavros Kavouras and William M. Adams

Received: 21 February 2021
Accepted: 15 April 2021
Published: 20 April 2021

Publisher's Note: MDPI stays neutral with regard to jurisdictional claims in published maps and institutional affiliations.

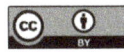

Copyright: © 2021 by the authors. Licensee MDPI, Basel, Switzerland. This article is an open access article distributed under the terms and conditions of the Creative Commons Attribution (CC BY) license (https://creativecommons.org/licenses/by/4.0/).

1. Introduction

Sweat evaporation is important for the dissipation of metabolic heat production, which may increase ten- to twenty-fold during exercise [1]. In hot environments, evaporative sweat cooling is the main avenue of heat loss, preventing rapid rises of core body temperature [2–5]. Hypohydration, experienced as a result of sweat loss, increases physiological strain and perception of effort, which can decrease endurance exercise performance [6,7]. In addition, sweat loss during exercise can also result in electrolyte imbalance such as hyponatremia. Thus, it is important to replace electrolyte losses as part of the rehydration process after exercise [3,8,9].

Running is a common form of exercise as it can be easily performed and does not require any specialised equipment. There are an estimated five to eight million individuals participating in running events globally. A 50% increase in participation in running has been tracked over the last decade. This growth has, in part, been driven by increased participation in Asia [10]. In tropical warm, high humidity environments, the evaporation of sweat may be compromised, leading to lower rates of body heat dissipation [11]. Thus, it is reasonable to suggest that appropriate hydration may be even more important for endurance running when in tropical Asian countries.

An athlete's sweat rate and sweat electrolyte concentration vary depending on individual characteristics, type and intensity of exercise, clothing, equipment worn as well as environmental conditions [12–20]. Therefore, the assessment of individual sweat rate and sweat electrolytes losses for specific exercise and environmental conditions is recommended to create individualised hydration strategies. This approach may reduce the risk of heat illness and optimise performance [21]. Despite the individuality in the response to dehydration, current guidelines advise limiting fluid deficits to no more than 2% body mass loss during exercise to avoid compromised cognitive function and aerobic exercise performances [21]. Further decrements in performance are associated with increasing levels of hypohydration (3–10%), particularly in hot weather typical in tropical climates [12,22]. Individualised drinking plans may also reduce the risk of over-drinking and exercise-associated hyponatremia [23–28].

Tropical natives are likely to be more heat-acclimatised than athletes who live in temperate or cool environments. Heat-acclimatised individuals have thermoregulatory adaptations such as lowered core body temperature, lowered heart rate, earlier onset of sweating and higher sweat rate [29–31]. Although variable, mean sweat sodium concentrations ([Na^+]) are reported to be approximately 50 mmol·L^{-1} [32]. To the authors' knowledge, there are limited data on sweat rate and sweat composition of tropical native athletes, which may impact on hydration strategies during and after exercise in this population. Knowledge of sweat responses and sweat composition of tropical native athletes will allow us to understand if consensus recommendations on hydration are also relevant to heat-acclimatised athletes.

Therefore, the purpose of the present study was to evaluate the hydration status, fluid intake, sweat rate, and sweat [Na^+] in recreational tropical native runners.

2. Materials and Methods

2.1. Study Design and Participants

This study adopted an observational cohort study design. A total of 102 males and 64 females were recruited to participate in this study. All measurements were made on a single day of practice sessions in various running groups. Ethics approval was obtained from the Centre of Ethical Reinforcement for Human Research, Mahidol University (MU-CIRB 2018/208.2311 and protocol no. 2018/198.0910). All participants provided written informed consent before participation.

2.2. Experimental Protocol

Resting heart rate, blood pressure and aural temperature were measured before and after running. Heart rate and blood pressure were measured using an upper arm blood pressure monitor (BM 28, Beurer GmbH, Ulm, Germany). Aural temperature was measured using an ear thermometer (FT 78, Beurer GmbH, Ulm, Germany). Participants with high resting blood pressure and/or high resting aural temperature (systolic blood pressure >180 mmHg and/or diastolic blood pressure >110 mmHg and/or aural temperature >38 °C) were excluded from the study.

Six running sessions were completed on separate days. Each session involved a warm-up of 10–15 min, followed by 30–70 min of running, and ended with 10–15 min of cool-down. Participants ran at their individual pace, with most participants running at a light to moderate intensity. Two running sessions were conducted in the morning, between 6 a.m. and 8 a.m., while four running sessions were conducted in the evening, between 5 p.m. and 8 p.m. The first five running sessions were conducted at Lumphini Park, Bangkok, Thailand while the sixth running session was conducted in a park within Mahidol University, Nakhon Pathom, Thailand. All six sessions were held in a public park with a 2.5 km running track. A water station was provided. Runners consumed plain water (Aquafina, PepsiCo, Harrison, NY, USA) *ad libitum* from individual water bottles. Water bottles were weighed before and after each running session to record the volume of fluid intake during running.

Before each running session, all participants voided their bladders. Mid-stream urine samples were collected to measure urine specific gravity (USG). Pre-exercise body mass was measured using a bench scale (N.V. Mettler-Toledo S.A., Zaventem, Belgium) while minimally clothed (T-shirts, shorts or tights, and without shoes), and recorded to the nearest 0.10 kg. For participants who needed to urinate during the run, body mass was measured before and after the excretion to estimate urine output. To collect sweat, the right or left forearm was cleaned with an alcohol pad (3M, Minneapolis, MN, USA), rinsed with distilled water, and dried with electrolyte-free gauze. An absorbent patch (9 cm × 10 cm) (3M™ Tegaderm™ + Pad Film Dressing with Non-Adherent Pad, 3M, Minneapolis, MN, USA) was then applied to the mid-forearm [33].

After each running session, the participants towel-dried themselves and post-exercise body mass was measured. The same bench scale was used and participants wore the same attire as during the pre-exercise body mass assessment. The absorbent patch was then removed from the forearm, placed in the barrel of a plastic syringe using clean forceps and squeezed with a plunger to collect sweat. Sweat samples were analysed for sweat $[Na^+]$ and sweat potassium concentration ($[K^+]$).

2.3. Measurement of Environmental Conditions

Ambient temperature and relative humidity were measured and recorded at 10-min intervals using a data logger (QUESTemp°34, 3M, Minneapolis, MN, USA) during each running session, and the mean value was calculated.

2.4. Urine Specific Gravity (USG)

USG from mid-stream urine samples were measured using a hand-held refractometer (PAL-10S, ATAGO®, Saitama, Japan). USG was assessed in duplicates and the average value was used for recording. USG was used an indicator of hydration status, with USG >1.020 indicating hypohydration and USG >1.030 indicating severe hypohydration [34].

2.5. Whole-Body Sweat Loss (WBSL) and Whole-Body Sweat Rate (WBSR)

WBSL and WBSR were calculated using Equations (1) and (2) respectively:

$$\text{WBSL (L)} = (\text{Pre-exercise body mass (kg)} - \text{Post-exercise body mass (kg)}) + \text{Fluid intake (L)} - \text{Urine output (L)}, \quad (1)$$

$$\text{WBSR (L·h}^{-1}) = \text{WBSL (L)}/\text{Exercise duration (h)}. \quad (2)$$

2.6. Whole-Body Sweat Sodium Concentration

Sweat $[Na^+]$ and sweat $[K^+]$ were analysed via ion-selective electrode (ISE) technology using Na^+ (LAQUAtwin Na-11, HORIBA Advanced Techno Co., Ltd., Kyoto, Japan) and K^+ analysers (LAQUAtwin K-11, HORIBA Advanced Techno Co., Ltd., Kyoto, Japan). Whole-body sweat $[Na^+]$ (mmol·L^{-1}) and whole-body sweat Na^+ loss (mmol) were calculated using Equations (3) and (4) respectively [33]:

$$\text{Predicted whole-body sweat }[Na^+]\text{ (mmol·L}^{-1}) = 0.57\text{ (forearm sweat }Na^+) + 11.05, \quad (3)$$

$$\text{Whole-body sweat }Na^+\text{ loss (mmol)} = \text{WBSL (L)} * \text{Predicted whole-body sweat }[Na^+]\text{ (mmol·L}^{-1}). \quad (4)$$

Sweat [Na$^+$] were classified into three groups: low ([Na$^+$] <30 mmol·L^{-1}), moderate ([Na$^+$] = 30–60 mmol·L^{-1}), and high ([Na$^+$] >60 mmol·L^{-1}) [35,36]. Additionally, 12 samples were randomly selected and analysed using the gold standard high-performance liquid chromatography (HPLC) method (Dionex ICS-5000, Thermo Fisher Scientific, Inc., Waltham, MA, USA).

2.7. Statistical Analysis

Statistical analysis was conducted using IBM SPSS Statistics version 19.0 (IBM, Armonk, NY, USA). Descriptive data were generally expressed as mean ± standard deviation (SD). All biochemical data were log-transformed to reduce non-uniformity of error. The data were back transformed before being expressed as parametric mean ± SD. Normality was determined using the Shapiro–Wilk test. Differences in age, running characteristics, body mass loss, fluid intake, and net fluid balance between males and female runners were analysed using independent *t*-test. Pearson correlation coefficient was used to analyse the correlation between parameters, including the correlation of whole-body sweat [Na$^+$] between ISE and HPLC methods. Correlation coefficients were interpreted based on the following thresholds: $r \leq 0.35$ = weak, $0.36 \leq r \leq 0.67$ = moderate, and $0.68 \leq r \leq 1.0$ = strong [37]. For all analyses, a *p*-value of < 0.05 was considered significant.

3. Results

3.1. Number of Subjects and Environmental Conditions for Each Running Session

There were 166 participants in total (102 males and 64 females). The number of participants for each running session is shown in Table 1, together with the mean ambient temperature and mean relative humidity. The mean (range) ambient temperature and relative humidity across the six running sessions were 29.6 (28.0–31.5) °C and 70 (55–87)% respectively.

Table 1. Time of day, time, environmental conditions and number of participants during each running session.

Session	Time of Day	Time	Mean Ambient Temperature (°C)	Mean Relative Humidity (%)	Participants	
					Male	Female
1	Morning	7.00 a.m. to 8.00 a.m.	28.5	75	9	6
2	Morning	6.00 a.m. to 8.00 a.m.	30	86	10	4
3	Evening	7.00 p.m. to 8.00 p.m.	29.5	63	16	8
4	Evening	7.00 p.m. to 8.00 p.m.	28	87	31	13
5	Evening	7.00 p.m. to 8.00 p.m.	29.8	56	12	12
6	Evening	5.00 p.m. to 6.00 p.m.	31.5	55	24	21

3.2. Participants' Age, Running Profile, and Body Mass Change across Running

Participants were aged between 21–68 years with running experience ranging from 6 months to more than 10 years. All runners were native to Thailand and had been within the country for 6 months, exercising in hot and humid environments, prior to the trial. The running durations of all participants during the running sessions were between 30–100 min. Male runners ran a further mean distance and at a faster mean pace than female runners ($p < 0.05$) (Table 2). However, the mean running duration did not differ between sexes. Both mean WBSL and mean WBSR among the male runners were greater than among the female runners ($p < 0.05$) (Table 2). While six male and four female runners had >2% body mass loss after the running session, percentage body mass loss did not differ between sexes ($p > 0.05$) (Table 2).

Table 2. Mean age, running profile, body mass change, sweat rate, and fluid intake of male and female runners across all running sessions. Data are presented as mean ± SD (range).

	Male (n = 102)	Female (n = 64)
Age (years)	36 ± 9 (21–68)	34 ± 9 (22–62)
Running duration (min)	43.7 ± 14.8 (33–97)	43.6 ± 13.6 (43–100)
Running distance (km)	6.4 ± 1.1 (2.5–12.5)	5.3 ± 1.1 * (2.5–10)
Running pace (min·km^{-1})	6.8 ± 3.7 (3.5–10.0)	8.2 ± 3.9 * (4.3–11.0)
Pre-running body mass (kg)	70.8 ± 10.6 (46.9–99.7)	56.7 ± 9.7 * (42.3–93.2)
Post-running body mass (kg)	70.2 ± 10.6 (46.6–99.0)	56.4 ± 9.6 * (42.3–92.8)
Percentage body mass loss (%)	1.3 ± 0.5 (0.2–3.6)	1.2 ± 0.5 (0.1–3.7)
Whole-body sweat loss (WBSL) (L)	0.9 ± 0.3 (0.2–2.6)	0.6 ± 0.3 * (0.1–1.9)
Whole-body sweat rate (WBSR) (L·h^{-1})	1.3 ± 0.5 (0.2–3.8)	0.9 ± 0.3 * (0.1–2.2)
Fluid intake (L)	0.3 ± 0.3 (0–1.1)	0.3 ± 0.2 (0–1.1)

* $p < 0.05$, compared to male participants.

3.3. Urine Specific Gravity

USG data were absent from 18 male and four female runners due to insufficient urine samples. Mean USG of runners who ran in the morning and evening were 1.015 ± 0.008 and 1.013 ± 0.007, respectively. There was no difference between the mean USG of runners from the morning and evening sessions ($p > 0.05$). The number of hypohydrated participants (USG > 1.020) did not differ between the morning or evening running session ($p > 0.05$). However, a greater percentage of participants were hypohydrated (USG > 1.020) before the run when the running session was conducted in the morning (28%) than in the evening (15%) (Table 3). A greater number of runners were severely hypohydrated (USG > 1.030) before the run when the session was conducted in the morning (4%) than in the evening (1%). In addition, when the running session was conducted in the morning, there is a moderate positive correlation between pre-exercise USG and fluid intake ($p < 0.05$, $r = 0.42$), and a moderate negative correlation between pre-exercise USG of male runners and WBSL ($p < 0.05$, $r = -0.54$).

Table 3. Level of dehydration between sexes (male vs. female) and time of day of running session (morning vs. evening) based on pre-exercise urine specific gravity (USG).

Time of Day of Session	Sex	Urine Specific Gravity (USG)		
		≤1.020	>1.020	>1.030
Morning	Male	11 (69%)	4 (31%)	1 (6%)
	Female	7 (78%)	2 (22%)	0 (0%)
	Total	18 (72%)	6 (28%)	1 (4%)
Evening	Male	59 (85%)	10 (15%)	1 (1%)
	Female	43 (84%)	8 (16%)	0 (0%)
	Total	102 (85%)	18 (15%)	1 (1%)

3.4. Relative Sweat Loss and Fluid Intake during Running

Mean WBSR during recreational running was higher in males than females ($p < 0.05$) (Table 2). Sweat loss relative to body mass was calculated and differences between sexes were compared. Males had higher sweat loss relative to body mass than female runners

(19 ± 8 vs. 16 ± 6 mL·kg^{-1}·h^{-1}, $p < 0.05$) (Figure 1). With regards to fluid intake during running, 15 of the 102 male runners (14.7%) did not drink any water during the run. However, only two of the 64 female runners (3.1%) did not drink any water during the run. Mean *ad libitum* fluid intake during running in males and females did not differ between sexes ($p > 0.05$) (Table 2). However, male runners had a lower fluid intake relative to body mass than female runners (6 ± 6 vs. 8 ± 7 mL·kg^{-1}·h^{-1}, $p < 0.05$) (Figure 1). Therefore, males had a greater negative fluid balance relative to body mass than female runners (-13 ± 8 mL·kg^{-1}·h^{-1} or -67.4% vs. -8 ± 7 mL·kg^{-1}·h^{-1} or -48.9%, $p < 0.05$) (Figure 1). Furthermore, running pace and sweat rate were found to have a moderate negative correlation ($r = -0.47$, $p < 0.01$).

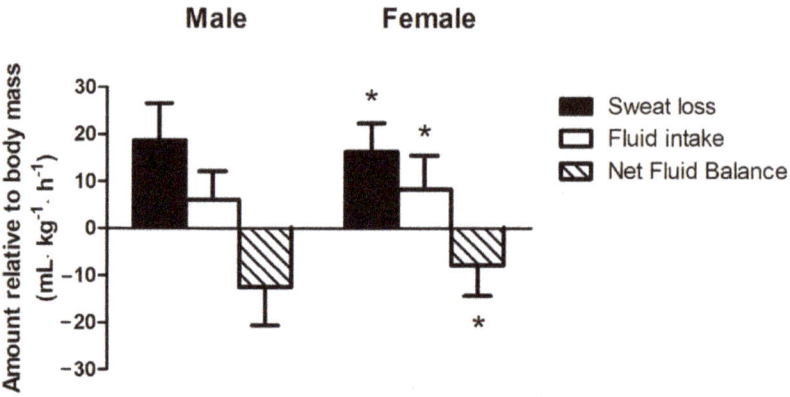

Figure 1. Relative sweat loss, fluid intake, and net fluid balance (mL·kg^{-1}·h^{-1}) between sexes. Data are presented as mean $\pm$ SD. * $p < 0.05$, compared to male participants.

3.5. Sweat Sodium and Potassium Concentration

Sweat data were absent from five male and 15 female participants due to insufficient volume of sweat sample. Figure 2A presents the distribution of sweat [Na$^+$] among the remaining 97 males and 49 female runners. Sweat [Na$^+$] did not correlate with sweat rate, USG, fluid intake, or running distance or pace ($p > 0.05$). A strong positive correlation was observed between sweat [Na$^+$] measured using ISE method and HPLC ($p < 0.001$, $r = 0.994$) (Figure 3). Mean rate of sweat Na$^+$ loss (54 ± 27 vs. 39 ± 22 mmol·h^{-1}) was higher in males than females (both $p < 0.05$) (Figure 2B) but no difference was observed in whole-body sweat [Na$^+$] losses between sexes ($p > 0.05$). The majority of runners' sweat [Na$^+$] were classified as moderate (male: 76%; female: 51%). High sweat [Na$^+$] was least prevalent as it was only observed in 8% and 16% of male and female runners respectively. Mean sweat [K$^+$] did not differ between the male (3.9 ± 1.1 mmol·L^{-1}) and female runners (3.5 ± 0.7 mmol·L^{-1}) ($p > 0.05$).

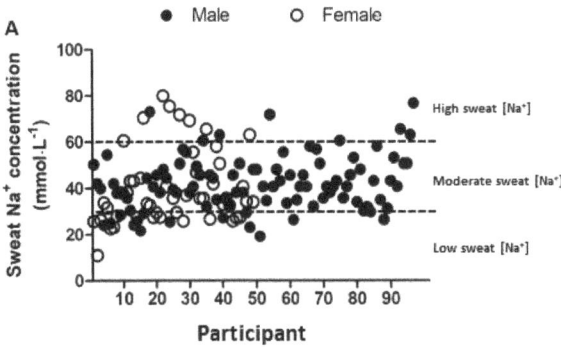

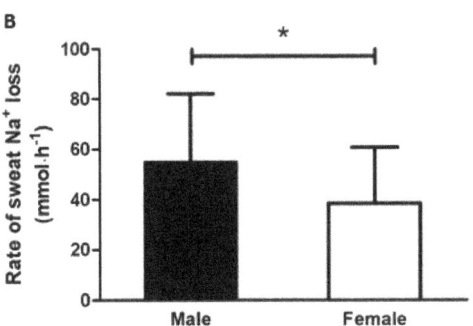

Figure 2. (**A**) Distribution of whole-body sweat Na$^+$ concentration (mmol·L^{-1}) among 97 male and 49 female participants; (**B**) rate of sweat Na$^+$ loss (mmol·h^{-1}) compared between male and female runners. Data are presented as mean ± SD. * $p < 0.05$, compared to male participants.

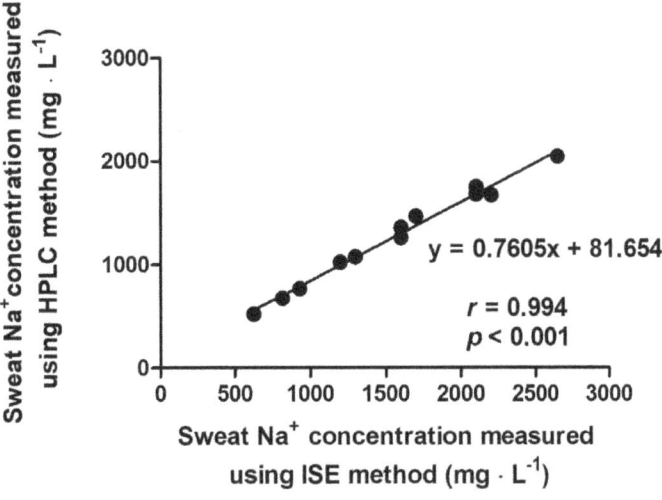

Figure 3. Relationship between sweat Na$^+$ concentration measured by ion-selective electrode (ISE) and high-performance liquid chromatography (HPLC) methods.

4. Discussion

The aim of this study was to evaluate the hydration status, fluid intake, sweat rate, and sweat [Na$^+$] in recreational tropical native runners. Consistent with previous studies, WBSR ranged between 0.3–2.5 L·h^{-1}, with male runners having higher WBSR and WBSL relative to body mass than female runners. Fluid intake was lower in male runners compared to females, who consumed more fluid relative to body mass than males. Predicted whole-body sweat [Na$^+$] did not vary between sexes and did not correlate with any other parameters. However, males had a higher sweat Na$^+$ loss and rate of sweat Na$^+$ loss as compared to female tropical native runners.

The mean WBSR (male: 1.3 ± 0.5 L·h^{-1} and female: 0.9 ± 0.3 L·h^{-1}) for tropical native runners was similar to those reported previously in American runners involving 275 male and 52 female adult endurance athletes (male: 1.4 ± 0.4 L·h^{-1} and female: 1.1 ± 0.6 L·h^{-1}) (16). Relative WBSL was also comparable to experienced marathon runners in a 16-km race (18.7 ± 7.9 vs. 21.6 ± 5.1 mL·kg^{-1}·h^{-1}), albeit the race being performed in an environment with cooler ambient temperature but similar relative humidity (29.6 ± 1.2 °C, $70 \pm 15\%$ vs. 20.5 ± 0.7 °C, $76.6 \pm 1.7\%$) [38]. These similar observations, despite differences in environmental conditions, could be caused by the effects of heat acclimatisation in experienced athletes [39]. Experienced athletes have thermoregulatory adaptations which include increased sudomotor function associated with acclimatisation [39].

The mean WBSR observed during our study is lower compared to another study involving male runners in a half-marathon, despite similar environmental conditions (1.3 ± 0.5 vs. 1.5 ± 0.3 L·h^{-1}) [40]. A reason for this observation is likely to be differences in exercise intensity. The running pace in the present study was slower than that performed in the half-marathon (6.8 vs. 5.6 min·km^{-1}). Both laboratory and field-based studies have reported the relationship between exercise intensity and sweat rate in various exercise types such as running, cycling, and football training [41,42]. However, it is important to note that despite the slower running speed, the relative intensity of exercise may have been similar between the two groups. Speculatively, runners completing a half-marathon distance would have a greater maximal aerobic capacity and faster submaximal running velocities compared to tropical native recreational runners. However, the relative intensity of the runs was not measured and hence, was a limitation of the present study.

Our study found that male runners had a higher WBSR than female runners, and that sweat loss relative to body mass was lower in female than male runners. Males generally have a higher sweat rate than females due to larger body size, musculature and higher metabolic rate [43]. The sex of the runner also plays a role in the peripheral control of sweat rate via the number of activated sweat glands (ASGs) and sweat gland output (SGO) [44]. While females have a higher number of ASGs than males during the early follicular phase, their sweat rate in dry and/or humid environments is still lower than males [45]. This may be related to SGO, as previous studies have reported lower SGO in females compared to males during passive heat stress [46]. Moreover, previous evidence on the difference in thermoregulatory adaptation mechanisms revealed that after training, males can only enhance SGO while females can enhance both SGO and ASGs. While trained athletes usually have a higher sweat rate than untrained athletes due to the thermoregulatory adaptations, sweat responses at the same exercise intensity showed that trained males still have higher sweat rates than trained females [44]. Thus, sex can play a role in determining fluid loss through sweat.

To support performance and reduce the risk of heat illness, the American College of Sports Medicine Position Stand advises to avoid body mass loss of >2% from pre-exercise body mass during exercise [12]. In this study, six male and four female runners experienced >2% body mass loss after the run. Consistent with previous research during a marathon race, the mean *ad libitum* fluid intake did not differ between male and female runners [47]. However, when expressed relative to body mass, fluid intake was higher in female runners compared to their male counterparts. As a result, we also observed that female runners experienced less negative net fluid balance relative to body mass. This could be due to the lower pre- and post-exercise body mass of female runners as compared to males. However, there remained a large range (-46–15 mL·kg^{-1}·h^{-1}) in net fluid balance after exercise in both males and females. This observation would suggest that runners should understand their individual fluid intake requirements to prevent excessive hypohydration, link levels of hypohydration with running performance, and reduce the risk of accumulating body mass through fluid intake during exercise [25]. It is important to note that, due to the nature of the field study, it was not possible to measure body mass in the ideal conditions (i.e., nude body mass) or weigh individual running attires after the run. Based on previous studies, a fully soaked running attire weighs approximately 0.26 kg [48,49]. Although accounting for a trapped sweat volume of 0.26 L or lower would not affect our overall conclusions, this is an acknowledged limitation of the present study.

Predicted whole-body sweat [Na$^+$] did not differ between sexes. However, male runners had higher mean rate of Na$^+$ loss than female runners. The likely reason for these observations is the higher mean WBSR and WBSL relative to body mass in males than females [50]. This indicates that runners who sweat more are at a greater risk of losing more Na$^+$ than runners who sweat less. The predicted whole-body sweat [Na$^+$] of tropical native runners ranged between 11–80 mmol·L^{-1}. These values are similar to a previous study in runners completing a marathon (7–95 mmol·L^{-1} [36]), albeit at a lower mean ambient temperature (24.4 $\pm$ 3.6 °C) and mean relative humidity (28 $\pm$ 5%). Our findings are also comparable to the sweat [Na$^+$] data collected from 506 athletes across various sports (12.6–104.8 mmol·L^{-1}) [16]. Asian populations have higher dietary Na$^+$ intake across all ages as compared to those from other parts of the world [51,52]. While the World Health Organisation recommends that sodium intake should not exceed 2 g/day, most Southeast Asian countries consume more than the recommended amount [53]. For example, the average sodium intake in Thailand is 3–5 g per day and the average sodium intake in Singapore is 3–4 g per day [53]. As high Na$^+$ intake has been shown to increase sweat [Na$^+$] [54], the higher predicted whole-body sweat [Na$^+$] in the present study may have been expected. The analysis of sweat [K$^+$] in the present provided a quality control for the analysis of sweat samples [15]. Therefore, we have confidence in the sweat [Na$^+$] values. A possible explanation for the similarity in sweat [Na$^+$] might be the effects of heat acclimatisation, which has been shown to reduce sweat sodium [55,56]. However, dietary intake and its associated Na$^+$ intake were not measured, and this is a limitation of the present study. Thus, it is not possible to ascertain if acclimatisation counteracted the impact of high Na$^+$ intake on sweat [Na$^+$]. Given the inter-individual variability of predicted whole-body sweat [Na$^+$] and that no correlation to age, exercise intensity, exercise duration or sweat rate was found, the results support recommendation of individualised fluid and electrolyte replacement strategies.

Runners were more likely to be hypohydrated before the morning run compared to the evening. It is recommended that participants should slowly drink approximately 5–10 mL per kg of their body mass at least 2 h before exercising to allow for fluid absorption and achieve euhydration [22]. The finding in the present study could be attributed to insufficient time to drink appropriate volumes of fluid and the ingestion of food in the morning. The moderate positive correlation between pre-exercise USG and fluid intake, and moderate negative correlation between pre-exercise USG and WBSL suggest that hypohydration may impair thermoregulatory function, which increases the risk of heat illness in hot climates [57]. This is of interest as endurance running events such as marathons typically begin early in the morning. Since achieving euhydration before exercise can reduce the risk of heat illnesses [9,12], runners are encouraged to adjust their pre-race wake-up time to ensure they can meet pre-exercise hydration guidelines when running in tropical climates.

Practical Implications and Future Directions

This study showed that the range of sweat rates and sweat [Na$^+$] of tropical native runners were similar to that reported previously in hydration literatures. Therefore, individual fluid recommendations also apply to tropical native runners. Future studies should aim to analyse the runners' dietary Na$^+$ intake to understand the impact on the sweat Na$^+$ losses. Finally, the data in the present study were collected during recreational running. Understanding the impact of hydration strategies before and during exercise on running performance in competitive tropical native runners is required. Correspondingly, these studies can ascertain if the threshold of hypohydration tolerance, i.e., 2% body mass loss on exercise performance, also applies to tropical native athletes.

5. Conclusions

These descriptive data gathered on recreational tropical native runners revealed the individual variability in hydration status, fluid intake, sweat rate, and sweat Na$^+$ loss during exercise. Female runners experienced less negative net fluid balance compared to males due to greater fluid intake per body mass and lower sweat loss. Whole-body sweat [Na$^+$] also varied between individuals independent of sex.

Author Contributions: Conceptualization, J.S., V.S., I.R., and J.K.W.L.; methodology, J.S., I.R., and J.K.W.L.; validation, I.R., and R.K.R.; investigation, J.S., V.S., K.N., and P.S.; data curation, J.S., V.S., K.N., and P.S.; writing—original draft preparation, J.S.; writing—review and editing, J.S., I.R., R.K.R., C.H.W.L., and J.K.W.L.; supervision, V.S., and J.K.W.L.; project administration, J.S.; funding acquisition, J.S., I.R., and J.K.W.L. All authors have read and agreed to the published version of the manuscript.

Funding: This work was supported by grants from Faculty of Physical Therapy, Mahidol University, Suntory PepsiCo Beverage Thailand Co., Ltd., and Gatorade Sports Science Institute.

Institutional Review Board Statement: The study was conducted according to the guidelines of the Declaration of Helsinki, and approved by the Centre of Ethical Reinforcement for Human Research, Mahidol University (MU-CIRB 2018/208.2311 and protocol no. 2018/198.0910, 23 November 2018)

Informed Consent Statement: Informed consent was obtained from all subjects involved in the study.

Data Availability Statement: The data presented in this study are available on request from the corresponding author and the permission of all parties involved in the study.

Acknowledgments: We would like to thank all participating runners and all those involved in data collection. We would also like to thank Corey Ungaro for completion of the sweat sodium concentration analysis using HPLC.

Conflicts of Interest: I.R. and R.K.R. are employees of the Gatorade Sports Science Institute, a division of PepsiCo, Incorporated. The views expressed in this article are those of the authors and do not necessarily reflect the position or policy of PepsiCo, Incorporated.

References

1. Cunha, F.; Midgley, A.; Monteiro, W.; Farinatti, P. Influence of cardiopulmonary exercise testing protocol and resting VO2 assessment on %HRmax, %HRR, %VO2max and %VO2R relationships. *Int. J. Sports Med.* **2010**, *31*, 319–326. [CrossRef]
2. Binkley, H.M.; Beckett, J.; Casa, D.J.; Kleiner, D.M.; Plummer, P.E. National Athletic Trainers' Association position statement: Exertional heat illnesses. *J. Athl. Train.* **2002**, *37*, 329.
3. McDermott, B.P.; Anderson, S.A.; Armstrong, L.E.; Casa, D.J.; Cheuvront, S.N.; Cooper, L.; Kenney, W.L.; O'Connor, F.G.; Roberts, W.O. National Athletic Trainers' Association position statement: Fluid replacement for the physically active. *J. Athl. Train.* **2017**, *52*, 877–895. [CrossRef]
4. Adams, W.; Fox, R.; Fry, A.; MacDonald, I. Thermoregulation during marathon running in cool, moderate, and hot environments. *J. Appl. Physiol.* **1975**, *38*, 1030–1037. [CrossRef] [PubMed]
5. Gagnon, D.; Jay, O.; Kenny, G.P. The evaporative requirement for heat balance determines whole-body sweat rate during exercise under conditions permitting full evaporation. *J. Physiol.* **2013**, *591*, 2925–2935. [CrossRef] [PubMed]
6. Lee, J.K.W.; Nio, A.Q.; Lim, C.L.; Teo, E.Y.; Byrne, C. Thermoregulation, pacing and fluid balance during mass participation distance running in a warm and humid environment. *Eur. J. Appl. Physiol.* **2010**, *109*, 887–898. [CrossRef] [PubMed]
7. Reeve, T.; Gordon, R.; Laursen, P.B.; Lee, J.K.W.; Tyler, C.J. Impairment of cycling capacity in the heat in well-trained endurance athletes after high-intensity short-term heat acclimation. *Int. J. Sports Physiol. Perform.* **2019**, *14*, 1058–1065. [CrossRef] [PubMed]
8. Murray, B. The role of salt and glucose replacement drinks in the marathon. *Sports Med.* **2007**, *37*, 358–360. [CrossRef]
9. Noakes, T. Fluid replacement during marathon running. *Clin. J. Sport Med.* **2003**, *13*, 309–318. [CrossRef]

10. Andersen, J.J. The State of Running 2019. Available online: https://runrepeat.com/state-of-running (accessed on 24 October 2020).
11. Gleeson, M. Temperature regulation during exercise. *Int. J. Sports Med.* **1998**, *19*, S96–S99. [CrossRef]
12. Sawka, M.N.; Burke, L.M.; Eichner, E.R.; Maughan, R.J.; Montain, S.J.; Stachenfeld, N.S. American College of Sports Medicine position stand. Exercise and fluid replacement. *Med. Sci. Sports Exerc.* **2007**, *39*, 377–390. [PubMed]
13. Armstrong, L.E. Assessing hydration status: The elusive gold standard. *J. Am. Coll. Nutr.* **2007**, *26* (Suppl. 5), 575S–584S. [CrossRef]
14. Amano, T.; Ichinose, M.; Koga, S.; Inoue, Y.; Nishiyasu, T.; Kondo, N. Sweating responses and the muscle metaboreflex under mildly hyperthermic conditions in sprinters and distance runners. *J. Appl. Physiol.* **2011**, *111*, 524–529. [CrossRef]
15. Baker, L.B. Sweating rate and sweat sodium concentration in athletes: A review of methodology and intra/interindividual variability. *Sports Med.* **2017**, *47*, 111–128. [CrossRef] [PubMed]
16. Baker, L.B.; Barnes, K.A.; Anderson, M.L.; Passe, D.H.; Stofan, J.R. Normative data for regional sweat sodium concentration and whole-body sweating rate in athletes. *J. Sports Sci.* **2016**, *34*, 358–368. [CrossRef]
17. Baker, L.B.; Ungaro, C.T.; Sopeña, B.C.; Nuccio, R.P.; Reimel, A.J.; Carter, J.M.; Stofan, J.R.; Barnes, K.A. Body map of regional vs. whole body sweating rate and sweat electrolyte concentrations in men and women during moderate exercise-heat stress. *J. Appl. Physiol.* **2018**, *124*, 1304–1318. [CrossRef]
18. Gonzalez, R.R.; Cheuvront, S.N.; Ely, B.R.; Moran, D.S.; Hadid, A.; Endrusick, T.L.; Sawka, M.N. Sweat rate prediction equations for outdoor exercise with transient solar radiation. *J. Appl. Physiol.* **2012**, *112*, 1300–1310. [CrossRef]
19. Kilding, A.; Tunstall, H.; Wraith, E.; Good, M.; Gammon, C.; Smith, C. Sweat rate and sweat electrolyte composition in international female soccer players during game specific training. *Int. J. Sports Med.* **2009**, *30*, 443–447. [CrossRef]
20. Patterson, M.J.; Galloway, S.D.; Nimmo, M.A. Variations in regional sweat composition in normal human males. *Exp. Physiol.* **2000**, *85*, 869–875. [CrossRef]
21. Maughan, R.J.; Shirreffs, S.M. Development of individual hydration strategies for athletes. *Int. J. Sport Nutr. Exerc. Metab.* **2008**, *18*, 457–472. [CrossRef] [PubMed]
22. Goulet, E.D. Dehydration and endurance performance in competitive athletes. *Nutr. Rev.* **2012**, *70* (Suppl. 2), S132–S136. [CrossRef]
23. Almond, C.S.; Shin, A.Y.; Fortescue, E.B.; Mannix, R.C.; Wypij, D.; Binstadt, B.A.; Duncan, C.N.; Olson, D.P.; Salerno, A.E.; Newburger, J.W.; et al. Hyponatremia among runners in the Boston Marathon. *N. Engl. J. Med.* **2005**, *352*, 1550–1556. [CrossRef] [PubMed]
24. Carter, R., III. Exertional heat illness and hyponatremia: An epidemiological prospective. *Curr. Sports Med. Rep.* **2008**, *7*, S20–S27. [CrossRef]
25. Chorley, J.; Cianca, J.; Divine, J. Risk factors for exercise-associated hyponatremia in non-elite marathon runners. *Clin. J. Sport Med.* **2007**, *17*, 471–477. [CrossRef] [PubMed]
26. Hew-Butler, T.; Loi, V.; Pani, A.; Rosner, M.H. Exercise-associated hyponatremia: 2017 update. *Front. Med.* **2017**, *4*, 21. [CrossRef]
27. Rosner, M.H. (Ed.) Exercise-associated hyponatremia. In *Seminars in Nephrology*; Elsevier: Amsterdam, The Netherlands, 2009.
28. Speedy, D.B.; Noakes, T.D.; Schneider, C. Exercise-associated hyponatremia: A review. *Emerg. Med.* **2001**, *13*, 17–27. [CrossRef] [PubMed]
29. Nadel, E.; Pandolf, K.; Roberts, M.; Stolwijk, J. Mechanisms of thermal acclimation to exercise and heat. *J. Appl. Physiol.* **1974**, *37*, 515–520. [CrossRef]
30. Roberts, M.F.; Wenger, C.B.; Stolwijk, J.A.; Nadel, E.R. Skin blood flow and sweating changes following exercise training and heat acclimation. *J. Appl. Physiol.* **1977**, *43*, 133–137. [CrossRef]
31. Shapiro, Y.; Hubbard, R.W.; Kimbrough, C.M.; Pandolf, K.B. Physiological and hematologic responses to summer and winter dry-heat acclimation. *J. Appl. Physiol.* **1981**, *50*, 792–798. [CrossRef]
32. Thomas, D.T.; Erdman, K.A.; Burke, L.M. Position of the Academy of Nutrition and Dietetics, Dietitians of Canada, and the American College of Sports Medicine: Nutrition and athletic performance. *J. Acad. Nutr. Diet.* **2016**, *116*, 501–528. [CrossRef]
33. Baker, L.B.; Stofan, J.R.; Hamilton, A.A.; Horswill, C.A. Comparison of regional patch collection vs. whole body washdown for measuring sweat sodium and potassium loss during exercise. *J. Appl. Physiol.* **2009**, *107*, 887–895. [CrossRef] [PubMed]
34. Bates, G.P.; Miller, V.S.; Joubert, D.M. Hydration status of expatriate manual workers during summer in the Middle East. *Ann. Occup. Hyg.* **2010**, *54*, 137–143.
35. Lara, B.; Salinero, J.; Areces, F.; Ruiz-Vicente, D.; Gallo-Salazar, C.; Abián-Vicén, J.; Del Coso, J. Sweat sodium loss influences serum sodium concentration in a marathon. *Scand. J. Med. Sci. Sports* **2017**, *27*, 152–160. [CrossRef] [PubMed]
36. Lara, B.; Gallo-Salazar, C.; Puente, C.; Areces, F.; Salinero, J.J.; Del Coso, J. Interindividual variability in sweat electrolyte concentration in marathoners. *J. Int. Soc. Sports Nutr.* **2016**, *13*, 31. [CrossRef]
37. Taylor, R. Interpretation of the correlation coefficient: A basic review. *J. Diagn. Med. Sonogr.* **1990**, *6*, 35–39. [CrossRef]
38. Passe, D.; Horn, M.; Stofan, J.; Horswill, C.; Murray, R. Voluntary dehydration in runners despite favorable conditions for fluid intake. *Int. J. Sport Nutr. Exerc. Metab.* **2007**, *17*, 284–295. [CrossRef] [PubMed]
39. Périard, J.; Racinais, S.; Sawka, M.N. Adaptations and mechanisms of human heat acclimation: Applications for competitive athletes and sports. *Scand. J. Med. Sci. Sports* **2015**, *25*, 20–38. [CrossRef]
40. Byrne, C.; Lee, J.K.W.; Chew, S.A.N.; Lim, C.L.; Tan, E.Y.M. Continuous thermoregulatory responses to mass-participation distance running in heat. *Med. Sci. Sports Exerc.* **2006**, *38*, 803–810. [CrossRef]

41. Hargreaves, M.; Dillo, P.; Angus, D.; Febbraio, M. Effect of fluid ingestion on muscle metabolism during prolonged exercise. *J. Appl. Physiol.* **1996**, *80*, 363–366. [CrossRef] [PubMed]
42. Sawka, M.N. Physiological consequences of hypohydration: Exercise performance and thermoregulation. *Med. Sci. Sports Exerc.* **1992**, *24*, 657–670. [CrossRef]
43. Bar-Or, O. Effects of age and gender on sweating pattern during exercise. *Int. J. Sports Med.* **1998**, *19*, S106–S107. [CrossRef]
44. Ichinose-Kuwahara, T.; Inoue, Y.; Iseki, Y.; Hara, S.; Ogura, Y.; Kondo, N. Sex differences in the effects of physical training on sweat gland responses during a graded exercise. *Exp. Physiol.* **2010**, *95*, 1026–1032. [CrossRef]
45. Morimoto, T.; Slabochova, Z.; Naman, R.; Sargent, F., 2nd. Sex differences in physiological reactions to thermal stress. *J. Appl. Physiol.* **1967**, *22*, 526–532. [CrossRef]
46. Inoue, Y.; Tanaka, Y.; Omori, K.; Kuwahara, T.; Ogura, Y.; Ueda, H. Sex-and menstrual cycle-related differences in sweating and cutaneous blood flow in response to passive heat exposure. *Eur. J. Appl. Physiol.* **2005**, *94*, 323–332. [CrossRef]
47. Hew, T.D. Women hydrate more than men during a marathon race: Hyponatremia in the Houston marathon: A report on 60 cases. *Clin. J. Sport Med.* **2005**, *15*, 148–153. [CrossRef]
48. Tan, X.R.; Low, I.C.C.; Byrne, C.; Wang, R.; Lee, J.K.W. Assessment of dehydration using body mass changes of elite marathoners in the tropics. *J. Sci. Med. Sport.* **2021**. [CrossRef] [PubMed]
49. Pugh, L.; Corbett, J.; Johnson, R. Rectal temperatures, weight losses, and sweat rates in marathon running. *J. Appl. Physiol.* **1967**, *23*, 347–352. [CrossRef] [PubMed]
50. Maughan, R. Fluid and electrolyte loss and replacement in exercise. *J. Sports Sci.* **1991**, *9*, 117–142. [CrossRef]
51. Powles, J.; Fahimi, S.; Micha, R.; Khatibzadeh, S.; Shi, P.; Ezzati, M.; Engell, R.E.; Lim, S.S.; Danaei, G.; Mozaffarian, D.; et al. Global, regional and national sodium intakes in 1990 and 2010: A systematic analysis of 24 h urinary sodium excretion and dietary surveys worldwide. *BMJ Open* **2013**, *3*, e003733. [CrossRef] [PubMed]
52. Elliott, P.; Brown, I. *Sodium Intakes around the World*; World Health Organization: Geneva, Switzerland, 2007.
53. Batcagan-Abueg, A.P.; Lee, J.J.; Chan, P.; Rebello, S.A.; Amarra, M.S.V. Salt intakes and salt reduction initiatives in Southeast Asia: A review. *Asia Pac. J. Clin. Nutr.* **2013**, *22*, 683.
54. Braconnier, P.; Milani, B.; Loncle, N.; Lourenco, J.M.; Brito, W.; Delacoste, J.; Maillard, M.; Stuber, M.; Burnier, M.; Pruijm, M. Short-term changes in dietary sodium intake influence sweat sodium concentration and muscle sodium content in healthy individuals. *J. Hypertens.* **2020**, *38*, 159–166. [CrossRef] [PubMed]
55. Buono, M.J.; Ball, K.D.; Kolkhorst, F.W. Sodium ion concentration vs. sweat rate relationship in humans. *J. Appl. Physiol.* **2007**, *103*, 990–994. [CrossRef] [PubMed]
56. Buono, M.J.; Kolding, M.; Leslie, E.; Moreno, D.; Norwood, S.; Ordille, A.; Weller, R. Heat acclimation causes a linear decrease in sweat sodium ion concentration. *J. Therm. Biol.* **2018**, *71*, 237–240. [CrossRef] [PubMed]
57. Kenefick, R.W.; Cheuvront, S.N. Physiological adjustments to hypohydration: Impact on thermoregulation. *Auton. Neurosci.* **2016**, *196*, 47–51. [CrossRef] [PubMed]

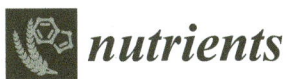

Article

Does the Minerals Content and Osmolarity of the Fluids Taken during Exercise by Female Field Hockey Players Influence on the Indicators of Water-Electrolyte and Acid-Basic Balance?

Joanna Kamińska [1,*], Tomasz Podgórski [1], Krzysztof Rachwalski [2] and Maciej Pawlak [1]

[1] Chair of Dietetics, Department of Physiology and Biochemistry, Poznań University of Physical Education, 61-871 Poznań, Poland; podgorski@awf.poznan.pl (T.P.); pawlak@awf.poznan.pl (M.P.)
[2] Chair of Theory and Methodology of Sport, Department of Theory and Methodology of Team Sport Games, Poznań University of Physical Education, 61-871 Poznań, Poland; rachwalski@awf.poznan.pl
* Correspondence: jkaminska@awf.poznan.pl; Tel.: +48-618-355-187

Abstract: Although it is recognized that dehydration and acidification of the body may reduce the exercise capacity, it remains unclear whether the qualitative and quantitative shares of certain ions in the drinks used by players during the same exertion may affect the indicators of their water–electrolyte and acid–base balance. This question was the main purpose of the publication. The research was carried out on female field hockey players ($n = 14$) throughout three specialized training sessions, during which the players received randomly assigned fluids of different osmolarity and minerals contents. The water–electrolyte and acid–base balance of the players was assessed on the basis of biochemical blood and urine indicators immediately before and after each training session. There were statistically significant differences in the values of all examined indicators for changes before and after exercise, while the differences between the consumed drinks with different osmolarities were found for plasma osmolality, and concentrations of sodium and potassium ions and aldosterone. Therefore, it can be assumed that the degree of mineralization of the consumed water did not have a very significant impact on the indicators of water–electrolyte and acid–base balance in blood and urine.

Keywords: hydration status; water–electrolyte balance; acid–base balance; fluids osmolarity; team sports; nutrition; women in sport

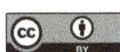

1. Introduction

Field hockey is a team sport practiced by women and men, both on a recreational and professional level [1]. At the elite level, field hockey players cover between 3.4 km and 9.5 km during training and competition depending on their position on the pitch [2,3], with 55% being low-intensity efforts (standing, walking), 38% moderate intensity (jogging, running), and the remaining 7% being high-intensity efforts (fast running, sprinting) [4]. Physical activity increases the body's internal temperature [5]. Compensating mechanisms, especially increased sweat production [6], cause a loss of water and the electrolytes contained in it [7]. Moreover, acidic compounds formed during exercise simultaneously contribute to disturbances in the acid–base balance [8,9], reducing sports performance, especially muscle endurance [10] or cognitive functions [11]. It is therefore important to control and, if necessary, replenish fluids of an appropriate qualitative and quantitative profile before or during exercise. The transport of fluids into the bloodstream and tissues depends, *inter alia*, on the speed at which they leave the stomach and on the effectiveness of their absorption in the small intestine. The above depends on the volume of fluid consumed, the content of energetic substances such as glucose in the fluid, and the concentration gradient on both sides of the intestinal barrier. Thus, the transport of water from the intestines into the bloodstream and tissues is greater for hypotonic than hypertonic drinks, since the latter support the movement of water from the tissues into the lumen of the gastrointestinal tract [12]. On the other hand, the ingestion of low-mineral water (hypotonic solutions) reduces plasma osmolality, which stimulates urine production and may increase dehydration [13,14].

The regulation of the concentration of sodium and potassium ion levels in the body depends on the renin–angiotensin–aldosterone system (RAA). Aldosterone inhibits the excretion of sodium in the urine, increasing the loss of potassium ions from body fluids. In addition, this hormone is secreted as a result of an increase in the concentration of hydrogen ions in the blood accompanying exercise [15]. Such an excess of hydrogen ions is excreted in the urine, and the speed of this process depends on the amount of urine excreted.

The volume of fluids consumed by humans is regulated not only by physiological factors, but also by subjective ones, whereby the taste attractiveness of liquids may prove to be an important factor in the hydration process, especially taking into account the volumes consumed by players [16]. In the case of water, its tastiness is influenced by an increase in the proportion of sodium ions, which stimulates physiological thirst and thus leads to better hydration [13]. Therefore, isotonic fluids most effectively compensate for water and electrolyte losses caused by physical exercise, while providing additional energy [17].

It has been hypothesized that consuming beverages with a higher osmolarity and/or content of minerals lead to a more favorable water–electrolyte and acid–base balance compared to the intake of low-mineralized water. To verify this hypothesis, taking into account the intensity and duration of training, ambient conditions and the athlete's individual physiological profile, during the standard training of female field hockey players, was the main purpose of the research. In the publication, the authors also set themselves the goal of describing changes in the water–electrolyte and acid–base balance indicators in terms of adapting the bodies of female field hockey players to standard training loads.

2. Materials and Methods

2.1. Experimental Approach

The levels of biochemical and hematological indicators in female field hockey players were assessed during three specialized training sessions, during which the players randomly received fluids of different osmolarities. The water–electrolyte and acid–base balance was assessed on the basis of blood and urine indicators, which were obtained immediately before and after each training session.

2.2. Participants

The research included 14 players training in field hockey, members of the women's national team and women's junior team. Players participated in training sessions five times per week. The weekly training time was, on average, 6.5 ± 1.0 h. Training was complemented with 1 match per week during the three weeks of the research period. The weekly framework of the training program is presented below:

Monday—active recovery training + static stretching
Tuesday—technical/tactical training session + interval run
Wednesday—technical/tactical training session (research measurements)
Thursday—training game/small side games
Friday—individual gym session
Saturday—free/passive recovery
Sunday—Polish League competition

Goalkeepers were excluded from the research due to the different nature of the effort they performed.

The average training experience of the female competitors was 12.5 ± 2.9 years. They were non-smokers, as evidenced by the mean contents of carboxyhemoglobin in the blood of female hockey players, amounting to $0.9\% \pm 0.2\%$. For 22 h before the tests, the contestants did not perform any intense physical effort. An hour before each test date, they ate a standard meal (porridge in milk with banana), the caloric content of which corresponded to 10% of the daily food ration of each of the competitors. Additionally, the competitors were not allowed to eat any food during the whole training.

The anthropometric data of the players were determined on the basis of measurements made before the start of each training session (Table 1). Their height and weight were measured using a medical scale WPT60/150 OW (Radwag®, Radom, Poland), while the waist circumference was measured using a tailor's tape measure. The mass of urine excreted was determined by comparing body mass immediately after exercise and body mass after urination (Figure 1).

Table 1. Somatic and physiological characteristics of female field hockey players ($n = 14$).

Characteristics	Low-Mineralized Water		High-Mineralized Water		Isotonic Drink		p Value
	$\overline{X} \pm SD$	95% CI	$\overline{X} \pm SD$	95% CI	$\overline{X} \pm SD$	95% CI	
Age (years)	21.9 ± 2.3	(20.6–23.2)	21.9 ± 2.3	(20.6–23.2)	21.9 ± 2.3	(20.6–23.2)	1.000
Body height (m)	1.70 ± 0.06	(1.67–1.74)	1.70 ± 0.06	(1.67–1.74)	1.70 ± 0.06	(1.67–1.74)	1.000
Body mass (kg)	65.3 ± 5.4	(62.2–68.4)	65.4 ± 5.4	(62.2–68.5)	65.2 ± 5.0	(62.3–68.1)	0.712
WHtR	42.9 ± 1.4	(42.1–43.7)	43.0 ± 1.4	(42.1–43.8)	42.9 ± 1.4	(42.1–43.7)	0.906
HR mean (bpm)	151.7 ± 3.0	(149.9–153.4)	152.0 ± 4.3	(149.5–154.5)	151.6 ± 2.1	(150.4–152.9)	0.962
Fluid intake (ml)	543.9 ± 270.0	(388.0–699.8)	535.7 ± 180.2	(431.7–639.8)	503.6 ± 224.7	(373.9–633.3)	0.800
Urine mass excreted after training (g)	157.1 ± 70.4	(116.5–197.8)	135.0 ± 104.6	(74.6–195.4)	115.7 ± 72.8	(73.7–157.8)	0.404

WHtR: waist-to-height ratio; HR: heart rate; $\overline{X}$: average; SD: standard deviation; CI: confidence interval.

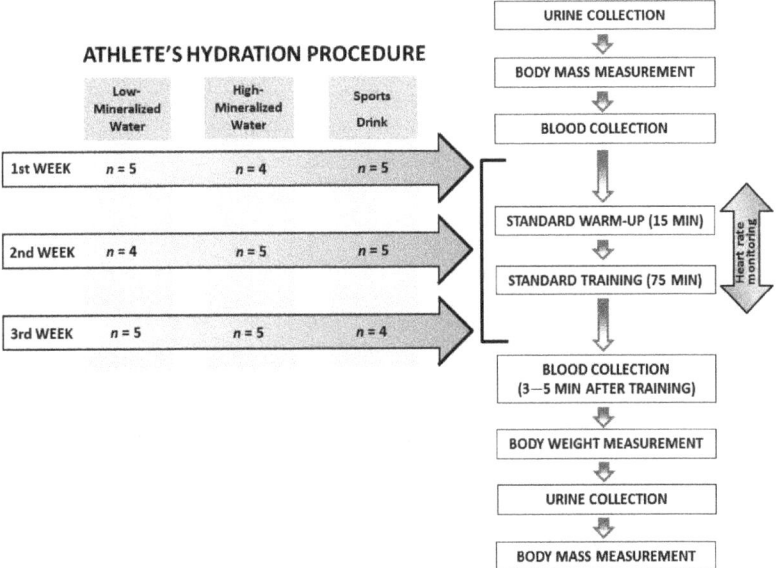

Figure 1. Flow chart of the study design.

2.3. Ethics Approval

The research related to human use complied with all relevant national regulations and institutional policies, has followed the tenets of the Declaration of Helsinki, and has been approved by the Bioethical Committee of the Poznan University of Medical Sciences (Approval No.: 140/15).

Informed consent was obtained from all individual participants included in the study.

2.4. Biochemical Analyses

The material for the research was capillary blood obtained from the fingertip of the non-dominant hand of the players, before and after the standard training unit. Blood was collected according to the applicable procedures, from the finger of the non-dominant hand using a Medlance® Red lancet-spike (HTL-Zone, Berlin, Germany) with a 1.5 mm blade and 2.0 mm penetration depth. In addition, each of the contestants was asked to submit a urine sample before and after training.

In blood collected from a heparinized capillary (65 µL), the concentration of electrolytes (Na^+, K^+, Ca^{2+}, Cl^-, HCO_3^-), lactate, plasma osmolality and pH, and standard base excess (BE), were determined using a gasometric analyzer (ABL90 FLEX, Radiometer, Copenhagen, Denmark). Additionally, 300 µL of capillary blood was collected in a Microvette® CB 300 tube (Sarstedt, Nümbrect, Germany) containing K2-EDTA (EDTA dipotassium salt) as an anticoagulant for hematocrit determination on a hematology reader (Mythic®18, Orphèe, Geneva, Switzerland). Another 300 µL of capillary blood was collected in a Microvette® CB 300 Z tube (Sarstedt, Nümbrect, Germany) with a clotting activator, in which the concentration of aldosterone was determined using an ELISA kit (DRG MedTek, Warsaw, Poland; Cat No. EIA-5298) and magnesium using the colorimetric method (Mg; Cormay, Łomianki, Poland; Cat No. 2-229). The absorbance readings were taken on a multi-detection microplate ELISA reader (Synergy 2 SIAFRT, BioTek, Winooski, VT, USA). Urine-specific gravity and pH were determined on a urine strip analyzer (URYXXON® Relax, Macherey-Nagel, Düeren, Germany).

2.5. Specialized Training

The three test dates were carried out at weekly intervals, in November and December 2016, in the hall, each time from 6:00 to 7:30 p.m. Each time, the contestants were randomly assigned to groups consuming fluids with different osmolality levels in a manner ensuring the consumption of each of the drinks (Figure 1). The competitors had free access to the randomly drawn fluid during each of the 1.5 h training sessions (Table 2) and decided on both the time and amount of intake (Table 1). The composition of the liquids, given by the producers on the packaging, is presented in Table 3, and the osmolality of these beverages was adopted based on the available literature: low-mineralized water ~20 (mOsm/kg water), highly mineralized water ~88 (mOsm/kg water), and isotonic drink ~279 (mOsm/kg water) [18].

During each training session, the air temperature and humidity were measured using data loggers located in the four corners of the pitch in the hall (EBI 310 TH, Ingolstadt, Germany). These indicators were not statistically significantly different on individual study dates.

Table 2. Framework training unit plan.

Training Group	Women's National Team and Women's Junior Team
Training duration	90 min
Venue	Indoor Hall 40 m × 20 m
Training objective	Preparation for indoor championship events according to the calendar of the European Field Hockey Federation
Warm-up	Warm-up incl. dynamic stretching + acceleration and speed drills—15 min Hockey-specific warm-up: various forms of passing and receiving the ball in motion (without the participation of a defender); shorter and longer passes, also with the use of a boards—5 min Scoring exercises (different zones of the shooting circle)—5 min
Training	Numerical advantage training—2 vs. 1 and 3 vs. 2/defensive organization in the numerical superiority of the opponent; cooperation with the goalkeeper—20 min Tactical cooperation in even numbers situation—3 vs. 3 on the side sector of the pitch (left and right board) with an emphasis on the transition phase (transition from defending to attacking)—15 min Build-up in 5 vs 4 superiority—4 × 3 min + 1 min break after every 3 min 5 vs. 4 game—2 × 5 min (change of teams after 5 min)

Table 3. The mineral composition of the fluids, specified by the manufacturer, consumed by female field hockey players during training.

Mineral	Low-Mineralized Water	High-Mineralized Water	Isotonic Drink + Low-Mineralized Water
		(mg/L)	
Ca^{2+}	48.10	319.00	288.10
Na^+	2.10	111.00	702.10
Mg^{2+}	6.68	47.90	126.68
K^+	1.20	49.50	261.20
HCO_3^-	166.30	1639.00	166.30
SO_4^{2-}	10.29	30.00	10.29
Cl^-	5.60	2.70	245.60
F^-	0.06	0.30	0.06
Total minerals	240.33	2199.40	1800.33
Glucose	0.00	0.00	52,600.00

All of the players participated in the training throughout its duration. At that time, their heart rate (HR) was monitored using the Polar Team2 PRO Heart Rate Monitoring System (Kempele, Finland) (Table 1). In all competitors, apart from the indicators measured in blood and urine, body mass and the amount of fluids consumed were also monitored before and after training. The complete study scheme is presented in Figure 1.

2.6. Statistical Analysis

Data are presented using the mean and standard deviation ($\overline{X} \pm SD$) and the confidence interval for the mean (95% CI). The values of the studied indices were statistically analyzed, and the variables were checked for normal distribution using the Shapiro–Wilk test. In order to compare the pre-training and post-training results obtained between the three study dates, repeated measures analysis of variance (ANOVA) was performed for normally distributed data, and Friedman ANOVA for indices without normal distribution. In order to compare the differences between the examined indices before and after training, the t-test for dependent samples was used for data with a normal distribution on individual test dates, and the Wilcoxon pair order test for data without normal distribution. Effect sizes (d) were calculated using means and standard deviations. To determine the effect size, Cohen's criteria were used [19], which say that values ≥ 0.2 and <0.5 are considered "small", ≥ 0.5 and <0.8 "medium", and ≥ 0.8 "large". The level of significance was set at $p < 0.05$. Statistical analysis was performed using a computer statistical package STATISTICA v13.1 (StatSoft, Inc., Tulsa, OK, USA).

3. Results

The resting values of the biochemical blood and urine indices of the players on the three study dates did not differ significantly from one another, which proves the homogeneity of the group in terms of the determined indicators. On the other hand, post-exercise differences between individual test terms were found. They concerned plasma osmolality, and the concentration of sodium and potassium ions and aldosterone (Table 4).

The comparison of the values of the examined indicators measured before and after exercise also showed statistically significant differences. They were related to all beverages (low-mineralized water, high-mineralized water, and isotonic drinks) and the indicators determined after their consumption: body mass, hematocrit value, concentration of calcium ions, aldosterone, bicarbonate ions, standard base excess, lactate and urine pH. In the case of consuming water, both low- and high-mineralized, differences in values before and after training were also observed for urine-specific gravity, potassium ion concentration and blood pH. However, the indicators that changed only when consuming isotonic drinks were plasma osmolality, and the concentrations of sodium and chloride ions (Table 4).

Table 4. Average values of the tested biochemical indicators of blood and urine in the examined persons after consuming beverages with different osmolarity levels ($n = 14$).

Indicator	Beverages	Pre-Exercise	Post-Exercise	p Value (Pre vs. Post)	Effect Size	p Value for ANOVA (Post-Exercise Differences between Beverages)
Body mass (kg)	Low High Isotonic	65.3 ± 5.4 65.4 ± 5.4 65.2 ± 5.0	65.1 ± 5.4 65.2 ± 5.5 65.0 ± 5.0	0.002 0.001 <0.001	0.04 0.03 0.04	0.706
Water Balance						
Hematocrit (l/L)	Low High Isotonic	0.377 ± 0.017 0.372 ± 0.020 0.367 ± 0.020	0.366 ± 0.021 0.360 ± 0.023 0.353 ± 0.021	0.048 <0.001 <0.001	0.56 0.59 0.71	0.212
Urine specific gravity (g/L)	Low High Isotonic	1.013 ± 0.006 1.014 ± 0.006 1.016 ± 0.009	1.019 ± 0.008 1.023 ± 0.009 1.019 ± 0.007	0.001 0.006 0.068	0.82 1.15 	0.108
Plasma osmolality (mOsm/kg)	Low High Isotonic	291.5 ± 2.1 291.6 ± 2.5 290.1 ± 2.9	290.1 ± 3.6 290.1 ± 3.6 285.3 ± 2.6	0.155 0.077 0.001	 1.73	<0.001 [a]
Electrolyte Balance						
Sodium ions (mmol/L)	Low High Isotonic	143 ± 1 143 ± 1 142 ± 2	142 ± 2 142 ± 2 140 ± 1	0.111 0.179 <0.001	 1.51	0.005 [a]
Potassium ions (mmol/L)	Low High Isotonic	4.4 ± 0.4 4.3 ± 0.3 4.5 ± 0.4	4.1 ± 0.4 3.9 ± 0.3 4.3 ± 0.3	0.024 <0.001 0.075	0.66 1.39 	0.022 [b]
Calcium ions (mmol/L)	Low High Isotonic	1.21 ± 0.03 1.20 ± 0.02 1.22 ± 0.03	1.19 ± 0.03 1.18 ± 0.04 1.19 ± 0.03	0.031 0.030 <0.001	0.76 0.60 1.06	0.624
Chloride ions (mmol/L)	Low High Isotonic	109 ± 1 108 ± 2 109 ± 2	108 ± 2 107 ± 2 107 ± 2	0.418 0.292 <0.001	 0.80	0.357
Magnesium (mmol/L)	Low High Isotonic	0.89 ± 0.01 0.89 ± 0.01 0.89 ± 0.02	0.89 ± 0.03 0.89 ± 0.02 0.90 ± 0.02	0.730 0.431 0.272		0.789
Aldosterone (pmol/L)	Low High Isotonic	125.8 ± 45.4 117.0 ± 53.9 112.2 ± 28.4	411.8 ± 184.0 424.2 ± 107.5 270.2 ± 104.6	0.001 <0.001 <0.001	2.13 3.61 2.06	0.005 [a]
Acid–Base Balance						
Bicarbonate ions (mmol/L)	Low High Isotonic	24.1 ± 1.6 24.7 ± 2.1 24.3 ± 1.4	22.4 ± 1.3 22.8 ± 1.5 22.3 ± 2.0	<0.001 0.005 <0.001	1.13 1.05 1.16	0.683
Standard base excess (mmol/L)	Low High Isotonic	−0.1 ± 1.3 0.9 ± 1.7 0.1 ± 1.7	−2.6 ± 1.8 −2.1 ± 2.0 −2.8 ± 2.8	<0.001 <0.001 <0.001	1.63 1.61 1.26	0.645
Blood pH	Low High Isotonic	7.40 ± 0.03 7.41 ± 0.02 7.40 ± 0.03	7.39 ± 0.03 7.39 ± 0.03 7.39 ± 0.03	0.024 0.012 0.102	0.45 0.82 	0.926
Urine pH	Low High Isotonic	6.2 ± 0.7 6.2 ± 0.7 6.0 ± 0.7	5.4 ± 0.6 5.6 ± 0.6 5.5 ± 0.6	0.002 0.005 0.018	1.31 0.89 0.81	0.313
Lactate (mmol/L)	Low High Isotonic	1.3 ± 0.4 1.3 ± 0.3 1.4 ± 0.4	5.8 ± 1.7 5.9 ± 2.6 5.9 ± 2.5	0.001 0.001 0.001	3.64 2.54 2.55	0.807

Low—low-mineralized water, High—high-mineralized water, Isotonic—sport drink; [a]—the average values for isotonic drinks are lower than for both waters; [b]—the average value for isotonic water is higher than for high-mineralized water.

4. Discussion

This is the first time that such extensive research describing post-training changes in water–electrolyte and acid–base balance in female field hockey players has been presented. Few publications have so far described the effects of fluids with heterogeneous mineral composition and different osmolarity on biochemical blood and urine parameters, adopted by the athletes, especially in women. Therefore, the authors decided to investigate this topic, including in the scope of their research a much wider range of indicators characterizing the water–electrolyte and acid–base balance than in other studies.

The values of the examined indicators, determined before and after the training unit, were in line with the ranges given in previous publications on the impact of exercise on the body. They describe post-exercise reductions in a number of indicators, including body mass [20,21], hematocrit value [22], osmolality [23], the concentration of sodium [21], potassium [24], calcium ions [24,25], magnesium [26], bicarbonate ions [24,27,28], standard base excess [8,28] and blood pH [27–29]. An increase in the value after exercise, in our own studies, was observed for urine-specific gravity [30], and the concentrations of aldosterone [31,32] and lactate [24,27–29]. However, there are no publications with results that can be related to the data on post-exercise blood chloride concentration and urine pH value in the presented study. It can therefore be assumed that the post-training changes found in the studied female field hockey players do not differ from the data found in other sports disciplines, such as beach volleyball [20], rugby [21,23,27], football [22,24], soccer [29], and basketball [25,30], as well as in swimming exercise [26] and in healthy untrained people after exercise on a treadmill [8] or an ergocyclometer [31,32]. Moreover, changes in the tested biochemical indices in the blood and urine are the result of physical exertion and the accompanying dehydration of the body.

The main question of the research, however, concerned the effect of the osmolarity of the fluids consumed by the athletes during exercise. The proposed arrangement of tests and assays performed for blood and urine biochemical indices made it possible to determine the hydration level of the players before the start of training, which was statistically the same at all times. Additionally, the monitoring of air temperature and humidity ensured that the ambient conditions did not affect the results of the experiment. The average values of air temperature in individual periods were, respectively, 20.9 ± 0.1 vs. 21.0 ± 0.1 vs. 20.8 ± 0.1, and air humidity was 52.5 ± 0.6 vs. 51.0 ± 0.8 vs. 52.0 ± 0.8. Moreover, the players, despite independently making decisions about the amount of fluids consumed during training, adopted a similar volume of experimental drinks on all test dates (Table 1). The above is also visible in the similar mass of urine output after training (Table 1). Such a lack of differences in the amount of urine output, up to 1 h after training, despite the use of fluids with different osmolarity levels, was recently demonstrated by Pence and Bloomer [33]. Their observations also show that drinking water increases urine output 2 to 4 h after drinking it, compared to drinks with a higher content of electrolytes.

The only statistically significant differences between liquids of different osmolarity levels were observed between biochemical markers after drinking water (regardless of the content of minerals in it) and isotonic drinks. These differences are expressed using indicators describing the water–electrolyte balance, such as plasma osmolality, the concentration of sodium and potassium ions, and aldosterone. No statistical differences were observed in the indicators characterizing the acid–base balance. The consumption of an isotonic drink that is rich in sodium caused the smallest increase in the concentration of aldosterone, which is responsible for the reabsorption of this element in the renal tubules, increasing the excretion of potassium ions in the urine [34,35]. As a consequence, the greatest post-exercise reduction in sodium ions and the lowest potassium ions were observed, which also translated into the highest reduction in blood osmolality. Moreover, the concentration of potassium ions measured post-exercise decreased the most in the plasma of players in the case of high-mineralized water, where the highest increase in aldosterone concentration was also noted (Table 4). The small number of publications on this issue and the heterogeneity of the data included therein do not favor a detailed analysis of the issue, especially in the absence of relevant data characterizing players in team games. The ambiguity of the results (Table 5) indicates the need for a more complete study of this issue. All authors analyzing plasma osmolality [36–38] and sodium and potassium ions [36,37] blood concentration after consuming fluids with different contents of minerals did not show a statistically significant difference between these fluids. This is in contrast to our research, wherein an isotonic drink was shown to decrease plasma osmolality and blood sodium ions concentration simultaneously, increasing the blood concentration of potassium more effectively than the analyzed waters. Among the publications presented in Table 5, only Powers et al. [36] examined the effect of the used fluids on the blood hydrogen ions' concentration. Although in our research we did not analyze the concentration of these ions, we did determine the pH values, which are coherent. Powers et al. [36] showed that the consumption of beverages containing electrolytes (EP, GP) more effectively stabilizes the concentration of hydrogen ions in the blood than liquids without electrolytes (NEP), especially during exercise. In our study, we did not observe any differences in the acid–base balance indicators determined in blood and urine, regardless of the used fluids. Due to the fact that we have the opportunity to compare our results only with one study [36], we are not able to clearly explain the reasons for the differences. This requires research involving a larger number of participants, as well as efforts (training loads) of varying intensity.

Table 5. Summary of publications on the impacts of drinks with different (indicated by the authors of the studies) osmolality levels on the biochemical and hematological indicators of people subjected to exercise tests.

Authors (Sport Discipline) (Kind of Effort) Sex	The Types of Beverages	Tested Biochemical Indicators	
		No Significant Differences	Significant Differences
Powers et al. [36] (cyclists; $n = 9$) (exercises with a constant load on a bicycle ergometer until fatigue) Men	Non-electrolyte placebo (NEP) (31 mOsm/kg) Electrolyte placebo drink without carbohydrate (EP) (48 mOsm/kg) Glucose polymer drink containing electrolytes (GP) (231 mOsm/kg)	Heart rate, plasma osmolality, concentration of lactate, potassium, calcium, sodium, and chloride in blood	The concentration of hydrogen ions in the blood was significantly lower after 30 min of exercise while using GP and EP compared to NEP
Gisolfi et al. [37] (wytrenowani; $n = 7$) (85 min 60%–65% VO_2max cycle ergometer) 5 Men, 2 Women	Water (1 ± 0.3 mOsm/kg) Hypertonic (197 ± 2 mOsm/kg) Isotonic (295 ± 6 mOsm/kg) Hypotonic (414 ± 2 mOsm/kg)	Osmolarity, sodium and potassium ions in plasma	There are no statistically significant differences
Suzuki et al. [38] (cyclists; $n = 6$) (cycling at 60% VO_2peak for 90 min in the hot conditions) Men	Plain water (no data) Hypotonic sports drink (193 mOsm/kg) Isotonic sports drink (317 mOsm/kg)	Plasma osmolality, lactate concentration	There are no statistically significant differences
Łagowska et al. [39] (rowers; $n = 11$) (80 min of exercises on a rowing ergometer) Men	Commercially available sports drink (258 mOsm/kg) Natural carbohydrate electrolyte drink (402 mOsm/kg)	Lactate concentration, hematocrit	There are no statistically significant differences
Our work (field hockey; $n = 14$) (90-min training unit) Women	Low-mineralized water (~20 mOsm/kg) High-mineralized water (~88 mOsm/kg) Isotonic drink (~279 mOsm/kg)	HR, hematocrit, concentration of lactate, calcium, chloride and bicarbonate ions, magnesium, standard base excess, blood and urine pH, and urine-specific gravity	Consumption of an isotonic drink caused the smallest increase in the concentration of aldosterone and potassium ions, and the greatest post-exercise reduction in sodium ions and blood osmolality

VO_2max: maximal oxygen uptake; VO_2peak: peak oxygen uptake.

However, our own research shows that the amount of fluids, but not the quality, is of greater importance for maintaining the correct water–electrolyte and acid–base balance.

Our study has some limitations, which include the lack of the consideration of ions in the urine and sweat. Analyses of the 24 h diet diaries before the performed tests were also not undertaken.

The essential point of this manuscript is that the research topic is related to the determination of the effect of fluids with different minerals contents on the water–electrolyte and acid–base balances. The available literature on this topic does not have homogeneous results and specific recommendations for hydration strategies in various sports disciplines, including field hockey. It was also the first time that such a wide range of blood and urine biochemical parameters was used. The benefit of this study is that the measurements were carried out in real training conditions, and not directly in isolated laboratory tests.

In the future, in order to more accurately assess the aim set in the study, we plan to repeat the research, increasing the number of female players, including testing players from other team games.

5. Conclusions

Based on a review of the available literature, we found that field hockey does not differ from other sports in terms of the biochemical blood and urine indicators characterizing the post-training changes of players.

The osmolarity of consumed fluids does not significantly affect the indicators of the water–electrolyte balance and acid–base balance during exercise. Such an effect is only noticeable after consuming an isotonic drink, manifesting itself in greater changes in the concentration of aldosterone, sodium and potassium ions and plasma osmolality than in the case of hypotonic drinks. Furthermore, the degree of mineralization of the water consumed by female field hockey players did not affect the indicators of water–electrolyte and acid–base balance in the blood and urine.

Isotonic drinks, unlike hypotonic drinks, most likely stabilize the RAA system during training, which ensures the best hydration as defined by plasma osmolality.

The wide spectrum of commercially available sports drinks and waters used by athletes raises the question of selecting those liquids that stabilize the water–electrolyte and acid–base balances. Moreover, they should positively affect the exercise capacity of athletes. The information contained in this publication discusses this issue in terms of the different osmolarity levels of beverages, making the applied knowledge useful for both players and coaches.

Author Contributions: Conceptualization, J.K. and T.P.; methodology, J.K., T.P. and K.R.; validation, J.K. and T.P.; formal analysis, J.K.; investigation, J.K. and T.P.; resources, T.P.; data curation, J.K.; writing—original draft, J.K.; writing—review and editing, J.K., T.P., K.R. and M.P.; visualization, J.K. and T.P.; supervision, J.K., T.P. and M.P.; project administration, T.P.; funding acquisition, T.P. All authors have read and agreed to the published version of the manuscript.

Funding: This research was funded by Development of Academic Sport, grant number N RSA3 03553.

Institutional Review Board Statement: The research related to human use has complied with all relevant national regulations and institutional policies, has followed the tenets of the Declaration of Helsinki, and has been approved by the Bioethical Committee of the Poznan University of Medical Sciences (Approval No.: 140/15).

Informed Consent Statement: Informed consent was obtained from all individual participants included in the study.

Data Availability Statement: The data presented in this study are available on request from the corresponding author. The data are not publicly available due to ethical restrictions.

Acknowledgments: The authors would like to thank Urszula Bartkowiak from Department of Physiology and Biochemistry, Poznań University of Physical Education, for her assistance with collecting material for research.

Conflicts of Interest: The authors declare no conflict of interest.

References

1. Barboza, S.D.; Joseph, C.; Nauta, J.; van Mechelen, W.; Verhagen, E. Injuries in Field Hockey Players: A Systematic Review. *Sports Med.* **2018**, *48*, 849–866. [CrossRef]
2. MacLeod, H.; Sunderland, C. Fluid balance and hydration habits of elite female field hockey players during consecutive international matches. *J. Strength Cond. Res.* **2009**, *23*, 1245–1251. [CrossRef]
3. Gabbett, T.J. GPS analysis of elite women's field hockey training and competition. *J. Strength Cond. Res.* **2010**, *24*, 1321–1324. [CrossRef] [PubMed]
4. Macutkiewicz, D.; Sunderland, C. The use of GPS to evaluate activity profiles of elite women hockey players during match-play. *J. Sports Sci.* **2011**, *29*, 967–973. [CrossRef] [PubMed]
5. González-Alonso, J.; Mora-Rodríguez, R.; Below, P.R.; Coyle, E.F. Dehydration markedly impairs cardiovascular function in hyperthermic endurance athletes during exercise. *J. Appl. Physiol.* **1997**, *82*, 1229–1236. [CrossRef] [PubMed]
6. Leiper, J.B.; Broad, N.P.; Maughan, R.J. Effect of intermittent high-intensity exercise on gastric emptying in man. *Med. Sci. Sports Exerc.* **2001**, *33*, 1270–1278. [CrossRef]
7. Shirreffs, S.M.; Maughan, R.J. Whole body sweat collection in humans: An improved method with preliminary data on electrolyte content. *J. Appl. Physiol.* **1997**, *82*, 336–341. [CrossRef]
8. Wiecek, M.; Maciejczyk, M.; Szymura, J.; Szygula, Z. Changes in oxidative stress and acid-base balance in men and women following maximal-intensity physical exercise. *Physiol. Res.* **2015**, *64*, 93–102. [CrossRef]
9. Hanon, C.; Bernard, O.; Rabate, M.; Claire, T. Effect of two different long-sprint training regimens on sprint performance and associated metabolic responses. *J. Strength Cond. Res.* **2012**, *26*, 1551–1557. [CrossRef]
10. Cunniffe, B.; Fallan, C.; Yau, A.; Evans, G.H.; Cardinale, M. Assessment of physical demands and fluid balance in elite female handball players during a 6-day competitive tournament. *Int. J. Sport Nutr. Exerc. Metab.* **2015**, *25*, 78–88. [CrossRef]
11. EFSA Panel on Dietetic Products, Nutrition and Allergies (NDA). Scientific opinion on dietary reference values for water. *EFSA J.* **2010**, *8*, 1459.
12. Maughan, R.J.; Leiper, J.B. Limitations to fluid replacement during exercise. *Can. J. Appl. Physiol.* **1999**, *24*, 173–187. [CrossRef]
13. Nose, H.; Mack, G.W.; Shi, X.R.; Nadel, E.R. Role of osmolality and plasma volume during rehydration in humans. *J. Appl. Physiol.* **1988**, *65*, 325–331. [CrossRef] [PubMed]
14. Shirreffs, S.M.; Aragon-Vargas, L.F.; Keil, M.; Love, T.D.; Phillips, S. Rehydration after exercise in the heat: A comparison of 4 commonly used drinks. *Int. J. Sport Nutr. Exerc. Metab.* **2007**, *17*, 244–258. [CrossRef] [PubMed]
15. Yamauchi, T.; Harada, T.; Kurono, M.; Matsui, N. Effect of exercise-induced acidosis on aldosterone secretion in men. *Eur. J. Appl. Physiol. Occup. Physiol.* **1998**, *77*, 409–412. [CrossRef] [PubMed]
16. Passe, D.H. Physiological and psychological determinants of fluid intake. In *Sports Drinks: Basic Science and Practical Aspects*; Maughan, R.J., Murray, R., Eds.; CRC Press: Boca Raton, FL, USA, 2001; pp. 45–87.
17. Ersoy, N.; Ersoy, G. Sports drinks for hydration and alternative drinks review. *Turk. Klin. J. Sports Sci.* **2013**, *5*, 96–100.
18. Sadowska, A.; Świderski, F.; Rakowska, R.; Waszkiewicz-Robak, B.; Żebrowska-Krasuska, M.; Dybkowska, E. Beverage osmolality as a marker for maintaining appropriate body hydration. *Rocz. Panstw. Zakl. Hig.* **2017**, *68*, 167–173.
19. Cohen, J. *Statistical Power Analysis for the Behavioral Sciences*, 2nd ed.; Lawrence Erlbaum Associates: Hillsdale, NJ, USA, 1988.
20. Zetou, E.; Giatsis, G.; Mountaki, F.; Komninakidou, A. Body weight changes and voluntary fluid intakes of beach volleyball players during an official tournament. *J. Sci. Med. Sport* **2008**, *11*, 139–145. [CrossRef]
21. Jones, B.; Till, K.; King, R.; Gray, M.; O'Hara, J. Are Habitual Hydration Strategies of Female Rugby League Players Sufficient to Maintain Fluid Balance and Blood Sodium Concentration During Training and Match-Play? A Research Note from the Field. *J. Strength Cond. Res.* **2016**, *30*, 875–880. [CrossRef]
22. O'Connell, S.M.; Woodman, R.J.; Brown, I.L.; Vincent, D.J.; Binder, H.J.; Ramakrishna, B.S.; Young, G.P. Comparison of a sports-hydration drink containing high amylose starch with usual hydration practice in Australian rules footballers during intense summer training. *J. Int. Soc. Sports Nutr.* **2018**, *15*, 1–10. [CrossRef]
23. Bargh, M.J.; King, R.F.; Gray, M.P.; Jones, B. Why do team-sport athletes drink fluid in excess when exercising in cool conditions? *Appl. Physiol. Nutr. Metab.* **2017**, *42*, 271–277. [CrossRef]
24. Karakoc, Y.; Duzova, H.; Polat, A.; Emre, M.H.; Arabaci, I. Effects of training period on haemorheological variables in regularly trained footballers. *Br. J. Sports Med.* **2005**, *39*, e4. [CrossRef]
25. Wang, L.; Zhang, J.; Wang, J.; He, W.; Huang, H. Effects of high-intensity training and resumed training on macroelement and microelement of elite basketball athletes. *Biol. Trace Elem. Res.* **2012**, *149*, 148–154. [CrossRef]
26. Laires, M.J.; Alves, F. Changes in plasma, erythrocyte, and urinary magnesium with prolonged swimming exercise. *Magnes. Res.* **1991**, *4*, 119–122. [PubMed]
27. Couderc, A.; Thomas, C.; Lacome, M.; Piscione, J.; Robineau, J.; Delfour-Peyrethon, R.; Borne, R.; Hanon, C. Movement Patterns and Metabolic Responses During an International Rugby Sevens Tournament. *Int. J. Sports Physiol. Perform.* **2017**, *12*, 901–907. [CrossRef] [PubMed]
28. Macutkiewicz, D.; Sunderland, C. Sodium bicarbonate supplementation does not improve elite women's team sport running or field hockey skill performance. *Physiol. Rep.* **2018**, *6*, e13818. [CrossRef]
29. Wiacek, M.; Andrzejewski, M.; Chmura, J.; Zubrzycki, I.Z. The changes of the specific physiological parameters in response to 12-week individualized training of young soccer players. *J. Strength Cond. Res.* **2011**, *25*, 1514–1521. [CrossRef]

30. Osterberg, K.L.; Horswill, C.A.; Baker, L.B. Pregame urine specific gravity and fluid intake by National Basketball Association players during competition. *J. Athl. Train.* **2009**, *44*, 53–57. [CrossRef] [PubMed]
31. Wolf, J.P.; Nguyen, N.U.; Dumoulin, G.; Berthelay, S. Plasma renin and aldosterone changes during twenty minutes' moderate exercise. Influence of posture. *Eur. J. Appl. Physiol. Occup. Physiol.* **1986**, *54*, 602–607. [CrossRef]
32. Mannix, E.T.; Palange, P.; Aronoff, G.R.; Manfredi, F.; Farber, M.O. Atrial natriuretic peptide and the renin-aldosterone axis during exercise in man. *Med. Sci. Sports Exerc.* **1990**, *22*, 785–789. [CrossRef] [PubMed]
33. Pence, J.; Bloomer, R.J. Impact of Nuun Electrolyte Tablets on Fluid Balance in Active Men and Women. *Nutrients* **2020**, *12*, 3030. [CrossRef] [PubMed]
34. Boone, C.H.; Hoffman, J.R.; Gonzalez, A.M.; Jajtner, A.R.; Townsend, J.R.; Baker, K.M.; Fukuda, D.H.; Stout, J.R. Changes in Plasma Aldosterone and Electrolytes Following High-Volume and High-Intensity Resistance Exercise Protocols in Trained Men. *J. Strength Cond. Res.* **2016**, *30*, 1917–1923. [CrossRef] [PubMed]
35. Morgan, R.M.; Patterson, M.J.; Nimmo, M.A. Acute effects of dehydration on sweat composition in men during prolonged exercise in the heat. *Acta Physiol. Scand.* **2004**, *182*, 37–43. [CrossRef] [PubMed]
36. Powers, S.K.; Lawler, J.; Dodd, S.; Tulley, R.; Landry, G.; Wheeler, K. Fluid replacement drinks during high intensity exercise: Effects on minimizing exercise-induced disturbances in homeostasis. *Eur. J. Appl. Physiol. Occup. Physiol.* **1990**, *60*, 54–60. [CrossRef] [PubMed]
37. Gisolfi, C.V.; Summers, R.W.; Lambert, G.P.; Xia, T. Effect of beverage osmolality on intestinal fluid absorption during exercise. *J. Appl. Physiol.* **1998**, *85*, 1941–1948. [CrossRef] [PubMed]
38. Suzuki, K.; Hashimoto, H.; Oh, T.; Ishijima, T.; Mitsuda, H.; Peake, J.M.; Sakamoto, S.; Muraoka, I.; Higuchi, M. The effects of sports drink osmolality on fluid intake and immunoendocrine responses to cycling in hot conditions. *J. Nutr. Sci. Vitam.* **2013**, *59*, 206–212. [CrossRef]
39. Łagowska, K.; Podgórski, T.; Celińska, E.; Kryściak, J. A comparison of the effectiveness of commercial and natural carbohydrate–electrolyte drinks. *Sci. Sports* **2017**, *32*, 160–164. [CrossRef]

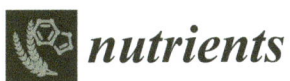

Review

Rehydration during Endurance Exercise: Challenges, Research, Options, Methods

Lawrence E. Armstrong

Human Performance Laboratory and Korey Stringer Institute, University of Connecticut, Storrs, CT 06269-1110, USA; Lawrence.Armstrong@Uconn.edu

Abstract: During endurance exercise, two problems arise from disturbed fluid–electrolyte balance: dehydration and overhydration. The former involves water and sodium losses in sweat and urine that are incompletely replaced, whereas the latter involves excessive consumption and retention of dilute fluids. When experienced at low levels, both dehydration and overhydration have minor or no performance effects and symptoms of illness, but when experienced at moderate-to-severe levels they degrade exercise performance and/or may lead to hydration-related illnesses including hyponatremia (low serum sodium concentration). Therefore, the present review article presents (a) relevant research observations and consensus statements of professional organizations, (b) 5 rehydration methods in which pre-race planning ranges from no advanced action to determination of sweat rate during a field simulation, and (c) 9 rehydration recommendations that are relevant to endurance activities. With this information, each athlete can select the rehydration method that best allows her/him to achieve a hydration middle ground between dehydration and overhydration, to optimize physical performance, and reduce the risk of illness.

Keywords: thirst; drinking; sweat; sodium; hyponatremia; overhydration; dehydration; marathon; triathlon

Citation: Armstrong, L.E. Rehydration during Endurance Exercise: Challenges, Research, Options, Methods. *Nutrients* **2021**, *13*, 887. https://doi.org/10.3390/nu13030887

Academic Editor: Ajmol Ali

Received: 11 February 2021
Accepted: 1 March 2021
Published: 9 March 2021

Publisher's Note: MDPI stays neutral with regard to jurisdictional claims in published maps and institutional affiliations.

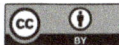

Copyright: © 2021 by the author. Licensee MDPI, Basel, Switzerland. This article is an open access article distributed under the terms and conditions of the Creative Commons Attribution (CC BY) license (https://creativecommons.org/licenses/by/4.0/).

1. Introduction

The essential components of central nervous system maintenance of body water volume and concentration include perceptions, behavior, nervous system responses, and the release of hormones (vasopressin, AVP; angiotensin II; atrial natriuretic peptide; apelin) [1–4]. Perturbations of whole-body water volume and concentration are monitored by the brain, the resulting thirst and oropharyngeal sensations modulate drinking, and neuroendocrine responses regulate water and electrolyte excretion or retention by the kidneys [1]. During typical daily activities that do not include exercise, these complex interactions act to maintain total body water volume and serum concentration within 1–3% of baseline each day [5–7]. However, the relative influence of these processes varies with different life activities [8]. Table 1 explains that, during sedentary daily pursuits in a mild environment, renal responses and thirst are the primary homeostatic regulators. During prolonged endurance exercise at low intensities (5–24 h duration), renal responses and thirst have minor-to-large effects on water regulation. As the duration of exercise increases, sweat losses become a major factor in whole-body water balance [9], regardless of the volume of fluid consumed.

This review article considers endurance exercise from the perspectives of body water and electrolyte balance, the negative effects that substantial fluid–electrolyte disturbances (i.e., both water loss and gain) have on competitive performance and health, and ways that endurance athletes can minimize performance decrements and mitigate the risk of exercise-associated illness. This is important because an endurance athlete can lose as much as 11–12% (7.8–8.5 kg) of body weight in the form of water, during a 12.3-h Ironman triathlon in a cool environment (3.8-km swim, 180-km bike, 42.2-km run) [10]. This also is important because day-long walking or hiking in a desert environment can result in extreme body mass losses of 14–18% when fluids are unavailable or restricted (Figure 1). Conversely, excessive fluid intake (i.e., water retention) can result in a body mass gain of more than 10% (7.8 kg) in 12.7 h while competing in an ultraendurance triathlon (ambient temperature, Tamb, 20.5 °C) [11]. These vastly different changes of body mass represent the primary problem and focus of this review paper: how to maintain a rehydration middle ground during prolonged exercise that reliably reduces the risk of illness by avoiding overhydration, and maintains exercise performance by avoiding significant dehydration.

Table 1. The relative effects of thirst, drinking, and physiological responses on fluid-electrolyte balance during ordinary daily activities and endurance exercise.

Activity	Thirst & Drinking Behavior	Sweat Gland Secretion of Hypotonic Fluid	Kidney Regulation of Water & Electrolytes	Neuroendocrine Homeostatic Responses [a]	Effects on Water & Electrolyte Balance
Sedentary daily activities (16 h)	Basal [b]	Negligible	Basal [b]	Basal [b]	CNS responses are sufficient to maintain water and electrolyte homeostasis
Brief exercise (5–30 min) at moderate-to-high intensity	Minor	Minor-to-moderate	Minor	Minor, brief	Water and electrolyte losses are minor
Endurance exercise (0.5–5 h) at low-to-high intensity	Minor-to-large	Moderate-to-large	Minor-to-moderate	Minor-to-large, prolonged	Moderate-to-large turnover [c] due to sweating and drinking
Ultraendurance exercise (5–24 h) at low-to-moderate intensity	Moderate-to-large	Large	Moderate-to-large	Large, prolonged	Water and electrolyte losses in sweat and urine exceed 24 h dietary intake

CNS, central nervous system (i.e., brain and spinal cord); TBW, total body water. [a], CNS effects involving nerves and hormones that regulate whole-body water volume and concentration, blood volume/pressure/osmolality, and thirst (see [9] for a review of this topic). [b], a standard low level maintenance of whole-body fluid-electrolyte balance with small turnover (intake versus loss) and minor perturbations. [c], turnover refers to the sum of gains and losses of water and electrolytes.

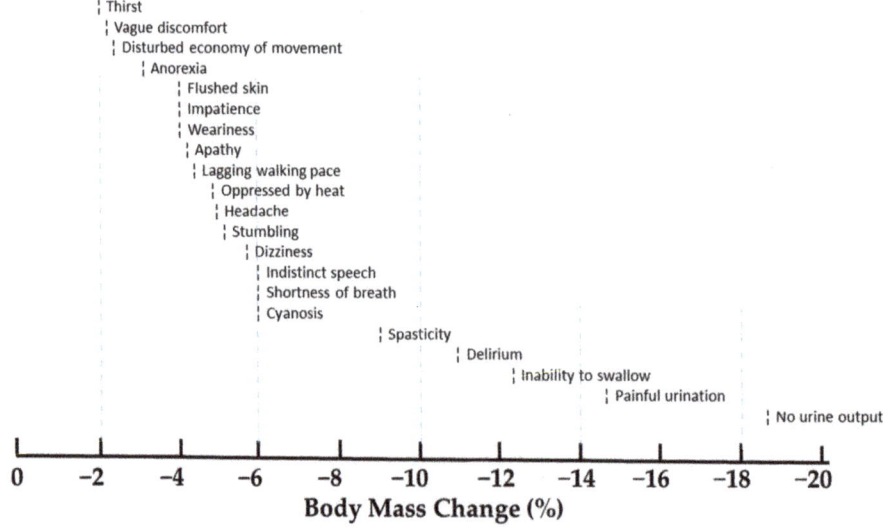

Figure 1. Signs and symptoms of dehydration in men who walked in the desert without drinking. The symbol which appears to the left of each sign or symptom identifies the approximate water deficit of its first report. Based on information from [12].

2. Problem: Water and Salt Losses during Endurance Exercise

Most ultraendurance competitors do not meet their fluid needs during competition [13], due primarily to three factors that interact to influence sweat volume and body mass during prolonged exercise [14]. The first of these factors is exercise intensity. Table 2 presents whole-body water balance measurements of 32 cyclists who completed a 164-km event in the state of Texas, USA during the month of August [15]. Cyclists have been grouped on the basis of time to complete 164 km: 9.6, 6.3, and 4.8 h. The total volume of sweat lost by these groups were similar (range of 7000–7200 g), demonstrating that the higher exercise intensities of groups 4.8 and 6.3 stimulated a greater sweat rate per hour ($p < 0.01$ to 0.0001) than that of group 9.6. Exercise intensity also affected body mass proportionally. The body mass change values for cyclist groups 9.6, 6.3, and 4.8 (columns 2–4, row 11) were −1800, −2300, and −2750 g. The second factor is exercise duration. As shown in Table 2, slower cyclists may be on the course at least twice as long as faster competitors. Not surprisingly, similar body mass losses occur commonly (Figure 2) during ultra-running, ultra-cycling, and ultra-triathlon events [16]. Environmental temperature represents a third factor that influences body water balance. During 42.2 km marathon running, mild ambient conditions of 7, 10–12, and 20 °C resulted in mean sweat rates of 0.81, 0.96, and 1.52 L/h, respectively [17]. In addition, researchers measured the sweat rates of athletes in a laboratory building (29 °C, 51% relative humidity; running and cycling protocols), a mobile laboratory (29 °C, 65% rh), or field environment (25 °C, 55% rh) [18]. The majority of these athletes competed in team/skill sports ($n = 1022$) and individual endurance sports ($n = 255$). The highest average sweat rates were observed in the sports of American football (1.51 L/h) and Endurance Sports (1.28 L/h), whereas the lowest occurred in baseball (0.83 L/h) and soccer (0.94 L/h).

Table 2. Characteristics of three groups of cyclists who completed a 164 km summer road cycling event in 4.8–9.6 h (modified from [15]). No drinking instructions or experimental interventions were involved.

Variables	Average Exercise Duration (h) [a]		
	9.6	6.3	4.8
Pre-event body mass [b] (kg)	81.90	82.05	82.55
Number of male cyclists	11	11	10
Ground speed (km/h)	17.2 [d]	26.6 [d]	34.0 [d]
Rating of perceived exertion at finish [c]	16	16	16
ad libitum total fluid intake [e] (g)	+6100	+4500	+3900 [f]
Rate of fluid intake (g/h)	+635	+715	+810
Sweat secreted [g] (g)	−7700	−7150	−7000
Sweat rate (g/h)	−800 [d]	−1135	−1460
Urine excreted [g] (g)	−1300	−550	−450 [d]
Solid food mass consumed [e] (g)	+423	+355	+350
Body mass change [b] (g)	−1800	−2300	−2750
Body mass change (%)	−2.0	−2.9	−3.4

Note: values are means or medians; negative values represent reduced mass or loss of fluid from the body; air temperature ranged from 24.4 °C (08:00 h) to 41.1 °C (15:00 h); for the purposes of this table, 1 g = 1 mL and 1 kg = 1 L. [a], cyclist groups 9.6 and 6.3 voluntarily stopped at 3 roadside aid stations for research measurements, elimination, drinking, and eating. Group 4.8 rode as part of a 5-h pace team and did not stop during the entire event. [b], measured with a calibrated floor scale (±100 g). [c], using a printed 6 (very, very light) to 20 (very, very hard) point perceptual rating scale [19]. [d], significantly different from all other groups ($p = 0.01$ to 0.0001). [e], based on cyclist diet records and confirmed by interviews. [f], significantly different from group 9.6 ($p = 0.04$). [g], detailed methods are described in the original publication [15].

Representing extreme points of reference, the following individual sweat rate values have been observed. First, an elite marathon runner (age, 26 y; height, 185 cm; body mass, 66.9 kg) produced 3.7 L of sweat per h during the 1984 Los Angeles Summer Olympics marathon (24–28 °C Tamb; time to complete 42.2-km race, 2 h 14.3 min; body mass change, 5.43 kg, −8.1%) [21]. Second, a runner (age, 30 y; height, 185 cm; body mass, 91.8 kg) who had experienced heatstroke twice previously was observed to have a sweat loss of 4.1 L during a 70-min laboratory race simulation (25 °C) [22]. Third, the sweat rate of a male tennis player (age, 26 y; height, 197 cm; body mass, 91.4 kg) was 4.3 L/h during a 60 min laboratory simulation (36.1 °C; brisk walking and jogging on a treadmill) [23]. The sweat sodium losses (i.e., calculated by multiplying the measured sweat volume times the sweat sodium concentration) during the two simulations were 5930 and 7610 mg Na+, respectively. Additionally, as noted above, extreme body mass losses of −11 to −12% were experienced by competitors in an Ironman triathlon that required an average of 12.3 h to complete [10].

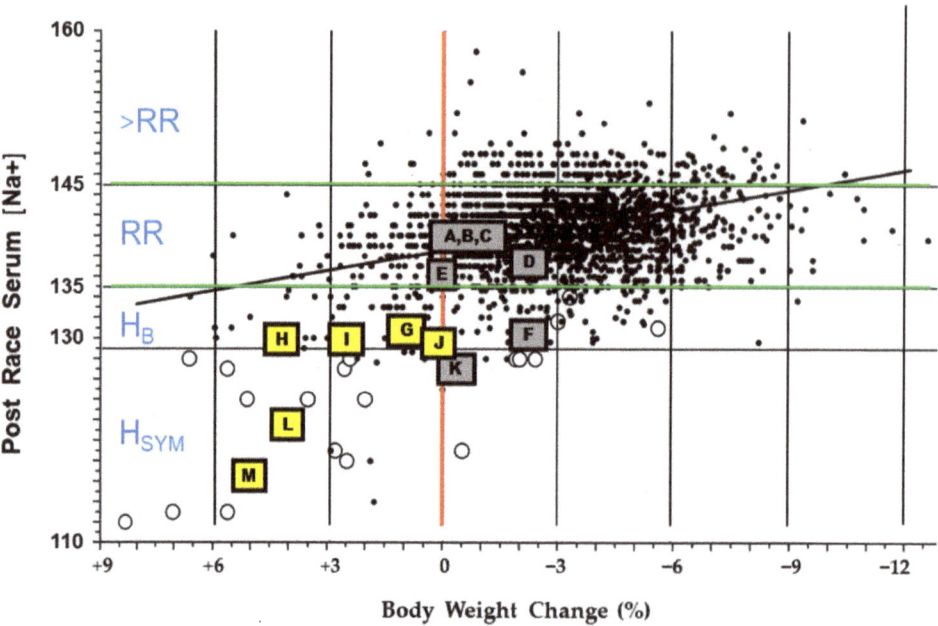

Figure 2. The relationship between body weight change (%) and serum Na+ after 4.0–13.3 h of exercise (n = 2135) as modified from [20]. Solid circles (●) represent asymptomatic marathon runners and Ironman triathletes. Open circles (○) depict athletes with severe symptoms including hyponatremic encephalopathy (central nervous system dysfunction due to brain swelling). Horizontal zone abbreviations: >RR, serum Na+ concentration above resting normal; RR, the laboratory reference range for healthy adults (green horizontal boundaries); H_B, biochemical hyponatremia which involves few or no symptoms; H_{SYM}, symptomatic hyponatremia. Symbols A–M were overlaid by the present author (see details below in Section 3.2.1). Gray highlighted symbols depict individuals with fluid intake rates of ≤700 mL/h and body mass losses of 0.1 to 2.6%. Yellow highlighted squares indicate exertional hyponatremia cases (each n = 1) with fluid intake rates ranging from 733–2061 L/h and body mass increases of +0.1 to +5.0%. Reprinted via the PNAS Open Access option from [20].

2.1. Effects of Dehydration on Endurance Exercise Performance

The negative influences of dehydration on exercise performance are recognized by professional sports medicine organizations [24–27] and sport governing bodies [28] in position statements regarding rehydration, exertional heat illness, and physical performance. Although the precise water deficit at which performance decrements occurs is difficult to determine because of inter-individual differences, there is overall consensus in the literature that dehydration of −2 to −4% represents the range in which endurance exercise performance declines [24–26,28–31]. This effect is illustrated in Figure 3, which presents a performance analysis of 34 published studies involving dehydration; a body water deficit of 1–3% was less likely to impair endurance exercise performance significantly ($p < 0.05$) than dehydration of 4–7% [32]. These 60 statistical comparisons involved outdoor track running, trail running, outdoor road cycling, indoor treadmill running, indoor rowing ergometry, and indoor cycle ergometry.

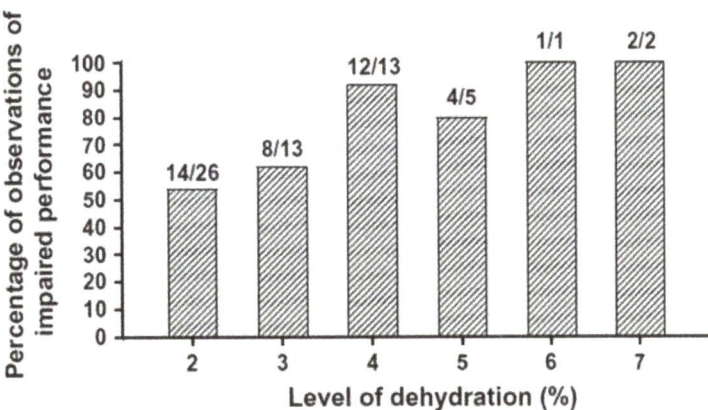

Figure 3. The effects of dehydration on exercise performance. Fractions represent the number of statistically significant ($p < 0.05$) observations out of the number at each level of body mass loss. Across all dehydration levels, 68% of comparisons indicated impairment. Reprinted from [32] via the Creative Commons Attribution 4.0 International License (http://creativecommons.org/licenses/by/4.0/) accessed on 2 March 2021.

It also is relevant that controlled field studies have reported statistically significant decrements of endurance exercise performance at lower levels of dehydration (−1.0 to −2.2%). These controlled protocols evaluated running competitions at (a) three distances on an outdoor all-weather track [33] and (b) an outdoor cycling hill-climbing performance competition [34]. Similar performance decrements were reported for two indoor cycling simulations [35,36] when dehydration ranged from 1.0–1.8%.

Decrements of outdoor cycling performance which occur at ≤4% body mass loss have been disputed in one meta-analysis [37] which evaluated 5 research articles (13 effect estimates). However, virtually all researchers agree that moderate-to-severe dehydration (e.g., 4–7% versus 1–2% body mass loss; Figure 3) results in greater physiologic strain and decreased aerobic exercise performance [24,26,29,30,32,38–41].

Physiologists agree that dehydration-induced aerobic performance decrements are greater in hot versus cool environments [24,29,41,42], due to greater thermal and cardiovascular strain (i.e., increased skin temperature and blood flow, greater plasma volume loss, decreased cardiac output) that becomes physiologically impactful in the dehydration range of 2–4% of body mass [43,44]. In terms of associated physiological effects, a summary of 8 relevant publications [29] noted that a 4–5% dehydration level reduced maximal oxygen consumption (VO_{2max}) more in a hot environment (−9 to −27% when $T_{amb} \geq 30\ °C$) than in a cool or mild environment (−3 to −7% when T_{amb} was 15–26 °C). The consequences of this dehydration included a shorter exercise time to exhaustion, an obligatory reduction in exercise intensity, or both.

2.2. Effects of Dehydration on Symptomatology and Illness

The classic desert field observations of Adolph and colleagues [12] during the mid-1940s were among the first descriptions of exercise-induced dehydration that approached and exceeded 10% body mass loss. Although Adolph's systematic observations of dehydrated soldiers walking in the desert ($T_{amb} > 37\ °C$) were not subject to statistical analyses, they provide a thorough description of the detrimental health effects of prolonged dehydration. Figure 1 presents a summary of the signs and symptoms that were reported when dehydration exceeded 2%. The following Section 2.2.1 through Section 2.2.3 describe disorders that result from water and salt deficiencies.

2.2.1. Exercise Associated Collapse

A patient classification and care matrix, developed after years of treating runners in t medical tent of the Twin Cities Marathon, Minnesota, USA [45] facilitates clinical decisio, making and expedites the transition of distressed runners through a field medical facility near the finish line. Treatment of exercise-associated collapse centers on fluid replacement and body cooling or warming if needed. For suspected dehydration after the marathon, oral fluid replacement is preferred (e.g., water, fluid-electrolyte beverage, or 200–300 mL of salty soup bouillon to aid fluid retention). Intravenous fluid is necessary when casualties are unable to tolerate oral intake, and when there are clinical indications of severe volume depletion or ongoing fluid losses from vomiting or diarrhea. During medical treatment, to avoid adding water to a runner who already is overhydrated, exertional hyponatremia (see Section 3.2) is ruled out before intravenous fluid administration by assessing the serum Na^+ concentration of runners who finish after 4 h [45].

2.2.2. Exertional Heat Illnesses

Water and salt losses in sweat have implications for the health of athletes who exercise in hot environments. Water and sodium deficits are recognized as predisposing factors for exertional heat stroke [46–48], exertional heat cramps [49], and exertional heat exhaustion [43,50]. Regarding the latter illness, research has shown that (a) mild exercise (40–50% VO_{2max}) in hot environments (34–39 °C) does not induce heat exhaustion unless a significant fluid-electrolyte loss and cardiovascular strain exist; (b) a moderate but cumulative dehydration across 3 days can result in exertional heat exhaustion [51,52]; and (c) 85% of heat exhaustion patients who presented at a deep metalliferous mine infirmary exhibited a urine specific gravity of 1.020–1.040, indicating mild-to-severe dehydration [53].

2.2.3. Kidney Dysfunction and Renal Stress

Failure of the kidneys to perform essential functions (i.e., the clinical disorder named acute renal failure) is possible but uncommon during marathon footraces of 42.2 km and dehydration less than 4% of body mass [54]. However, both immediate (during and post-race) and delayed effects (i.e., 1–5 d after the event) of dehydration have been reported as abnormal values for urine flow rate, osmolar clearance, creatinine clearance, and protein in the renal filtration apparatus [54]. When no renal dysfunction is observed, considerable renal concentrating stress is possible. For example, 11 out of 33 cyclists who finished a summer 164 km ultraendurance event exhibited marked urine concentration, verified with specific gravity > 1.030 [55].

3. Problem: Overhydration during Endurance Exercise

3.1. Hyperhydration and Exercise Performance

No evidence suggests that deliberate pre-exercise consumption of excess pure water has an ergogenic effect on exercise performance [24,56]. Glycerol, however, often is ingested prior to exercise (e.g., 1.2 g/kg body mass with a volume of fluid equal to 26 mL/kg body mass) to hyperhydrate athletes by increasing water retention and plasma volume while decreasing urine volume [57]. This act delays reaching a level of dehydration that degrades exercise performance. Research results are not conclusive, in that studies have shown both an ergogenic effect and no effect on exercise performance [58,59]. However, one caveat should be noted. As glycerol dilutes both intracellular and extracellular fluids prior to exercise, it may predispose athletes to low serum Na^+ as described in the next paragraph, especially if aggressive drinking occurs during exercise. A similar predisposition to low serum Na^+ has been reported for deliberate overhydration with water and dilute fluids [24,60,61].

3.2. Exertional Hyponatremia (EHN): A Potential Medical Emergency

When overhydration during exercise dilutes blood, an osmotic pressure gradient causes water to move into cells. The resulting cell swelling can result in EHN, one of the few illnesses that is potentially fatal to otherwise healthy athletes during exercise.

Recognizable symptoms appear in most athletes at a serum concentration of approximately 130–135 mmol Na$^+$/L [26,62] and include lightheadedness, dizziness, nausea, puffiness (e.g., hands and feet), and body weight gain from baseline [63]. The majority of athletes whose serum Na$^+$ is below 130 mmol/L (Figure 2) experience symptoms; these may include headache, vomiting, frothy sputum, difficulty breathing, pulmonary edema (i.e., fluid accumulation with swelling), and altered mental status such as confusion or seizure that results from cerebral edema [10,64].

The signs and symptoms of EHN do not necessarily correlate with the serum Na+ in the range shown in Table 3 ($\geq$130 mmol Na$^+$/L). The total symptoms score (column 10), rated with a validated Environmental Symptoms Questionnaire [65], was not related to the change of serum Na$^+$ (column 5). Indeed, the self-rated symptoms of hyponatremic cyclists LC and AM (serum Na+ of 130 mmol/L) ranked among the lowest in this subject sample [66]. Thus, the severity of symptoms and not the absolute value of serum Na$^+$ concentration guide the course of medical treatment [63].

Table 3. Athlete physiological and perceptual responses during a summer road cycling event (7.1–10.9 h duration). Data are rank-ordered on the basis of serum Na$^+$ change (column 5). Modified from [66] with unpublished data added.

Cyclists	Total Fluid Intake (L) [a,b]	Total Fluid Intake (ml/kg) [a,b]	Sodium Intake (mg) [a,b]	Change of Serum Na$^+$ (mmol/L) [a]	Pre-Event Body Mass (kg)	Body Mass Change (%) [a]	Urine Specific Gravity at Finish Line	Rating of Thirst at Finish Line [c]	Environmental Symptoms Questionnaire [d] Total Score at Finish Line
A	3.7	42	356	+6	88.6	−4.6	1.021	4	13
B	5.3	75	194	+4	71.0	+1.4	1.024	8	10
C	3.0	48	328	+3	61.8	−4.2	1.030	6	11
D	4.7	62	149	+1	75.2	−1.2	1.026	8	27
E	10.9	139	1166	+1	78.5	−1.5	1.020	7	25
F	4.6	54	124	−1	85.5	+0.1	1.021	6	21
G	4.1	50	261	−2	82.0	−1.8	1.030	5	13
H	3.4	41	263	−2	82.9	−0.1	1.023	4	11
I	9.5	103	823	−2	91.8	−4.6	1.034	6	25
J	9.6	124	1259	−3	77.2	−1.9	1.016	4	17
K	10.5	101	1182	−3	104.7	+1.0	1.026	5	21
L	9.2	109	1601	−6	84.7	+1.1	1.003	5	12
LC [e]	13.7	191	1179	−11	72.0	+4.3	1.003	2	4
AM [e]	14.7	189	3292	−11	77.5	+0.1	1.010	2	11

[a], during the 164-km ride; [b], consumed in water, beverages, sport drinks, solid foods, bars, gels, tablets, capsules; [c], a visual rating scale presented thirst levels of increasing intensity, ranging from 1(not thirsty) to 9 (very, very thirsty); [d], see reference [65]; [e], cyclists LC and AM experienced exertional hyponatremia, both with a serum Na$^+$ of 130 mmol/L.

Table 3 includes data regarding two recreational cyclists (LC and AM) who began a summer 164-km event (Tamb, 34 ± 5 °C) with normal serum electrolytes but finished the ride with a serum sodium concentration of 130 mmol/L, indicative of mild EHN. The data of 12 other finishers (A–L, column 1) are presented to allow comparisons. Although they did not ride together, both cyclists consumed a large and similar relative volume of fluid (191 and 189 mL/kg), experienced an identical 11 mmol/L decrease of serum sodium, and reported low thirst sensations. However, one (LC) gained 3.1 kg (+4.3% of body mass) during 8.9 h of exercise (i.e., suggesting a dilutional effect) and the other (AM) maintained body mass (+0.1 kg, +0.1%, 10.6 h), suggesting that no excess fluid was retained. Thus, Table 3 suggests a complex, individualized EHN etiology [66].

After exercise, fluids should be consumed judiciously because symptoms of EHN may develop hours after excess fluid consumption, as described in two published case reports. The first involved a 21-year old man who had aggressively consumed water and gained 5.25 kg of body weight during 5 h of treadmill exercise in a hot environment [61]. He was asymptomatic until he experienced nausea and malaise late that evening, and was transferred to a nearby hospital with a serum Na$^+$ of 122 mmol/L. After a night of observation, fluid restriction, and large urine output, he was released at 11:00 a.m. the next morning without symptoms. A more serious EHN case with delayed symptom onset involved a 49-year old runner who finished a 42.2 km marathon in 4 h 22 min then boarded an airline flight to return home [67]. Approximately 5 h after he finished the race, he became ill and experienced a grand mal seizure in the aisle of the cabin. The pilots diverted the aircraft to a nearby city for an emergency landing. The runner was transported to a hospital, where he experienced two additional seizures while unconscious with a serum Na$^+$ of 129 mmol/L. A chest x-ray indicated pulmonary edema and a brain scan revealed cerebral edema; he also was diagnosed with renal insufficiency and liver damage. During the ensuing 18 months, this runner learned that he was unable to mentally process information that had previously been routine, and he was unable to perform his professional duties.

3.2.1. Predisposing Factors for EHN

Exercise duration greater than 4 h, high sweat rate, high sweat Na$^+$, and small body size have been identified as predisposing factors for EHN [63,68–70]. Table 4 allows consideration of other risk factors; data are rank-ordered on the basis of final serum Na$^+$ (column 5). As the severity of EHN increased (i.e., moving from top to bottom as serum Na$^+$ decreased), both body mass change (column 6) and the rate of fluid intake (column 8) trended toward increasing. The individuals and groups in Table 4 (labeled A through M in column 1) also are depicted in Figure 2, allowing comparisons to a large data base of marathon runners and Ironman triathletes. The open symbols (○) in Figure 2 represent individuals who sought medical care for symptomatic EHN.

Table 4. Factors that influence exertional hyponatremia. Letters in column 1 refer to the symbols embedded in Figure 2.

Symbols in Figure 2	Men	Women	Scenario (Ambient Temperature, °C)	Final Serum Na$^+$ (mmol/L)	Body Mass Change (%)	Exercise Duration (h)	Rate of Fluid Intake (ml/h)	Mean Initial Body Mass (kg)	Source
Background data points	a	a	11 endurance events [a]	See Figure 3	See Figure 3	b	b	b	[20]
A	42		164 km cycling (34.4)	141	−0.8	9.1	649	85.9	[55]
B	31		164 km cycling (24.4–39.5)	141	−1.4	9.0	700	85.4	[66]
C		6	164 km cycling (34.4)	140	−0.1	9.0	520	67.3	[55]
D	50		100 km run (15.6–21.7)	138	−2.6	12.2	600	74.9	[71]
E	7		Treadmill walk (41.0) [c]	136	−0.1	4.0 [c]	640	77.9	[61]
F	5		44 km trail run (15–34)	131	−2.2	9.3	290 [d]	81.9	[72]
G		1	Ironman triathlon (21.0) [e,f]	131	+0.9	13.3	733	57.5	[73]
H	1		164 km cycling (24.4–39.5) [g]	130	+4.3	8.9	1,500	72.0	[66]
I		1	Ironman triathlon (21.0) [e,f]	130	+2.5	12.0	764	59.0	[73]
J	1		164 km cycling (24.4–39.5) [g]	130	+0.1	10.6	1,400	77.5	[66]
K	2	5	Ironman triathlon [e]	128	−0.5	12.3	b	62.5	[74]
L	1		Treadmill walk (41.0) [c]	122	+4.0	4.0 [c]	2,061 [h]	82.2	[61]
M	1		Ironman triathlon [e]	116	+5.0	14.0	1,642	b	[75]

Note: values are means or medians (columns 5–9) when the number of subjects is ≥ 2. [a], 3 Ironman triathlons, 6 marathon footraces (42.2 km), a 109 km cycling tour, and a 160 km footrace (2,135 athletes); [b], not reported; [c], 5.6 km/h, 5% grade, 30 min walking and 30 min seated rest per hour; [d], runners were allowed to drink and eat only fluids and food provided by the race organizing committee, at 11 intermediate checkpoint stations, positioned every 3–5 km; they did not drink when thirsty or ad libitum; [e], triathlon stages were 3.8 km swim, 180 km cycle, 42.2 km run; [f], this athlete stopped during the cycling stage due to hyponatremic illness; [g], identical to cyclists LC and AM in Table 4 (column 1); [h], this individual purposefully overhydrated.

A few athletes possess a "perfect storm" of characteristics in which a high sweat rate (e.g., 2.0–3.0 L/h) coexists with a high sweat sodium concentration (e.g., 40–80 mmol Na$^+$/L; 2.3–4.6 g NaCl/L). These athletes may be identified by white salt deposits on a shirt, jersey, or shorts. Due to their relatively large sodium loss in sweat, they are at increased risk of developing EHN. In a hypothetical calculation, Hiller [68] noted that an Ironman triathlete with a sweat rate of 1.5 L/h could lose 36 g of NaCl (14,040 mg of sodium) in 12 h. This observation is supported by the mathematical prediction model of Montain et al. [76], which demonstrates that a high sweat sodium concentration is an important etiological factor.

3.2.2. EHN Etiologies

Multiple EHN origins have been described [20,61,66,67,71], and consensus regarding a single etiology is difficult to reach because some cases reportedly involve hyponatremia with body mass gain (i.e., hypervolemic hyponatremia, water retention that exceeds sweat and urine losses) [10,77–79], whereas other EHN cases involve hyponatremia with body mass loss due to partially replaced sweat water and sodium losses (hypovolemic hyponatremia) [10,68,77,80]. Importantly, a 2015 consensus document noted that all known EHN fatalities to that date had involved overconsumption of dilute fluids [63].

3.2.3. EHN Cases Involve Variable Vasopressin Responses

Vasopressin (antidiuretic hormone) is the body's principal water-regulating hormone. It functions to maintain body water balance, in conjunction with thirst, by regulating serum osmolality within narrow limits [81]. Although dehydration with elevated serum osmolality is the primary stimulus for the release of vasopressin from the pituitary, non-osmotic factors also are known, including plasma volume decrease, hypoglycemia, nausea, and vomiting [82].

In an unknown percentage of EHN cases, serum vasopressin increases abnormally during overhydration, facilitating water retention. This inappropriately high serum vasopressin also stimulates sodium excretion by the kidneys, reducing serum Na^+. As vasopressin has a brief half-life and laboratory analysis is technically difficult, this hormone rarely is analyzed in cases of EHN. Nevertheless, this condition was verified during a marathon field study [83] in which 43% of runners with a serum Na^+ < 130 mmol/L exhibited inappropriately high serum vasopressin levels (range, 3–17 pg/mL), and during a case of symptomatic EHN that developed during a laboratory investigation [61]. A notable exception to these reports occurred among 7 symptomatic Ironman triathletes [74] who finished 12 h of exercise with a median body weight loss of 0.5%, post-exercise plasma Na^+ of 128 mmol/L, and a post-exercise plasma vasopressin concentration of 1.6 pmol/L; these values represented symptomatic EHN with a low serum vasopressin concentration. A control group of 11 asymptomatic triathletes exhibited the following comparison values: body weight loss of 3.9%, plasma Na^+ of 141 mmol/L, and a plasma vasopressin concentration of 4.6 pmol/L; these levels represented a typical hormonal response to moderate dehydration. These variable vasopressin responses illustrate why it is difficult to attain consensus regarding the role of arginine vasopressin in EHN.

A coherent explanation for variable vasopressin responses was published by Hew-Butler [82]. Her review article distinguished intense (brief, >90% of maximal oxygen consumption), steady state (sustained at 40–60% of maximal oxygen uptake), and prolonged endurance (>1 h) exercise. During the former, an obvious and statistically significant increase of plasma vasopressin occurs that exceeds the expected increase due to increased plasma osmolality. Steady state exercise also generally stimulates a statistically significant vasopressin increase. During prolonged competitive endurance exercise, a similar vasopressin increase occurs, with or without significant increases of serum Na^+ or osmolality; this elevation persisted for 2 h after a 24 h competitive track race and for 31 h after a 38 km non-competitive run. In all of these exercise types, it appears that published vasopressin responses are difficult to interpret because of differences in exercise intensity [82].

3.2.4. Evidence for an EHN Drinking Rate Threshold

A previous analysis of 6 groups of runners and triathletes reported that no case of symptomatic EHN occurred (serum sodium < 130 mmol/L during continuous exercise that lasted 3.2–12.3 h) among 270 athletes who consumed less than 750 mL of fluid per hour [67]. In addition, case reports of two female ultradistance triathletes [73] observed that their post-race hyponatremia (130 and 131 mmol Na+/L) was accompanied by weight gain (0.5 and 1.5 kg). They consumed fluids during competition at a rate of 730 and 760 mL/h. Figure 2 also supports this drinking rate threshold for the onset of EHN, in that all yellow highlighted square symbols represent individuals who consumed fluids at a rate > 700 mL/h, and gained weight during their respective exercise bouts. These individuals are clustered in the lower left quadrant of Figure 2, among symptomatic athletes (open symbols, ○). These observations suggest that endurance athletes who consume fluids at a rate < 700 mL/h have a decreased risk of EHN. This theoretical 700 mL/h fluid consumption rate threshold is consistent with the 400 to 800 mL/h recommendations of both the International Marathon Medical Directors Association [84], the American College of Sports Medicine [24], and a mathematical model that was designed to clarify the etiology of EHN [76].

3.2.5. Does Sodium Intake Counteract a Low Serum Na^+?

It is widely recognized that salt (sodium chloride, NaCl) capsules are consumed during triathlons and marathons. Exploring this trend within endurance sports, Hoffman & Stuempfle [80] reported that 90–96% of runners consumed sodium supplements during a 161-km ultramarathon footrace because they believed that it prevented muscle cramps and hyponatremia. However, there is little evidence to support this belief. For example, Table 3 shows that cyclists J, K, L, LC and AM consumed the largest amounts of sodium but experienced the greatest decrease of serum Na^+, whereas cyclists A, B, C and D consumed small amounts of sodium and experienced an increased serum Na^+ [61]. Therefore, sodium consumption did not prevent EHN from occurring in cyclists LC and AM, and low sodium intake by other cyclists was not associated with EHN. Similar conclusions have been published regarding ultramarathon competitors by Speedy et al. [85], Hew-Butler et al. [86], Hoffman and Stuempfle [80], and Hoffman and Myers [87].

Two controlled laboratory studies also have quantified the effects of sodium consumption on serum Na^+. The first provided 3911 mg of sodium during 6 h of exercise in a 34 °C environment [88], and the second provided 1409 mg sodium during 3 h of exercise at 30 °C [89]. Post-exercise measurements detected a mean serum Na^+ increase of 3 mmol/L (i.e., supplemented versus control experiments) in both studies, indicating that sodium supplementation had a minor influence on serum Na^+ levels.

4. The Complexity of Thirst and Drinking

Thirst prompts seeking and consuming water, and is measured with a subjective rating scale. Drinking behavior is distinct from thirst, is measured as the volume of fluid consumed, and may involve fluid selection on the basis of preferred or required characteristics (i.e., temperature, palatability, ingredients, energy content) [90].

During sedentary daily activities (i.e., producing a small 24-h water turnover), the perception of thirst, the act of drinking, renal regulation of water and electrolytes, and neuroendocrine responses (Table 1) adequately regulate total body water volume and serum concentration within 1–3% of each individual's baseline, from one day to the next [5–7]. During prolonged endurance exercise, however, the relationship between perception of thirst and whole-body fluid–electrolyte balance can be distorted by physiological challenges [32,91] such as sizeable water and sodium losses in sweat, movement of water between the intracellular and extracellular spaces, or plasma volume depletion [6].

4.1. Multiple Factors Influence Drinking during Endurance Exercise

Figure 4 presents several factors that influence thirst and drinking behavior, each of which is monitored and regulated continuously by the central nervous system. Thus, the phrase dynamic complexity applies to the vast, integrated, brain-wide network of nerve circuits and brain regions that regulate thirst, drinking, body water volume, and fluid concentration [92]. The findings of two recent human studies [93,94] suggest that thirst is one of multiple conscious perceptions and subconscious autonomic responses (Figure 4) that evolve simultaneously during dehydration and rehydration to influence drinking behavior. Simply stated, the internal motivation to consume water is influenced by multiple factors that reinforce the perception of thirst.

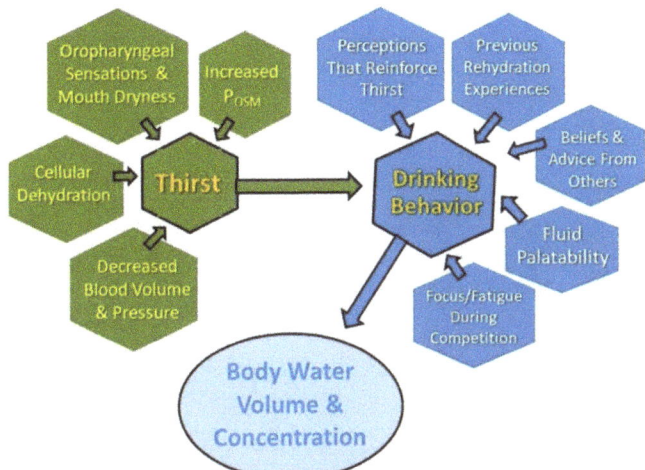

Figure 4. Influences on thirst and drinking behavior during endurance exercise. All factors in this diagram are perceived, monitored, and/or regulated by the brain.

As dehydration concentrates extracellular fluid, plasma osmolality (P_{osm}) is recognized as the primary factor that stimulates thirst [2,81,95]. However, as shown in Figure 5, the P_{osm} threshold at which thirst is perceived varies greatly across individuals (range, 274–293 mOsm/kg) and may be lower than the range of laboratory reference values for P_{osm} (285–295 mOsm/kg) [96]. The data in Figure 5 were compiled from 5 published human studies; the shape of this frequency distribution implies that the thirst threshold is a multifactorial (polygenic) characteristic [97]. Although inter-individual differences of the P_{osm} threshold for thirst have not been studied during exercise, Figure 5 suggests that the level of dehydration (i.e., increased P_{osm}) that initiates drinking during exercise might differ considerably among athletes.

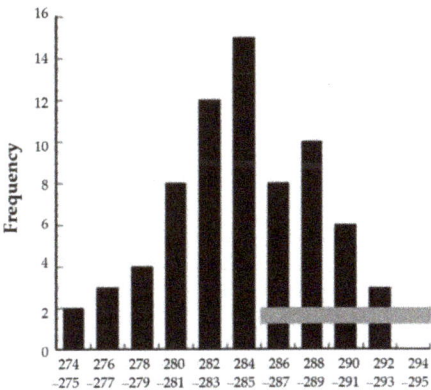

Figure 5. Frequency distribution of the plasma osmolality (P_{osm}) threshold for the onset of thirst. The horizontal gray bar delineates the laboratory reference range of P_{osm} values (285–295 mOsm/kg) for healthy adults. Reprinted under the terms and conditions of the Creative Commons Attribution (CC BY) license (http://creativecommons.org/licenses/by/4.0/) accessed on 2 March 2021. Modified from [97].

4.2. Inter-Individual Differences

Figure 6 illustrates six factors that influence the change of body mass and serum Na$^+$. Interactions of these factors with inherited characteristics and endurance training regimens produce great differences among athletes. In Figure 2, for example, if a male athlete experienced a body mass change of only—0.5% (0.35 kg) during a 13 h Ironman triathlon, his serum Na$^+$ could range from 119 (symptomatic EHN) to 157 mmol/L (severe hypernatremia). Conversely, if a male athlete finished with a serum Na$^+$ of 140 mmol/L (i.e., in the center of the reference range for healthy adults), his body weight change could range from +5.5% (+3.9 kg) to −12.5% (−8.8 kg). These large serum Na$^+$ and body mass ranges represent the effects of numerous perceptual, behavioral, hereditary and fluid-electrolyte variables (Figures 4–6), but are influenced mostly by the total volume of sweat produced (e.g., 15.6 L/13 h at a sweat rate of 1.2 L/h) and the total volume of fluid consumed (e.g., 9.1 L/13 h at a drinking rate of 700 mL/h).

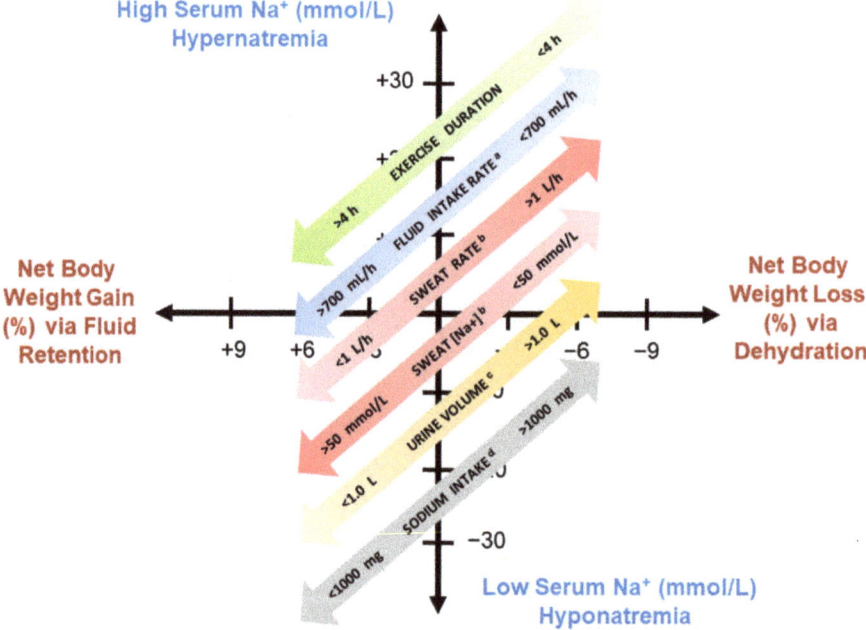

Figure 6. Factors that influence the relationship between body weight gain/loss and serum Na$^+$ during endurance exercise. The largest effects on whole body fluid–electrolyte balance are the volume of sweat lost and the volume of fluid consumed. Notes: ^{a}, water and low-sodium fluids promote dilution of body fluids; ^{b}, physical training and heat acclimatization increase sweat rate and decrease sweat sodium concentration; ^{c}, urine production decreases during exercise; ^{d}, increased dietary sodium encourages water retention but affects only a minor increase of serum Na$^+$.

Large inter-individual differences also exist among elite runners. Fluid intake rates were determined for 10 men who placed 1st or 2nd (range of finish times, 2:03:59 to 2:10:55) during prestigious city marathons [98]. Each runner's drinking behavior was recorded on videotape and fluid intake was estimated by multiplying drinking time by 45.2 mL/s (i.e., a value determined by laboratory drinking simulations). Half of these runners consumed fluids at rates that ranged from 30–300 mL/h (73–631 mL total), whereas the rate of fluid intake of the other 5 elite runners ranged from 420–1040 mL/h (886–2205 mL total). Clearly, these data indicate that elite marathon runners (a) ingest fluid at rates that span a wide range during competition (30–1040 mL/h), and (b) some individuals greatly exceed the proposed drinking rate threshold at which symptomatic EHN appears (700 mL/h), described above in Section 3.2.4.

4.3. Personal Beliefs and Sources of Rehydration Information

Personal beliefs about drinking may predispose an athlete to EHN, according to the findings of two case reports. The first [66] involved cyclists LC and AM in Table 3 (who also are designated as athletes H and J in Table 4). Their urine specific gravity measurements on Day-1 (LC, 1.006; AM, 1.004; 31 control cyclists, 1.017) and the morning of the road ride (LC, 1.003; AM, 1.005; controls, 1.019) indicated that both had overhydrated before prolonged exercise. The authors suggested that their pre-event hydration behavior, coupled with high rates of fluid intake during the ride (LC, 1500 mL/h; AM, 1400 mL/h), resulted in both cyclists experiencing asymptomatic EHN. The second publication [61] involved a controlled case report of EHN (serum Na^+, 122 mmol/L) observed during 5 h of intermittent treadmill walking in a hot environment (Tamb, 41 °C). A physically fit, 21 year-old male began exercise with blood values (serum Na^+, 134 mmol/L; osmolality, 282 mOsm/kg) slightly below the laboratory reference ranges for healthy males, because he had voluntarily overhydrated throughout the previous day. Overhydration prior to exercise is known to lower serum Na^+ and therefore increase the risk of dilutional hyponatremia if fluids are aggressively consumed during exercise [24]. This man acknowledged that his pre-exercise overhydrated state, and his high rate of fluid intake during exercise (2061 mL/h; 10.31 L total), were purposeful. He believed that drinking a large volume of water would decrease his risk of exertional heat exhaustion and heatstroke.

To understand the factors that guide drinking behavior, Winger and colleagues [99] surveyed 106 female and 97 male runners who had competed in road races (average experience, 13.0 and 8.3 y, respectively) at distances ranging from 5 to 42.2 km. Seven years later, Wilson [100] surveyed 223 female and 199 male marathon runners (average number completed by both groups, 4). Both studies focused on runner perceptions of fluid replacement, their beliefs about rehydration during exercise, and drinking behaviors. Winger et al. [99] observed that the most important influences on the drinking behavior of runners were: trial and error/personal history, recommendations from running groups or clubs, and advice from friends; sport drink companies were the least influential sources of information. Among marathon runners, Wilson [100] reported that the following sources of information were considered to be the most reliable: social media, print magazines, a personal trainer, and a fellow runner; scientific journals, dietitians/nutritionists, and running coaches were rated as the least reliable sources of information.

4.4. Unique Characteristics of Competitive Events

Distinctive aspects of different sporting events also can influence an athlete's rate of fluid intake; three examples follow. First, the possibility of inhaling water when respiratory ventilation rate is high (e.g., 120–155 L/min), and potentially having to stop to clear both lungs [21], may deter runners from drinking. Second, whereas fluid intake during endurance footraces is generally limited to the number of aid stations along a race course or a water bottle in hand, cyclists can consume fluids whenever desired because containers are attached to the bicycle frame or held in jersey pockets. Third, during the water stage of a triathlon, endurance swimmers have no access to fluids except the water they inadvertently consume during competition. These factors explain, in part, the consistent observation that endurance competitors replace $\leq$ 50% of sweat losses when allowed liquids ad libitum [101–103].

5. Rehydration Options

Table 5 describes five approaches to rehydration that endurance athletes employ: drink when thirsty, ad libitum drinking, individualized planned drinking, drink nothing, and drink as much as possible. In the following paragraphs, these approaches will be named options 1 through 5. The percentage of athletes who employ each option during endurance exercise is unknown.

Table 5. Five options for rehydration during endurance exercise.

Description	Objective/Rationale	Relevant Publications
1. Drink when thirsty. Fluid intake occurs only when thirst is sensed.	Primary focus: to prevent exertional hyponatremia. Secondary goal: to prevent a level of dehydration that impairs exercise performance. Proponents of this method assert that increased extracellular concentration triggers thirst to naturally protect athletes from the negative consequences of both fluid excess and severe dehydration. However, no randomized, controlled study confirms that drinking when thirsty successfully prevents exertional hyponatremia. Rationale: drinking when thirsty preserves serum Na^+ and osmolality within the normal laboratory reference range.	[55,84,104–110]
2. Ad libitum drinking. Consuming fluid whenever and in whatever volume desired, without specific focus on thirst.	Primary focus: to prevent exertional hyponatremia. Secondary goal: to prevent a level of dehydration that impairs exercise performance. Ad libitum drinking often is viewed as being identical to drinking when thirsty (above), however it is subtly different. See text for details.	[6,55,101,110,111]
3. Individualized planned drinking. This involves drinking a predetermined fluid volume that is determined by measuring sweat rate.	Primary focus: to prevent excessive dehydration that impairs exercise performance and to prevent exertional hyponatremia. Secondary goals: to decrease the risk of heat illness (heat exhaustion, heat stroke), and reduce cardiovascular/thermoregulatory strain associated with dehydration. Rationale: because there is considerable inter-individual variability of sweat rate and sweat electrolyte concentration, a customized fluid replacement plan meets each athlete's individual rehydration needs.	[24,26,32,66,108,112,113]
4. Purposefully drink nothing during exercise.	No professional sport medicine or sport nutrition organization recommends this extreme option for prolonged endurance exercise.	
5. Purposefully drink as much as possible, in excess of thirst.	No professional sport medicine or sport nutrition organization recommends this extreme option for prolonged endurance exercise. Nevertheless, a 2011 survey of runners (5 to 42.2 km finishers) determined that 8.9% plan to drink as much as possible during racing and training.	[99]

5.1. Options 1 and 2

The distinction between option 1 (using perceived thirst as the only signal to drink) and option 2 (consuming fluid whenever and in whatever volume desired) is subtle [101]. In fact, some professional organizations and experts have not recognized these as distinct behaviors and some authors use these terms synonymously [6,26,84,98,99,101]. However, a 2014 field study determined that cyclists could identify whether they typically used option 1 or 2 and self-selected into one of two study groups (n = 12 in each). Despite the fact that cyclists understood options 1 and 2 as distinct rehydration behaviors, no between-group differences were observed in the following measurements: total fluid intake (L), body mass change (%), time to ride 164 km (h), urine specific gravity, and rating of thirst at the finish line [110]. Thus, the greatest value of distinguishing options 1 and 2 may exist in communications among athletes.

During prolonged endurance exercise, the effectiveness of thirst and drinking in maintaining whole-body fluid–electrolyte balance is challenged [32] by large water and sodium losses in sweat, perturbations of intracellular volume or concentration, and plasma volume depletion [6]. As one example of several in the literature, Greenleaf et al. [91] reported that test subjects who drank ad libitum during exercise-heat stress, were not thirsty and felt fully recovered despite a body water deficit of 4–5 L. This phenomenon was named involuntary dehydration [6,12] because thirst was not sufficient to maintain body water and fluid intake did not match the level of dehydration. Voluntary dehydration is observed in most endurance athletes [17,102].

A field study involving 26 ultraendurance cyclists explored thirst during exercise [114]. Ratings of thirst were statistically compared to several other variables during 7 h of exercise (mean ground speed, 25.4 km/h; Tamb, 35.5 °C). The total fluid intake of these male cyclists varied greatly, ranging from 2.1 to 10.5 L during the 164 km ride. Post-event ratings of thirst were not significantly correlated with any measured variable, including total fluid intake (i.e., a measure of drinking behavior), body mass index, height, ground speed, body water balance (ingested fluid volume—volume of fluid lost), and change of body mass. In other words, the intensity of thirst did not represent the degree of dehydration or the volume of fluid consumed. This observation is consistent with the known effects of oropharyngeal sensations on drinking behavior. These sensory signals (e.g., mouth dryness, swallowing fluid) rapidly reduce and limit fluid intake by modulating satiety and opposing overdrinking [115]. Thus, whenever fluid is consumed, even if the volume is small, oropharyngeal signals diminish the sensation of thirst [93,115] and theoretically reduce the risk of EHN by reducing fluid intake.

5.2. Option 3

Individualized planned drinking appeals to athletes who prefer to design their exercise rehydration systematically. This approach to rehydration is recommended by the National Athletic Trainer's Association [26] and the American College of Sports Medicine [24]. The accuracy of this method relies on an objective measurement of sweat rate during outdoor exercise. After sweat rate is determined, the athlete can design a customized fluid replacement plan for use during endurance exercise, realizing that the predetermined rate of fluid intake always should be less than sweat rate, to avoid overhydration and body weight gain.

5.2.1. Determining Sweat Rate

The method to determine sweat rate involves voiding the bowel and bladder, weighing body mass before exercise on a digital floor scale with a precision of 0.1 kg (i.e., 0.2 lb), simulating a future competitive event (i.e., considering environmental conditions, exercise intensity), and measuring body weight after exercise [116,117]. Sweat rate equals the body mass change per hour. If fluid is consumed or if urine is excreted between the pre- and post-exercise body weight measurements, the final sweat rate should be corrected as follows: sweat rate (L/h) = body weight difference (1 kg = 1 L) + water intake (L)—urine volume (L). All factors are measured over a 1-h or half-hour period; the latter is corrected to 1 h mathematically.

5.2.2. Determining a Morning Baseline Body Mass

As body mass measurements may be impractical or impossible at the event site, it is valuable for each athlete to determine his/her baseline body mass approximately 1 week before an event. This is done by measuring body weight upon waking, on 3–5 consecutive days, using an accurate digital floor scale ($\pm$0.1 kg or lb). The median (middle) or average body mass serves as a useful baseline [116]. The important comparison is made between this baseline value and the body mass measured on the morning after an endurance event [118,119]. If the post-event body mass is notably less or greater than baseline, fluid intake should be adjusted accordingly (i.e., avoiding overconsumption and underconsumption) for 1–2 days; thirst and urine color changes will assist this adjustment of fluid intake [5,118,119]. Three other details are important. First, wear little or no clothing each time that body mass is recorded. Second, if dietary carbohydrate "loading" is used during the days prior to competition, body mass may increase (0.5–1.5 kg) because water is stored with glycogen in skeletal muscles. This extra water temporarily inflates body mass measurements, and these values should not be used to determine one's baseline. Third, this technique may not be valid after an event lasting 7–24 h because loss of muscle mass and/or fat mass may confound interpretation of body water status for several days after an ultraendurance event [16].

5.2.3. Interpreting Body Mass Changes

During exercise lasting 0.5–4.0 h, body mass change (ΔM_b) is the most commonly used representation of body water change [120,121] because most of body weight loss is water loss, muscle and adipose tissue losses are negligible, and ΔM_b has a measurement resolution of $\pm$0.1 L (e.g., 100 mL out of a 42–47 L total body water volume) when using a floor scale that reads to $\pm$100 g. Within the time frame of 0.5–4.0 h, ΔM_b essentially equals water loss (i.e., when corrected for the mass of fluid and food intake, urine output, and sweat loss), because no other body constituent is lost at a similar rate [120,122]. Option 3 in Table 5 is the only approach to rehydration that incorporates a known sweat rate value (calculated using ΔM_b measurements) and a planned rate of fluid intake (personally monitored during competition).

When endurance exercise lasts longer than 4 h, the contributions of other factors confound the interpretation of ΔM_b [13]. These include mass loss due to carbohydrate or fat oxidation, cellular water generated during metabolic reactions, and skeletal muscle and/or adipose tissue catabolism [15,16,71]. However, because athletes seldom know the technical methods to calculate these internal gains and losses of water, measurements of ΔM_b remain the only realistic surrogate measure of dehydration for athletes and field-based practitioners [15,77,119,122].

5.3. Options 4 and 5

The practices of drinking as much as possible (i.e., increasing the risk of EHN) and drinking nothing (i.e., increasing the likelihood of a performance decrement) are discouraged. No professional sports medicine or sports nutrition organization recommends these extreme options during endurance exercise.

6. Rehydration Recommendations for Endurance Athletes

Attempting to control all of the factors that influence thirst, drinking behavior, exercise performance, and health (described in the paragraphs above) is a formidable and unreasonable task. Nevertheless, the aim of rehydration should be to consume a volume of fluid that not only avoids dehydration greater than 2–4% of body mass, but also avoids overhydration. Although no single recommendation will suffice for all individuals (e.g., across a range of ambient temperatures, and with varied sweat rates, body masses, and exercise durations/intensities) [123], the following 9 recommendations are appropriate for most endurance and ultraendurance activities.

1. Measure body weight before and after exercise (Section 5.2.1). Change of body mass during exercise is a reasonable, albeit not perfect, surrogate measure of water gain or loss [15,77,119,122]. If body weight cannot be assessed on the day of endurance exercise, measure body weight on the morning after and compare this weight to a pre-determined baseline morning body weight [119]. Detailed methods are described above in Sections 5.2.2 and 5.2.3.
2. Do not gain weight during endurance exercise. Weight gain typically indicates fluid retention and increased risk of EHN [32,63].
3. Consume fluid at a rate less than 700 mL/h to reduce the risk of EHN. The proposed rationale for this recommendation is described in Section 3.2.4, Table 4 (column 8, symbols A–E), and Figure 2 (gray and yellow highlighted symbols). This recommendation is consistent with the 2001 guidelines of the International Marathon Medical Directors Association [84], and the 2007 fluid replacement position stand of the American College of Sports Medicine [24]. Both organizations recommend a 400 to 800 mL/h rate of fluid intake during endurance exercise.
4. Be alert for physiologic and perceptual cues that discourage drinking. When stomach fullness, bloating, or vomiting are experienced, decrease fluid intake [84].
5. Guide drinking behavior with this in mind: modest levels of dehydration up to 2–3% of body weight are tolerated well, with little risk of morbidity, symptoms, or a decline in exercise performance (Figure 1; Figure 3) [77].
6. According to the International Marathon Medical Directors Association [84], a weight loss that exceeds 4% of body mass justifies a medical consultation. The number of athletes affected by at least a 4% loss of body mass during prolonged endurance exercise is considerable, as shown in Figure 2.
7. After endurance exercise, white salt deposits on a shirt, jersey, or shorts indicate both a high sweat rate and a high sweat sodium concentration [124]. Consecutive days of profuse sweating (e.g., during lengthy training sessions) or a day-long utraendurance event in a hot environment may lead to whole-body salt deficiency [125,126] due to large sweat sodium losses, inadequate sodium intake, or both [46]. If salt depletion is suspected (e.g., increased salt appetite or salt craving), it is prudent to consider adding specific dietary food items to ensure that daily sodium intake replaces exercise-

8. induced sodium loss. Refer to [97] to identify the amount of sodium in common food items. Sodium supplementation during meals should be guided by dietary recommendations for daily sodium intake [127], and by considering the potential negative health effects of chronic high dietary salt intake [128].
   8. Sodium consumption in solid food or capsules has a minor influence on serum Na^+ and whole-body sodium balance during endurance exercise (Section 3.2.5) [88,89]. Athletes should be aware that sodium intake, while not discouraged, may provide little or no defense against EHN during prolonged exercise and the effects are unpredictable (see Table 3). This recommendation is supported by observations of ultramarathon runners [80]. Multiple regression analysis indicated that the amount of sodium consumed during a 161 km race accounted for only 6–8% of the variance in post-race serum Na^+. This recommendation also is supported by the Wilderness Medical Society Clinical Practice Guidelines [123], which advise that sodium and/or salty snacks be consumed along with an appropriate fluid volume. Salt intake should not be combined with overdrinking, which increases the risk of EHN despite sodium consumption; see recommendations 2–4 above.
   9. Experiment with rehydration options (Table 5) during training sessions, before using them in competition or in hot environments.

Funding: This research received no external funding.

Institutional Review Board Statement: Not applicable.

Informed Consent Statement: Not applicable.

Data Availability Statement: No new data were created or analyzed in this study. Data sharing is not applicable to this article.

Conflicts of Interest: The author declares no conflict of interest.

References

1. Thornton, S.N. Thirst and hydration: Physiology and consequences of dysfunction. *Physiol. Behav.* **2010**, *100*, 15–21. [CrossRef] [PubMed]
2. Fitzsimons, J.T. The physiological basis of thirst. *Kidney Int.* **1976**, *10*, 3–11. [CrossRef]
3. Galanth, C.; Hus-Citharel, A.; Li, B.; Llorens-Cortes, C. Apelin in the control of body fluid homeostasis and cardiovascular functions. *Curr. Pharm. Des.* **2012**, *18*, 789–798. [CrossRef] [PubMed]
4. Azizi, M.; Iturrioz, X.; Blanchard, A.; Peyrard, S.; De Mota, N.; Chartrel, N.; Vaudry, H.; Corvol, P.; Llorens-Cortes, C. Reciprocal regulation of plasma apelin and vasopressin by osmotic stimuli. *J. Am. Soc. Nephrol.* **2008**, *19*, 1015–1024. [CrossRef] [PubMed]
5. Cheuvront, S.N.; Kenefick, R.W. Am I drinking enough? Yes, no, and maybe. *J. Am. Coll. Nutr.* **2016**, *35*, 185–192. [CrossRef] [PubMed]
6. Greenleaf, J.E. Problem: Thirst, drinking behavior, and involuntary dehydration. *Med. Sci. Sports Exerc.* **1992**, *24*, 645–656. [CrossRef]
7. Bartoli, W.P.; Davis, J.M.; Pate, R.R.; Ward, D.S.; Watson, P.D. Weekly variability in total body water using ^2H_2O dilution in college-age males. *Med. Sci. Sports Exerc.* **1993**, *25*, 1422–1428. [CrossRef]
8. Armstrong, L.E. Assessing hydration status: The elusive gold standard. *J. Am. Coll. Nutr.* **2007**, *26*, 575S–584S. [CrossRef]
9. Armstrong, L.E.; Johnson, E.C. Water Intake, Water Balance, and the Elusive Daily Water Requirement. *Nutrients* **2018**, *10*, 1928. [CrossRef]
10. Speedy, D.B.; Noakes, T.D.; Rogers, I.R.; Thompson, J.M.; Campbell, R.G.; Kuttner, J.A.; Boswell, D.R.; Wright, S.; Hamlin, M.A. Hyponatremia in ultradistance triathletes. *Med. Sci. Sports Exerc.* **1999**, *31*, 809–815. [CrossRef]
11. Hew-Butler, T.; Collins, M.; Bosch, A.; Sharwood, K.; Wilson, G.; Armstrong, M.; Jennings, C.; Swart, J.; Noakes, T. Maintenance of plasma volume and serum sodium concentration despite body weight loss in ironman triathletes. *Clin. J. Sport Med.* **2007**, *17*, 116–122. [CrossRef]
12. Adolph, E.F. Signs and symptoms of desert dehydration. In *Physiology of Man in the Desert*; Adolf, E.F., Ed.; Interscience Publishers: Cummings Park, MA, USA, 1947.
13. Rehrer, N.J. Fluid and electrolyte balance in ultra-endurance sport. *Sports Med.* **2001**, *31*, 701–715. [CrossRef]
14. Barr, S.I.; Costill, D.L. Water: Can the endurance athlete get too much of a good thing? *J. Am. Diet. Assoc.* **1989**, *89*, 1629.
15. Armstrong, L.E.; Johnson, E.C.; Ganio, M.S.; Judelson, D.A.; Vingren, J.L.; Kupchak, B.R.; Kunces, L.J.; Muñoz, C.X.; McKenzie, A.L.; Williamson, K.H. Effective body water and body mass changes during summer ultra-endurance road cycling. *J. Sports Sci.* **2015**, *33*, 125–135. [CrossRef] [PubMed]

16. Knechtle, B.; Knechtle, P.; Wirth, A.; Rüst, C.A.; Rosemann, T. A faster running speed is associated with a greater body weight loss in 100-km ultramarathoners. *J. Sports Sci.* **2012**, *30*, 1131–1140. [CrossRef]
17. Rehrer, N.J.; Burke, L.M. Sweat losses during various sports. *Nutr. Diet.* **1996**, *53* (Suppl. S4), S13–S16.
18. Barnes, K.A.; Anderson, M.L.; Stofan, J.R.; Dalrymple, K.J.; Reimel, A.J.; Roberts, T.J.; Randell, R.K.; Ungaro, C.T.; Baker, L.B. Normative data for sweating rate, sweat sodium concentration, and sweat sodium loss in athletes: An update and analysis by sport. *J. Sports Sci.* **2019**, *37*, 2356–2366. [CrossRef] [PubMed]
19. Borg, G. Perceived exertion as an indicator of somatic stress. *Scand. J. Rehabil. Med.* **1970**, *2*, 92–98.
20. Noakes, T.D.; Sharwood, K.; Speedy, D.; Hew, T.; Reid, S.; Dugas, J.; Almond, C.; Wharam, P.; Weschler, L. Three independent biological mechanisms cause exercise-associated hyponatremia: Evidence from 2135 weighed competitive athletic performances. *Proc. Natl. Acad. Sci. USA* **2005**, *102*, 18550–18555. [CrossRef]
21. Armstrong, L.E.; Hubbard, R.W.; Jones, B.; Daniels, J.T. Preparing Alberto Salazar for the Heat of the 1984 Olympic Marathon. *Phys. Sportsmed.* **1986**, *14*, 73–81. [CrossRef]
22. Roberts, W.O.; Dorman, J.C.; Bergeron, M.F. Recurrent Heat Stroke in a Runner: Race Simulation Testing for Return to Activity. *Med. Sci. Sports Exerc.* **2016**, *48*, 785–789. [CrossRef] [PubMed]
23. Bergeron, M.F.; SIVOTEC Analytics, Boca Raton, FL, USA. Personal communication, 2021.
24. Sawka, M.N.; Burke, L.M.; Eichner, E.R.; Maughan, R.J.; Montain, S.J.; Stachenfeld, N.S. American College of Sports Medicine position stand. Exercise and fluid replacement. *Med. Sci. Sports Exerc.* **2007**, *39*, 377–390. [PubMed]
25. Armstrong, L.E.; Casa, D.J.; Millard-Stafford, M.; Moran, D.S.; Pyne, S.W.; Roberts, W.O. Exertional heat illness during training and competition. *Med. Sci. Sports Exerc.* **2007**, *39*, 556–572. [CrossRef] [PubMed]
26. McDermott, B.P.; Anderson, S.A.; Armstrong, L.E.; Casa, D.J.; Cheuvront, S.N.; Cooper, L.; Kenney, W.L.; O'Connor, F.G.; Roberts, W.O. National athletic trainers' association position statement: Fluid replacement for the physically active. *J. Athl. Train.* **2017**, *52*, 877–895. [CrossRef]
27. Casa, D.J.; DeMartini, J.K.; Bergeron, M.F.; Csillan, D.; Eichner, E.R.; Lopez, R.M.; Ferrara, M.S.; Miller, K.C.; O'Connor, F.; Sawka, M.N.; et al. National Athletic Trainers' Association position statement: Exertional heat illnesses. *J. Athl. Train.* **2015**, *50*, 986–1000. [CrossRef]
28. Collins, J.; Maughan, R.J.; Gleeson, M.; Bilsborough, J.; Jeukendrup, A.; Morton, J.P.; Phillips, S.M.; Armstrong, L.; Burke, L.M.; Close, G.L.; et al. UEFA expert group statement on nutrition in elite football. Current evidence to inform practical recommendations and guide future research. *Br. J. Sports Med.* **2020**, 01961. [CrossRef]
29. Cheuvront, S.N.; Kenefick, R.W. Dehydration: Physiology, assessment, and performance effects. *Compr. Physiol.* **2014**, *4*, 257–285.
30. Judelson, D.A.; Maresh, C.M.; Anderson, J.M.; Armstrong, L.E.; Casa, D.J.; Kraemer, W.J.; Volek, J.S. Hydration and muscular performance: Does fluid balance affect strength, power and high-intensity endurance? *Sports Med.* **2007**, *37*, 907–921. [CrossRef]
31. Sawka, M.N. Physiological consequences of hypohydration: Exercise performance and thermoregulation. *Med. Sci. Sports Exerc.* **1992**, *24*, 657–670. [CrossRef] [PubMed]
32. Kenefick, R.W. Drinking strategies: Planned drinking versus drinking to thirst. *Sports Med.* **2018**, *48*, S31–S37. [CrossRef]
33. Armstrong, L.; Costill, D.; Fink, W. Influence of diuretic-induced dehydration on competitive running performance. *Med. Sci. Sports Exerc.* **1985**, *17*, 456–461. [CrossRef]
34. Bardis, C.N.; Kavouras, S.A.; Arnaoutis, G.; Panagiotakos, D.B.; Sidossis, L.S. Mild dehydration and cycling performance during 5-kilometer hill climbing. *J. Athl. Train.* **2013**, *48*, 741–747. [CrossRef]
35. Bardis, C.N.; Kavouras, S.A.; Kosti, L.; Markousi, M.; Sidossis, L.S. Mild hypohydration decreases cycling performance in the heat. *Med. Sci. Sports Exerc.* **2013**, *45*, 1782–1789. [CrossRef]
36. Walsh, R.M.; Noakes, T.D.; Hawley, J.A.; Dennis, S.C. Impaired High-Intensity Cycling Performance Time at Low Levels of Dehydration. *Int. J. Sports Med.* **1994**, *15*, 392–398. [CrossRef] [PubMed]
37. Goulet, E.D. Effect of exercise-induced dehydration on time-trial exercise performance: A meta-analysis. *Br. J. Sports Med.* **2011**, *45*, 1149–1156. [CrossRef] [PubMed]
38. Sawka, M.N.; Pandolf, K.B. Effects of body water loss on physiological function and exercise performance. In *Fluid Homeostasis during Exercise*; Gisolfi, C.V., Lamb, D.R., Eds.; Benchmark Press: Carmel, IN, USA, 1990; pp. 1–38. ISBN 0-936157-52-6.
39. Sawka, M.N.; Young, A.J.; Francesconi, R.P.; Muza, S.R.; Pandolf, K.B. Thermoregulatory and blood responses during exercise at graded hypohydration levels. *J. Appl. Physiol.* **1985**, *59*, 1394–1401. [CrossRef]
40. Armstrong, L.E.; Maresh, C.M.; Gabaree, C.V.; Hoffman, J.R.; Kavouras, S.A.; Kenefick, R.W.; Castellani, J.W.; Ahlquist, L.E. Thermal and circulatory responses during exercise: Effects of hypohydration, dehydration, and water intake. *J. Appl. Physiol.* **1997**, *82*, 2028–2035. [CrossRef]
41. Cheuvront, S.N.; Carter, R.I.; Castellani, J.W.; Sawka, M.N. Hypohydration impairs endurance exercise performance in temperate but not cold air. *J. Appl. Physiol.* **2005**, *99*, 1972–1976. [CrossRef]
42. Sawka, M.N.; Leon, L.R.; Montain, S.J.; Sonna, L.A. Integrated physiological mechanisms of exercise performance, adaptation, and maladaptation to heat stress. *Compr. Physiol.* **2011**, *1*, 1883–1928. [PubMed]
43. Armstrong, L.E. Heat Exhaustion. In *Exertional Heat Illness: A Clinical and Evidence-Based Guide*; Adams, W.M., Jardine, J., Eds.; Springer Nature: New York, NY, USA, 2020; pp. 81–115. ISBN 978-3-030-27804-5.
44. Kenefick, R.W.; Cheuvront, S.N.; Palombo, L.J.; Ely, B.R.; Sawka, M.N. Skin temperature modifies the impact of hypohydration on aerobic performance. *J. Appl. Physiol.* **2010**, *109*, 79–86. [CrossRef]
45. Roberts, W.O. Exercise-associated collapse care matrix in the marathon. *Sports Med.* **2007**, *37*, 431–433. [CrossRef]

46. Gaffin, S.L.; Hubbard, R.W. Pathophysiology of heatstroke. In *Medical Aspects of Harsh Environments*; Pandolf, K.B., Burr, R.E., Eds.; Office of the Surgeon General, U.S. Army: Washington, DC, USA, 2001; Volume 1, pp. 161–209. ISBN 978-0-160-51071-7.
47. Lambert, G.P.; Lang, J.; Bull, A.; Pfeifer, P.C.; Eckerson, J.; Moore, G.; Lanspa, S.; O'Brien, J. Fluid restriction during running increases GI permeability. *Int. J. Sports Med.* **2008**, *29*, 194–198. [CrossRef] [PubMed]
48. Armstrong, L.E.; Lee, E.C.; Armstrong, E.M. Interactions of gut microbiota, endotoxemia, immune function, and diet in exertional heatstroke. *J. Sports Med.* **2018**, 5724575. [CrossRef] [PubMed]
49. Bergeron, M.F. Heat cramps: Fluid and electrolyte challenges during tennis in the heat. *J. Sci. Med. Sport* **2003**, *6*, 19–27. [CrossRef]
50. King, B.A.; Barry, M.E. The physiological adaptations to heat-stress with a classification of heat illness and a description of the features of heat exhaustion. *S. Afr. Med. J.* **1962**, *36*, 451–455.
51. Armstrong, L.E.; Hubbard, R.W.; Szlyk, P.C.; Sills, I.V.; Kraemer, W.J. Heat intolerance, heat exhaustion monitored: A case report. *Aviat. Space Environ. Med.* **1988**, *59*, 262–266.
52. Sawka, M.N.; Young, A.J.; Latke, W.A.; Neufer, P.D.; Quigley, M.D.; Pandolf, K.B. Human tolerance to heat strain during exercise: Influence of hydration. *J. Appl. Physiol.* **1992**, *73*, 368–375. [CrossRef]
53. Donoghue, A.M.; Sinclair, M.J.; Bates, G.P. Heat exhaustion in a deep underground metalliferous mine. *Occup. Environ. Med.* **2000**, *57*, 165–174. [CrossRef]
54. Irving, R.A.; Noakes, T.D.; Irving, G.A.; Van Zyl-Smit, R. The immediate and delayed effects of marathon running on renal function. *J. Urol.* **1986**, *136*, 1176–1180. [CrossRef]
55. Armstrong, L.E.; Casa, D.J.; Emmanuel, H.; Ganio, M.S.; Klau, J.F.; Lee, E.C.; Maresh, C.M.; McDermott, B.P.; Stearns, R.L.; Vingren, J.L.; et al. Nutritional, Physiological and Perceptual Responses During a Summer Ultra-Endurance Cycling Event. *J. Strength Cond. Res.* **2012**, *26*, 307–318. [CrossRef]
56. Hillman, A.R.; Turner, M.C.; Peart, D.J.; Bray, J.W.; Taylor, L.; McNaughton, L.R.; Siegler, J.C. A comparison of hyperhydration versus ad libitum fluid intake strategies on measures of oxidative stress, thermoregulation, and performance. *Res. Sports Med.* **2013**, *21*, 305–317. [CrossRef]
57. Kavouras, S.A.; Armstrong, L.E.; Maresh, C.M.; Casa, D.J.; Herrera-Soto, J.A.; Scheett, T.P.; Stoppani, J.; Mack, G.W.; Kraemer, W.J. Rehydration with glycerol: Endocrine, cardiovascular, and thermoregulatory responses during exercise in the heat. *J. Appl. Physiol.* **2006**, *100*, 442–450. [CrossRef] [PubMed]
58. Van Rosendal, S.P.; Osborne, M.A.; Fassett, R.G.; Coombes, J.S. Guidelines for glycerol use in hyperhydration and rehydration associated with exercise. *Sports Med.* **2010**, *40*, 113–139. [CrossRef] [PubMed]
59. Kerksick, C.M.; Wilborn, C.D.; Roberts, M.D.; Smith-Ryan, A.; Kleiner, S.M.; Jäger, R.; Collins, R.; Cooke, M.; Davis, J.N.; Galvan, E.; et al. ISSN Exercise & Sports Nutrition Review Update: Research & Recommendations. *J. Int. Soc. Sports Nutr.* **2018**, *15*, 1–57.
60. Montain, S.J. Strategies to prevent hyponatremia during prolonged exercise. *Curr. Sports Med. Rep.* **2008**, *7*, S28–S35. [CrossRef]
61. Armstrong, L.E.; Curtis, W.C.; Hubbard, R.W.; Francesconi, R.P.; Moore, R.O.; Askew, E.W. Symptomatic hyponatremia during prolonged exercise in heat. *Med. Sci. Sports Exerc.* **1993**, *25*, 543–549. [CrossRef]
62. Armstrong, L.E.; McDermott, B.P. Exertional hyponatremia. In *Emergency Management for Sport and Physical Activity*; Casa, D.J., Stearns, R., Eds.; Jones & Bartlett Learning: Burlington, MA, USA, 2015; pp. 169–180. ISBN 978-1-284-02216-2.
63. Hew-Butler, T.; Rosner, M.H.; Fowkes-Godek, S.; Dugas, J.P.; Hoffman, M.D.; Lewis, D.P.; Maughan, R.J.; Miller, K.C.; Montain, S.J.; Rehrer, N.J.; et al. Statement of the Third International Exercise-Associated Hyponatremia Consensus Development Conference, Carlsbad, California, 2015. *Clin. J. Sport Med.* **2015**, *25*, 303–320. [CrossRef] [PubMed]
64. Weschler, L.B. Exercise-associated hyponatraemia. *Sports Med.* **2005**, *35*, 899–922. [CrossRef] [PubMed]
65. Kobrick, J.L.; Sampson, J.B. New inventory for the assessment of symptom occurrence and severity at high altitude. *Aviat. Space Environ. Med.* **1979**, *50*, 925–929.
66. Armstrong, L.E.; Lee, E.C.; Casa, D.; Johnson, E.C.; Ganio, M.S.; McDermott, B.; Vingren, J.; Oh, H.M.; Williamson, K.H. Exertional Hyponatremia and Serum Sodium Change During Ultraendurance Cycling. *Int. J. Sport Nutr. Exerc. Metab.* **2017**, *27*, 139–147. [CrossRef]
67. Armstrong, L.E. Exertional hyponatremia. In *Exertional Heat Illnesses*; Armstrong, L.E., Ed.; Human Kinetics: Champaign, IL, USA, 2003; pp. 103–136. ISBN 0-7360-3771-3.
68. Hiller, W.D. Dehydration and hyponatremia during triathlons. *Med. Sci. Sports Exerc.* **1989**, *21* (Suppl. S5), S219–S221.
69. Armstrong, L.E.; Casa, D.J. Predisposing Factors for Exertional Heat Illnesses. In *Exertional Heat Illnesses*; Armstrong, L.E., Ed.; Human Kinetics: Champaign, IL, USA, 2003; pp. 162–167. ISBN 0-7360-3771-3.
70. Seal, A.D.; Anastasiou, C.A.; Skenderi, K.P.; Echegaray, M.; Yiannakouris, N.; Tsekouras, Y.E.; Matalas, A.L.; Yannakoulia, M.; Pechlivani, F.; Kavouras, S.A. Incidence of hyponatremia during a continuous 246-km ultramarathon running race. *Front. Nutr.* **2019**, *6*, 161. [CrossRef]
71. Rüst, C.A.; Knechtle, B.; Knechtle, P.; Wirth, A.; Rosemann, T. Body mass change and ultraendurance performance: A decrease in body mass is associated with an increased running speed in male 100-km ultramarathoners. *J. Strength Cond. Res.* **2012**, *26*, 1505–1516. [CrossRef] [PubMed]
72. Arnaoutis, G.; Anastasiou, C.A.; Suh, H.; Maraki, M.; Tsekouras, Y.; Dimitroulis, E.; Echegaray, M.; Papamichalopoulou, D.; Methenitis, S.; Sidossis, L.S.; et al. Exercise-Associated Hyponatremia during the Olympus Marathon Ultra-Endurance Trail Run. *Nutrients* **2020**, *12*, 997. [CrossRef] [PubMed]

73. Speedy, D.B.; Noakes, T.D.; Rogers, I.R.; Hellemans, I.; Kimber, N.E.; Boswell, D.R.; Campbell, R.; Kuttner, J.A. A prospective study of exercise-associated hyponatremia in two ultradistance triathletes. *Clin. J. Sport Med.* **2000**, *10*, 136–141. [CrossRef]
74. Speedy, D.B.; Rogers, I.R.; Noakes, T.D.; Wright, S.; Thompson, J.M.; Campbell, R.; Hellemans, I.; Kimber, N.E.; Boswell, D.R.; Kuttner, J.A.; et al. Exercise-induced hyponatremia in ultradistance triathletes is caused by inappropriate fluid retention. *Clin. J. Sport Med.* **2000**, *10*, 272–278.
75. Speedy, D.B.; Rogers, I.; Safih, S.; Foley, B. Hyponatremia and seizures in an ultradistance triathlete. *J. Emerg. Med.* **2000**, *18*, 41–44. [CrossRef]
76. Montain, S.J.; Cheuvront, S.N.; Sawka, M.N. Exercise associated hyponatremia: Quantitative analysis for understand the aetiology. *Br. J. Sports Med.* **2006**, *40*, 98–106. [CrossRef]
77. Hew-Butler, T.; Loi, V.; Pani, A.; Rosner, M.H. Exercise-associated hyponatremia: 2017 update. *Front. Med.* **2017**, *4*. [CrossRef]
78. Noakes, T.D.; Goodwin, N.; Rayner, B.L.; Branken, T.R.; Taylor, R.K. Water intoxication: A possible complication during endurance exercise. *Med. Sci. Sports Exerc.* **1985**, *17*, 370–375. [CrossRef] [PubMed]
79. Frizzell, R.T.; Lang, G.H.; Lowance, D.C.; Lathan, S.R. Hyponatremia and ultramarathon running. *JAMA* **1986**, *255*, 772–774. [CrossRef]
80. Hoffman, M.D.; Stuempfle, K.J. Sodium Supplementation and Exercise-Associated Hyponatremia during Prolonged Exercise. *Med. Sci. Sports Exerc.* **2015**, *47*, 1781–1787. [CrossRef] [PubMed]
81. Bankir, L.; Bichet, D.G.; Morgenthaler, N.G. Vasopressin: Physiology, assessment and osmosensation. *J. Intern. Med.* **2017**, *282*, 284–297. [CrossRef] [PubMed]
82. Hew-Butler, T. Arginine vasopressin, fluid balance and exercise. *Sports Med.* **2010**, *40*, 459–479. [CrossRef]
83. Siegel, A.J.; Verbalis, J.G.; Clement, S.; Mendelson, J.H.; Mello, N.K.; Adner, M.; Shirey, T.; Glowacki, J.; Lee-Lewandrowski, E.; Lewandrowski, K.B. Hyponatremia in marathon runners due to inappropriate arginine vasopressin secretion. *Am. J. Med.* **2007**, *120*, 461.e11–461.e17. [CrossRef]
84. Hew-Butler, T.; Verbalis, J.G.; Noakes, T.D. Updated fluid recommendation: Position statement from the International Marathon Medical Directors Association (IMMDA). *Clin. J. Sport Med.* **2006**, *16*, 283–292. [CrossRef] [PubMed]
85. Speedy, D.B.; Thompson, J.M.; Rodgers, I.; Collins, M.; Sharwood, K. Oral salt supplementation during ultradistance exercise. *Clin. J. Sport Med.* **2002**, *12*, 279–284. [CrossRef]
86. Hew-Butler, T.D.; Sharwood, K.; Collins, M.; Speedy, D.; Noakes, T. Sodium supplementation is not required to maintain serum sodium concentrations during an Ironman triathlon. *Br. J. Sports Med.* **2006**, *40*, 255–259. [CrossRef]
87. Hoffman, M.D.; Myers, T.M. Symptomatic Exercise-Associated Hyponatremia in an Endurance Runner Despite Sodium Supplementation. *Int. J. Sport Nutr. Exerc. Metab.* **2015**, *25*, 603–606. [CrossRef]
88. Barr, S.I.; Costill, D.L.; Fink, W.J. Fluid replacement during prolonged exercise: Effects of water, saline, or no fluid. *Med. Sci. Sports Exerc.* **1991**, *23*, 811–817. [CrossRef]
89. Vrijens, D.M.J.; Rehrer, N.J. Sodium-free fluid ingestion decreases plasma sodium during exercise in the heat. *J. Appl. Physiol.* **1999**, *86*, 1847–1851. [CrossRef]
90. Armstrong, L.E.; Kavouras, S.A. Thirst and drinking paradigms: Evolution from single factor effects to brainwide dynamic networks. *Nutrients* **2019**, *12*, 2864. [CrossRef]
91. Greenleaf, J.E.; Sargent, F. Voluntary dehydration in man. *J. Appl. Physiol.* **1965**, *20*, 719–724. [CrossRef]
92. Allen, W.E.; Chen, M.Z.; Pichamoorthy, N.; Tien, R.H.; Pachitariu, M.; Luo, L.; Deisseroth, K. Thirst regulates motivated behavior through modulation of brainwide neural population dynamics. *Science* **2019**, *364*, 6437. [CrossRef]
93. Armstrong, L.E.; Giersch, G.E.W.; Dunn, L.; Fiol, A.; Muñoz, C.X.; Lee, E.C. Inputs to Thirst and Drinking during Water Restriction and Rehydration. *Nutrients* **2020**, *12*, 2554. [CrossRef]
94. Armstrong, L.E.; Giersch, G.E.; Colburn, A.T.; Lopez, V.; Sekiguchi, Y.; Muñoz, C.X.; Lee, E.C. Progression of human subjective perceptions during euhydration, mild dehydration, and drinking. *Physiol. Behav.* **2021**, *229*, 113211. [CrossRef] [PubMed]
95. Fitzsimons, J.T. Angiotensin, thirst, and sodium appetite. *Physiol. Rev.* **1998**, *78*, 583–686. [CrossRef] [PubMed]
96. Kratz, A.; Ferraro, M.; Sluss, P.M.; Lewandrowski, K.B. Laboratory Reference Values. *N. Engl. J. Med.* **2004**, *35*, 1548–1563. [CrossRef]
97. Armstrong, L.E.; Muñoz, C.X.; Armstrong, E.M. Distinguishing Low and High Water Consumers: A Paradigm of Disease Risk. *Nutrients* **2020**, *12*, 858. [CrossRef]
98. Beis, L.Y.; Wright-Whyte, M.; Fudge, B.; Noakes, T.; Pitsiladis, Y.P. Drinking behaviors of elite male runners during marathon competition. *Clin. J. Sport Med.* **2012**, *22*, 254–261. [CrossRef] [PubMed]
99. Winger, J.M.; Dugas, J.P.; Dugas, L.R. Beliefs about hydration and physiology drive drinking behaviours in runners. *Br. J. Sports Med.* **2011**, *45*, 646–649. [CrossRef] [PubMed]
100. Wilson, P.B. Nutrition behaviors, perceptions, and beliefs of recent marathon finishers. *Phys. Sportsmed.* **2016**, *44*, 242–251. [CrossRef] [PubMed]
101. Cheuvront, S.N.; Haymes, E.M. Ad libitum fluid intakes and thermoregulatory responses of female distance runners in three environments. *J. Sports Sci.* **2001**, *19*, 845–854. [CrossRef]
102. Cheuvront, S.N.; Haymes, E.M. Thermoregulation and marathon running: Biological and environmental influences. *Sports Med.* **2001**, *31*, 743–762. [CrossRef]

103. Noakes, T.D. Fluid replacement during exercise. In *Exercise and Sport Science Reviews, Holloszy, J., Ed.*; Williams & Wilkins: Philadelphia, PA, USA, 1993; Volume 21, pp. 297–330. ISBN 978-0-683-00035-1.
104. Hoffman, M.D.; Cotter, J.D.; Goulet, É.D.; Laursen, P.B. View: Is drinking to thirst adequate to appropriately maintain hydration status during prolonged endurance exercise? Yes. *Wilderness Environ. Med.* **2016**, *27*, 192–195. [CrossRef]
105. Hoffman, M.D.; Cotter, J.D.; Goulet, É.D.; Laursen, P.B. Rebuttal from "Yes". *Wilderness Environ. Med.* **2016**, *27*, 198–200. [CrossRef]
106. Hoffman, M.D. Comment on "Drinking Strategies: Planned Drinking Versus Drinking to Thirst". *Sports Med.* **2019**, *49*, 1133–1134. [CrossRef]
107. Noakes, T.D. Hydration in the Marathon. Using Thirst to Gauge Safe Fluid Replacement. *Sports Med.* **2007**, *37*, 463–466. [CrossRef] [PubMed]
108. Kenefick, R.W. Author's Reply to Goulet: Comment on: "Drinking Strategies: Planned Drinking Versus Drinking to Thirst". *Sports Med.* **2019**, *49*, 635–636. [CrossRef]
109. Dion, T.; Savoie, F.A.; Asselin, A.; Gariepy, C.; Goulet, E.D. Half-marathon running performance is not improved by a rate of fluid intake above that dictated by thirst sensation in trained distance runners. *Eur. J. Appl. Physiol.* **2013**, *113*, 3011–3020. [CrossRef]
110. Armstrong, L.E.; Johnson, E.C.; Kunces, L.J.; Ganio, M.S.; Judelson, D.A.; Kupchak, B.R.; Vingren, J.L.; Munoz, C.X.; Huggins, R.A.; Hydren, J.R.; et al. Drinking to thirst versus drinking ad libitum during road cycling. *J. Athl. Train.* **2014**, *49*, 624–631. [CrossRef] [PubMed]
111. Hubbard, R.W.; Szlyk, P.C.; Armstrong, L.E. Influence of thirst and fluid palatability on fluid ingestion during exercise. In *Perspectives in Exercise Sciences and Sports Medicine. Fluid Homeostasis during Exercise*; Gisolfi, C.V., Lamb, D.R., Eds.; Benchmark Press: Indianapolis, IN, USA, 1990; Volume 1, pp. 39–95. ISBN 978-0-697-14816-2.
112. Armstrong, L.E.; Johnson, E.C.; Bergeron, M.F. Counterview: Is drinking to thirst adequate to appropriately maintain hydration status during prolonged endurance exercise? No. *Wilderness Environ. Med.* **2016**, *27*, 195–198. [CrossRef] [PubMed]
113. Armstrong, L.E.; Johnson, E.C.; Bergeron, M.F. Rebuttal from "No". *Wilderness Environ. Med.* **2016**, *27*, 200–202. [CrossRef] [PubMed]
114. Armstrong, L.E.; Johnson, E.C.; McKenzie, A.L.; Ellis, L.A.; Williamson, K.H. Ultraendurance Cycling in a Hot Environment: Thirst, Fluid Consumption and Water Balance. *J. Strength Cond. Res.* **2015**, *29*, 869–876. [CrossRef]
115. Figaro, M.K.; Mack, G.W. Regulation of fluid intake in dehydrated humans: Role of oropharyngeal stimulation. *Am. J. Physiol. Regul. Integr. Comp. Physiol.* **1997**, *272*, R1740–R1746. [CrossRef]
116. Armstrong, L.E.; Casa, D.J. Methods to evaluate electrolyte and water turnover of athletes. *Athl. Train. Sports Health Care* **2009**, *1*, 169–179. [CrossRef]
117. Casa, D.J. Proper hydration for distance running: Identifying individual fluid needs. *Track Coach* **2004**, *167*, 5321–5328.
118. Armstrong, L.E. Hydration assessment techniques. *Nutr. Rev.* **2005**, *63 Pt 2* (Suppl. S6), S40–S54. [CrossRef]
119. Ganio, M.S.; Armstrong, L.E.; Kavouras, S.A. Hydration. In *Sport and Physical Activity in the Heat*; Casa, D.J., Ed.; Springer: Cham, Switzerland, 2018; pp. 83–100. ISBN 978-3-319-70216-2.
120. Kavouras, S. Assessing hydration status. *Curr. Opin. Clin. Nutr. Metab. Care* **2002**, *5*, 519–524. [CrossRef] [PubMed]
121. Shirreffs, S.M. Markers of hydration status. *Eur. J. Clin. Nutr.* **2003**, *57* (Suppl. S2), S6–S9. [CrossRef]
122. Maughan, R.J.; Shirreffs, S.M.; Leiper, J.B. 2007. Errors in the estimation of sweat loss and changes in hydration status from changes in body mass during exercise. *J. Sports Sci.* **2007**, *25*, 797–804. [CrossRef] [PubMed]
123. Bennett, B.L.; Hew-Butler, T.; Rosner, M.H.; Myers, T.; Lipman, G.S. Wilderness Medical Society clinical practice guidelines for the management of exercise-associated hyponatremia: 2019 update. *Wilderness Environ. Med.* **2020**, *31*, 50–62. [CrossRef] [PubMed]
124. Kavouras, S.A. Sodium balance during exercise and hyponatremia. In *Fluid Balance, Hydration, and Athletic Performance*; Meyer, F., Szygula, Z., Wilk, B., Eds.; CRC Press: Boca Raton, FL, USA, 2015; pp. 23–31. ISBN 978-1-4822-2328-6.
125. Marriott, H. Water and salt depletion. *Br. Med. J.* **1942**, *2*, 285–290.
126. Taylor, H.L.; Henschel, A.; Mickelsen, O.; Keys, A. The effect of the sodium chloride intake on the work performance of man during exposure to dry heat and experimental heat exhaustion. *Am. J. Physiol.* **1943**, *140*, 439–451. [CrossRef]
127. National Academies of Sciences, Engineering, and Medicine. *Dietary Reference Intakes for Sodium and Potassium*; The National Academies Press: Washington, DC, USA, 2019. [CrossRef]
128. Diet, Nutrition and the Prevention of Chronic Diseases: Report of a Joint WHO/FAO Expert Consultation. Geneva, 28 January–1 February 2002. Available online: https://www.who.int/publications-detail-redirect/924120916X (accessed on 10 February 2021).

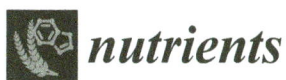

Article

A Case-Series Observation of Sweat Rate Variability in Endurance-Trained Athletes

JohnEric W. Smith *, Marissa L. Bello and Ffion G. Price

Department of Kinesiology, Mississippi State University, Starkville, MS 39762, USA; mlb1221@msstate.edu (M.L.B.); fgp13@msstate.edu (F.G.P.)
* Correspondence: jws597@msstate.edu; Tel.: +1-941-592-5575

Abstract: Adequate fluid replacement during exercise is an important consideration for athletes, however sweat rate (SR) can vary day-to-day. The purpose of this study was to investigate day-to-day variations in SR while performing self-selected exercise sessions to evaluate error in SR estimations in similar temperature conditions. Thirteen endurance-trained athletes completed training sessions in a case-series design 1x/week for a minimum 30 min of running/biking over 24 weeks. Body mass was recorded pre/post-training and corrected for fluid consumption. Data were split into three Wet-Bulb Globe Thermometer (WBGT) conditions: LOW (<10 °C), MOD (10–19.9 °C), HIGH (>20 °C). No significant differences existed in exercise duration, distance, pace, or WBGT for any group ($p > 0.07$). Significant differences in SR variability occurred for all groups, with average differences of: LOW = 0.15 L/h; MOD = 0.14 L/h; HIGH = 0.16 L/h ($p < 0.05$). There were no significant differences in mean SR between LOW-MOD ($p > 0.9$), but significant differences between LOW-HIGH and MOD-HIGH ($p < 0.03$). The assessment of SR can provide useful data for determining hydration strategies. The significant differences in SR within each temperature range indicates a single assessment may not accurately represent an individual's typical SR even in similar environmental conditions.

Keywords: hypohydration; hyperhydration; hyponatremia; fluid loss; fluid balance

1. Introduction

The lean tissue of the human body is composed of approximately 73% water [1]. Variations in body fat will result in individual body water levels ranging from ~50–70% of total body mass. This water is critically important for cardiovascular function and thermoregulation. When the body has adequate fluid intake to match fluid losses individuals are considered to be in a state of euhydration. When fluid intake is in excess of fluid loss individuals can become hyperhydrated and when fluid loss exceeds fluid intake individuals become hypohydrated.

Hypohydration is the term used to describe a state of suboptimal body water. At rest, internal factors that influence the body's water status are mainly body composition, hormonal activity, and sweating [2]. External factors with the greatest influence on body water levels include fluid intake, medications, medical conditions, physical activity, environmental conditions, and clothing [3]. Many athletes, from youth to professional, initiate training in hypohydrated states [4–6], and dehydration through sweat loss with insufficient fluid replacement will exacerbate this hypohydrated condition. As a result of hypohydration there is increased cardiovascular strain [7], thermal strain [8], perceived exertion [9], and reduced oxygen and nutrient delivery to the exercising muscle [8,10,11]. Due to these physiological responses to reductions in body water, exercise performance has been shown to be diminished with as little as 2% hypohydration [12–18].

Hyperhydration is the term used to describe a state of overhydration. At rest excess fluid consumption typically leads to increased urine output allowing for the maintenance of a euhydrated state. In individuals with compromised kidney function, unnecessary

Citation: Smith, J.W.; Bello, M.L.; Price, F.G. A Case-Series Observation of Sweat Rate Variability in Endurance-Trained Athletes. *Nutrients* **2021**, *13*, 1807. https://doi.org/10.3390/nu13061807

Academic Editors: Douglas J. Casa and Stavros Kavouras

Received: 15 April 2021
Accepted: 24 May 2021
Published: 26 May 2021

Publisher's Note: MDPI stays neutral with regard to jurisdictional claims in published maps and institutional affiliations.

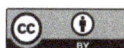

Copyright: © 2021 by the authors. Licensee MDPI, Basel, Switzerland. This article is an open access article distributed under the terms and conditions of the Creative Commons Attribution (CC BY) license (https://creativecommons.org/licenses/by/4.0/).

increases in fluid intake above fluid loss can lead to fluid retention [19]. Similarly, exercising individuals can experience fluid retention due to the increased actions of antidiuretic hormone and aldosterone upregulation during exercise [20,21]. Studies have demonstrated hyperhydration does not aid in exercise performance or heat tolerance [22–26]. While hyperhydration does not benefit exercise it can be detrimental to health. Uncompensable fluid intake can lead to dilution of electrolytes, particularly sodium, leading to hyponatremia, and if untreated can result in cerebral or pulmonary edema leading to death [8].

The evaporation of sweat can remove ~580 kcal/L and serves as a valuable tool to dissipate heat produced through metabolic processes [27]. As we exercise or perform physical work, metabolic heat production increases to match the increased work output. Sweat rate also increases in an effort to combat the increases in body temperature associated with increased metabolic rate. Unfortunately, sweat that drips from the body and does not evaporate does not provide a significant source of heat loss. In environments with higher humidity, sweat rates can be elevated significantly without fully corresponding to estimated metabolic heat production due to reductions in evaporative cooling as a result of moisture in the air [28].

There have been numerous studies exploring average sweat rates and the impact of intensity, duration, environmental conditions, and clothing [29,30]. Typical sweat rates are reported between 0.5–2.0 L/h during activity [31], although due to the large number of variables influencing sweat rate there is significant variability in the sweat rates reported across and within sports. It has been previously reported that about 2% of athletes have sweat rates that can exceed 3 L/h with the highest reported sweat rate during exercise is 5.73 L/h [29]. Within the extremes of the sweat rate range, little to no sweat is produced as a result of conditions such as hypohidrosis and anhidrosis, while hyperhidrosis can lead to extremely high sweat rates [32]. Reporting an average sweat rate when such large ranges exist can result in athletes incorrectly using and applying the information as the foundation for their individual hydration needs.

The most frequently used method to assess sweat loss in both laboratory and field settings is through pre- and post-exercise body mass changes during exercise. This technique is recommended as a viable method of assessing exercise sweat rate by the American College of Sports Medicine [31] and National Athletic Trainers Association [8]. Limited research has explored the within-subject variability of sweat rate, with day-to-day variation reported to be 5–7% in well-controlled settings. Due to the ease of measuring changes in body mass pre- and post-exercise this technique is commonly recommended to professional and recreational athletes. While athletes have been exposed to this technique, many athletes use it without the full understanding of the controls in place for laboratory-based studies likely resulting in increases in sweat rate variation on a day-to-day basis. Therefore, the purpose of this study was to determine the variability observed in day-to-day sweat rate within endurance trained individuals carrying out regular training without artificially controlled preparation, environmental, and exercise guidelines.

2. Materials and Methods

2.1. Study Participants

Individuals training as recreational runners and triathletes along with collegiate cross-country runners were recruited from the local area to explore the variability in sweat rate throughout multiple seasons. Data collection trials began in September and concluded in February as a result of COVID-19 restrictions. Thirteen endurance-trained males ($n = 3$) and females ($n = 10$) were included in the present study and were currently running a minimum of 120 min per week for the previous three months. All participants provided written consent prior to participating. This study was approved by the Institutional Review Board at Mississippi State University.

2.2. Experimental Design

Participants completed training sessions once per week for a minimum duration of 30 min in a case-series design. Sessions included either running or biking at a self-selected pace and intensity between 5:30 and 9:30 am. Duration and distance were measured using the athlete's GPS watches, pace was then calculated from these values. Environmental conditions were recorded using a Wet-Bulb Globe Thermometer (WBGT; QUESTemp 32, 3M, St. Paul, MN, USA) at exercise initiation and every 15 min during the training. Sweat rates were calculated from the change in body mass measured (Defender 3000, OHAUS, Parsippany, NJ, USA) before and after training, with correction for fluid intake. Immediately prior to the initiation of exercise athletes weighed dry exercise clothes and shoes alone, were asked to void their bladder, and then athlete body mass was collected while wearing dry exercise clothes and shoes. To account for sweat trapped by clothes [33], immediately post-exercise athletes' body mass was collected while wearing exercise clothes and shoes, athletes then changed to allow sweaty clothes and shoes to be weighed alone.

Sweat rate was calculated by:

$$\text{Sweat Rate} = \frac{(CBW_{PRE} - CBW_{POST}) + (CS_{WET} - CS_{DRY}) + (FB_{PRE} - FB_{POST})}{\text{Time(h)}} \quad (1)$$

where, CBW = clothed body weight (kg); CS = exercise clothing and shoes (kg); FB = food/beverage (kg).

Due to the short duration of exercise no adjustments were made to account for respiratory fluid losses.

Data collection took place outdoors in natural environmental conditions over 7 months except during times of precipitation. The natural environmental conditions were separated into three WBGT ranges: LOW (less than 10 °C), MOD (between 10–20 °C) and HIGH (above 20 °C).

2.3. Statistical Analysis

All data were analyzed using SPSS v26 statistical software (IBM, Armonk, NY, USA). Participant comparisons were included if a minimum of two sessions were completed for LOW, MOD, or HIGH conditions, and the highest and lowest sweat rates were used for analysis, as well as the mean sweat rates. A Shapiro-Wilks test of normality was conducted, there were no outliers, and the significance was above an alpha level of 0.05, therefore the data is normal and is parametric. Not all participants completed multiple training sessions in each range, therefore independent sample T-tests were used for comparisons between WBGT, duration, distance, and pace for each temperature range. Analysis of variance (ANOVA) tests with Tukey's Honestly Significant Difference (HSD) pairwise comparisons were used to analyze differences in mean sweat rates between temperatures. The participants who completed multiple training sessions in all three temperature ranges ($n = 4$) were included for subsequent analysis. A Friedman's Rank test was performed to test for differences between temperature ranges. Post-hoc analysis with Wilcoxon Signed-Rank test was conducted with a Bonferroni correction applied. Significance was set a priori at $p < 0.05$.

3. Results

Participants displayed no significant change between first and last training session (68.2 ± 14.7 kg vs. 68.4 ± 14.9 kg respectively; $p = 0.61$). Participant sessions were split into WBGT ranges for analysis. There were no significant differences in duration, distance, pace, and WBGT for any of the groups ($p > 0.07$). These data are shown in Table 1.

There were significant differences in sweat rate variability for all groups. LOW WBGTs demonstrated an average difference of 0.15 L/h in sweat rate between highest and lowest recordings ($p < 0.01$). MOD WBGTs showed an average difference of 0.14 L/h in sweat rate ($p < 0.05$). HIGH WBGTs revealed an average difference in sweat rate of 0.16 L/h ($p < 0.01$). Individual sweat rates are shown in Table 2 for each temperature range. Sweat rates for the four participants who completed training sessions within each WBGT range are represented in Table 3.

Table 1. Differences in duration, distance, pace, and Wet-Bulb Globe Thermometer between temperature ranges. (mean ± stdev).

Range	WBGT (°C)	Duration (Minutes)	Running Distance (Miles)	Running Pace (Min/Mile)	Cycling Distance (Miles)	Cycling Velocity (Miles/Hour)
<10 °C	5.7 ± 3.2	42.67 ± 13.33 (n = 9)	6.05 ± 4.67 (n = 8)	8.40 ± 2.39 (n = 8)	21.04 ± 0.03 (n = 1)	17.43 ± 0.16 (n = 1)
10–20 °C	13.5 ± 2.2	40.63 ± 11.29 (n = 6)	5.19 ± 1.82 (n = 6)	8.07 ± 1.10 (n = 6)		
>20 °C	22.5 ± 1.4	43.29 ± 14.11 (n = 11)	6.84 ± 5.60 (n = 10)	7.62 ± 1.67 (n = 10)	24.41 ± 4.53 (n = 1)	19.34 ± 0.83 (n = 1)

Table 2. Participant sweat rates (L/h) separated into highest, lowest, and mean values. 2A denotes Wet-Bulb Globe Thermometer values below 10 °C, 2B values between 10–20 °C, and 2C values above 20 °C.

2A.

<10 °C

Subject	Low (L/h)	High (L/h)	Mean (L/h)	Relative Mean (mL·kg^{-1}·h^{-1})	High-Low (L/h)	Maximal Variation from Mean (%)
1	0.84	0.90	0.87	13.5	0.06	3.4
2	0.43	0.52	0.48	8.5	0.09	9.4
3	0.41	0.56	0.48	7.2	0.15	15.5
4	0.65	0.95	0.84	8.7	0.30	17.8
5	0.97	1.00	0.99	9.6	0.03	1.5
8	0.54	0.61	0.57	9.1	0.07	6.2
9	0.57	0.75	0.66	10.2	0.18	13.7
11	0.39	0.52	0.45	5.2	0.13	14.4
12	0.67	0.90	0.78	12.6	0.23	14.8

2B.

10–20 °C

Subject	Low (L/h)	High (L/h)	Mean (L/h)	Relative Mean (mL·kg^{-1}·h^{-1})	High-Low (L/h)	Maximal Variation from Mean (%)
1	1.13	1.23	1.18	11.6	0.10	4.2
2	0.43	0.68	0.60	9.0	0.25	21.0
3	0.58	0.78	0.64	11.9	0.20	15.5
4	0.83	0.84	0.84	10.2	0.01	0.6
6	0.46	0.79	0.57	9.2	0.33	29.1
10	0.49	0.49	0.49	8.5	0.00	0.0

2C.

>20 °C

Subject	Low (L/h)	High (L/h)	Mean (L/h)	Relative Mean (mL·kg^{-1}·h^{-1})	High-Low (L/h)	Maximal Variation from Mean (%)
1	1.32	1.35	1.33	13.44	0.03	1.2
2	0.81	1.10	0.90	13.9	0.29	16.1
3	0.75	0.96	0.85	16.1	0.21	12.3
4	1.16	1.16	1.16	13.0	0.00	0.0
5	1.62	1.70	1.67	23.0	0.08	2.4
6	0.63	0.81	0.72	12.5	0.18	12.5
7	0.76	0.91	0.82	13.8	0.15	9.2
8	0.64	0.74	0.69	11.9	0.10	7.2
9	1.01	1.22	1.11	17.6	0.21	9.4
10	0.58	0.59	0.59	10.4	0.01	0.9
13	0.79	0.81	0.80	11.6	0.02	0.1

Table 3. Participant sweat rates (L/h) for the four participants that completed multiple training sessions within each Wet-Bulb Globe Thermometer range. Sweat rate values shown as highest, lowest, and mean values for each range.

Subject	Temperature	Low	High	Mean
	<10 °C	0.84 L/h	0.90 L/h	0.87 L/h
1	10–20 °C	1.13 L/h	1.23 L/h	1.18 L/h
	>20 °C	1.32 L/h	1.35 L/h	1.33 L/h
	<10 °C	0.43 L/h	0.52 L/h	0.48 L/h
2	10–20 °C	0.43 L/h	0.68 L/h	0.60 L/h
	>20 °C	0.81 L/h	1.10 L/h	0.90 L/h
	<10 °C	0.41 L/h	0.56 L/h	0.48 L/h
3	10–20 °C	0.58 L/h	0.78 L/h	0.64 L/h
	>20 °C	0.75 L/h	0.96 L/h	0.85 L/h
	<10 °C	0.65 L/h	0.95 L/h	0.84 L/h
4	10–20 °C	0.83 L/h	0.84 L/h	0.84 L/h
	>20 °C	1.16 L/h	1.16 L/h	1.16 L/h

Pairwise comparisons revealed no significant differences in sweat rate between LOW and MOD temperatures ($p > 0.9$), but significant sweat rate differences were found between LOW and HIGH ($p < 0.03$) and between MOD and HIGH ($p < 0.01$). These differences are represented in Figure 1. In the four participants who completed sessions in each range, there was a statistically significant difference in mean sweat rate depending on temperature condition, $\chi^2(2) = 6.500$, $p = 0.039$. Post hoc analysis revealed changes in temperature conditions did not elicit a significant change in mean sweat rate (Low-Mod, $p = 0.144$; Mod-High, $p = 0.68$; Low-High, $p = 0.68$). However it should be noted the differences in mean sweat rate mirrored those seen in the group totals. The differences between temperature ranges are shown in Figure 2.

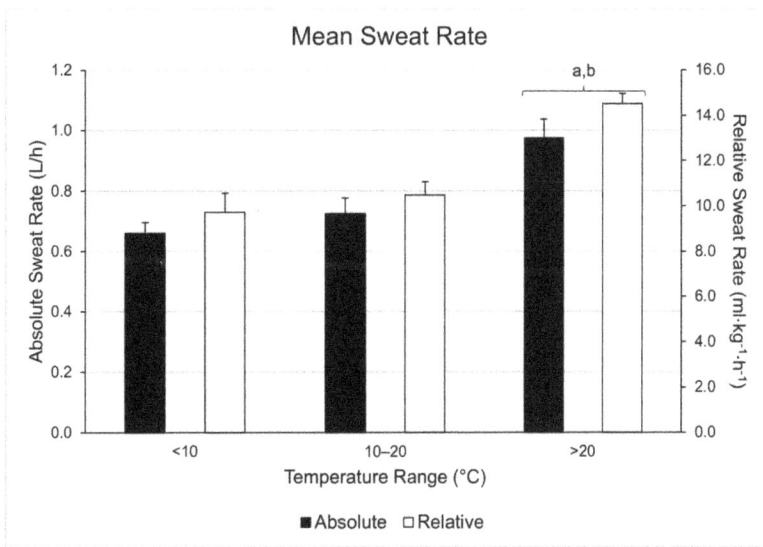

Figure 1. Mean sweat rates (absolute: L/h; relative: mL·kg^{-1}·h^{-1}) within each temperature range. a = significantly different from LOW, b = significantly different than MOD.

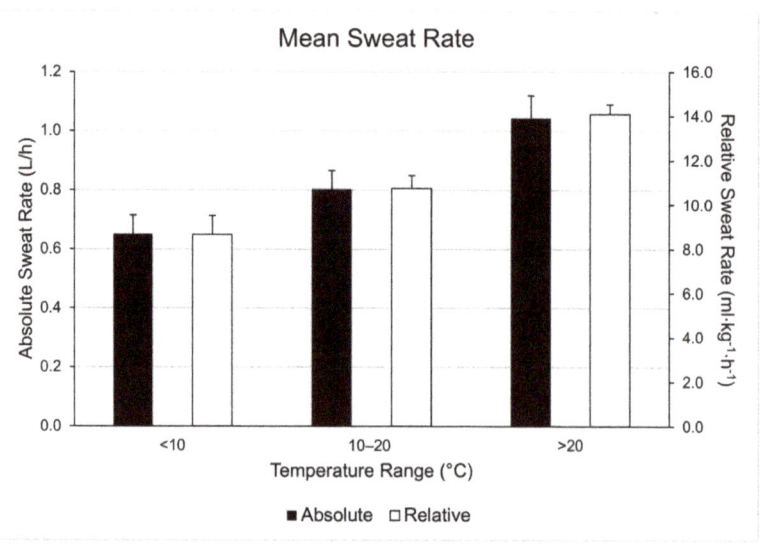

Figure 2. Mean sweat rates (L/h) for four participants that completed training sessions within each temperature range.

4. Discussion

Hypohydration resulting from the avoidance of fluid ingestion during exercise resulted in a number of publications and position stands in the 1990s promoting fluid ingestion in an effort to prevent related detrimental effects [34]. These positions have been updated as new data are released, moving away from statements such as "... consume the maximal amount that can be tolerated [34]." Initially, athletes used this guideline to unexpected levels, consuming fluid at greater levels than needed to replace fluid losses. This hyperhydration resulted in a number of deaths related to hyponatremia [35]. Due to these unfortunate events, the update to the American College of Sports Medicine in 2007 changed their recommendation to drinking to prevent dehydration and acknowledged the risk of hyponatremia with overdrinking. This position stand recommended the use of body weight changes during exercise to create an individualized hydration plan [31]. The 2016 Position Stand for "Nutrition for Athletic Performance" [36], while stating the prevalence of hypohydration and hypernatremia is thought to be greater, further expounded on the greater risks associated with hyponatremia and again suggested the use of exercise-related body mass changes for the development of an individualized hydration plan. The current study found the variation in day-to-day sweat rate (±7.9–11.7% from the individual's average in those conditions) is greater than what has previously been reported [37,38].

Hypohydration is a result of inadequate replacement of body water lost mainly through urine, feces, respiration, and sweat at rest. As the degree of hypohydration increases, the subsequent increases in cardiovascular strain [7], thermal strain [8], and perceived exertion [9] are exacerbated. Further, the reduction of oxygen and nutrient delivery to the exercising muscle increase correspondingly as a result of reductions in plasma volume [8,10,11]. Typically these responses do not significantly affect physical activity performance until reaching a threshold of a 2% change in body mass [36]. However, as plasma volume declines, heart rate increases to maintain cardiac output and blood flow to the skin is reduced leading to more rapid elevations in body temperature [8,10].

The ingestion of hypotonic fluids (sports drinks) disproportionately to fluid losses can lead to hyponatremia [39], defined as blood sodium levels below 135 mmol/L with or without the presence of symptoms [40]. While hyperhydration and hyponatremia can occur at rest, in team sports, and during shorter events, they are more commonly seen in endurance and ultra-endurance events. This hyperhydration is largely the result of overzealous efforts to prevent the previously mentioned deleterious effects resulting from hypohydration [40] and lack of exposure to the updated findings and takeaways in the scientific publications on the topic.

The prevention of hyponatremia and hypohydration are both critically important. It has been suggested that athletes primarily rely on thirst as a means to determine fluid ingestion in relation to exercise-associated fluid losses [41]. Contrary to this position, research has suggested that the reliance on thirst as a mechanism for fluid ingestion can lead to hypohydration, therefore, athletes should approach activity or exercise with an appropriate hydration plan [42]. Recommendations from the American College of Sports Medicine and the National Athletic Trainers Association both recommend the monitoring of body mass changes during exercise as a method to prevent detrimental levels of hypohydration while ensuring hyperhydration is also not occurring [8,31]. Through the simplicity of body weight assessment even recreational athletes can develop an individualized hydration plan.

A number of variables within and outside athlete's control affect sweat rate. Athletes can often dictate the time of training, their hydration status at the beginning of exercise, clothing, intensity, duration, and some medications. Outside of their control are environmental conditions, hormonal activity, medical conditions, and the action of some medications. During competitive events the variables that are under the athlete's control are typically reduced as a result of racing regulations and in an effort to remain competitive. Most of our understanding related to the variability of sweat rate in athletes is based on research in which athletes received guidance in preparation and execution. This results in a basic understanding of the physiological responses for comparative purposes but offers limited insight into the variability seen in athletes carrying out training in a more practical and real-world setting.

This study reported relative sweat rates in the HIGH condition (14.5 ± 3.8 mL·kg^{-1}·h^{-1}) similar to the 15.3 ± 6.8 mL·kg^{-1}·h^{-1} sweat rates reported by Baker et al. [29]. However, this study also found higher day-to-day sweat rate variations (± 7.9–11.7% from the individuals' average in those conditions) compared to previous research showing 5–7% variation [37,38]. This data also demonstrates that estimations could differ by as much as 23.4% between the lowest compared to the highest sweat rate. While it would be expected to see increased variation compared to more precisely controlled laboratory conditions, the values observed in this study represent potential day-to-day variability experienced by well-trained athletes in situations without well-defined preparatory guidelines.

The variable most frequently considered when assessing sweat rate is the environment, as sweat rate typically increases with elevations in environmental temperature, radiative heat load, and reductions in wind velocity [43]. Increases in humidity result in reductions in heat transfer from the evaporation of sweat causing sweat remaining on the skin or dripping off the athlete to result in reductions in heat removal. Prolonged exposure to this wet skin and a still, humid environment can lead to the blockage of sweat glands (hidromeiosis) resulting in a reduction in sweat rate [43,44]. Clothing is altered in response to environmental conditions and sporting needs, these changes can influence the sweating response due to the ability or inability to dissipate heat to the surrounding environment as well as the microenvironment created by the clothing shell [3,45,46]. This clothing shell will result in increased humidity around the athlete's skin inhibiting evaporative cooling [47]. Cooler environmental conditions also lead to athletes increasing the clothing coverage creating a microenvironment inside the clothing shell warmer than the surrounding atmospheric air [47]. The current study found increases in sweat rate in the HIGH environment but similar sweat rate responses to the LOW and MOD conditions. As the athletes were given the freedom to choose exercise apparel it is likely that alterations in athlete clothing in response to LOW conditions resulted in a microenvironment that resulted in similar heat stress and sweating response to the MOD conditions.

As an individual acclimatizes to their training environment the body adapts to be more efficient in its sweating response. As the thermal load was lower in the LOW and

MOD conditions, athletes only required a percentage of the sweat rates seen in the HIGH conditions. Adaptations to exercise in hot conditions lead to reductions in sweat sodium concentration, earlier onset of sweating [43], and increases in sweat rate [48,49]. While these adaptations were not assessed in this study, it would be expected that sweat sodium content and maximal sweat rate shifted throughout the study as a result of seasonal variations in environmental conditions and the corresponding sweat rates.

Another unaccounted-for variable in this study was hydration status at the beginning of exercise. As mentioned previously, hypohydration at levels greater than 2% performance decrements can be seen. Along with the declines in performance when an individual becomes more than 2% hypohydrated [8], they may experience a decline in sweat rate [50], assuming an initial euhydration status. Similarly, most research studies are conducted with defined initial hydration levels as a requirement to participate, while without defined guidelines a majority of athletes begin exercise in a hypohydrated state [8]. As a result of hypohydration the sweating response can be altered resulting in an increased threshold for onset of sweating [51] and reduced sweating sensitivity [52]. This study allowed athletes to arrive at assessments as they would to any other workout or training session. As a result, it is likely a majority of the athletes were hypohydrated at the initiation of exercise which may partially explain the increase in variability reported in this study as compared to previous studies.

Additionally, exercise intensity plays a role in the sweat response, as studies have found higher sweat rates during competition and high-intensity exercise compared with prolonged lower intensity [29,50,53]. This study found similar exercise intensities and durations across the three environmental conditions. As athletes are developing hydration strategies for training and competition attention needs to be given to the variations in intensity in the different settings. As a means to develop a competitive hydration strategy athletes may find it advantageous to perform mock races or training sessions at competitive intensities on a number of occasions within various conditions. While a few athletes in this study that had very little variation in estimates of hourly sweat rate, care needs to be taken in extrapolating sweat rate to longer duration events.

More static factors such as age, sex, tattoos, and medications/medical conditions have also been suggested or shown to also play a role in sweat rate. Adults have higher sweat rates compared to adolescents due to adolescents producing less sweat in the sweat glands [29,54,55]. Males have been shown to have higher absolute sweat rates as compared to females largely driven by higher body mass [29]. When corrected for body mass the increased sweat rate was seen to still be present based on age, but the sex differences disappeared [29]. Some studies have suggested variations in sweat rate in females as a result of menstrual cycle however, a majority of studies reports no difference in sweat rate as a result of menstrual phase [56–58]. There is conflicting data in regards to the impact of tattooed skin on sweat rate. Some studies have demonstrated a detrimental effect on sweat rate with tattoos [59,60] while other studies have reported no significant alterations in sweat rate as a result of tattoos [61,62]. Milaria rubia (heat rash), sunburn [63], diabetes mellitus [64], and spinal cord injuries [65,66] highlight a small number (but a large range in severity) of the medical conditions that can influence sweat rate. Likewise the medications that treat many illnesses also can influence sweat rates both positively and negatively [32,67]. While each of these variables can influence sweat rate and should be considered with changes, changes will likely be infrequent but likely result in new sweat rate estimates being needed when changes occur.

This study was observational leading to significant limitations. This study was conducted as an observation of athletes in the normal activity without influence on their training duration, intensity, initial hydration status, or clothing. The only disruption to the athletes typical training was the requirement for exercise to initiate Monday through Friday between 5:30 and 9:30 am beginning and ending at the laboratory to allow for body mass assessment and changing of clothes. Additionally, only asking athletes to carry out their exercise within these parameters resulted in some athletes not having sessions within all of the environmental (LOW, MOD, HIGH) conditions and resulted in varying numbers of observations within participants due to missed weeks. Finally, the only control for environmental conditions was the lack of trials during periods of precipitation. The use of post exercise clothing mass was used to calculate sweat trapped in clothing or shoes, fluid volume associated with precipitation invalidated this assessment. Environmental variations associated with radiative, convective, humidity, and dry temperature were combined into WBGT for comparisons. Future studies should investigate the variations in sweat rate throughout the various annual seasons within laboratory-controlled assessment conditions mirroring external environmental conditions.

Estimating fluid needs by assessing body mass changes during exercise is a valid technique and a useful tool for athletes [68,69]. However, even following the best practice recommendations [28], a single assessment can result in over and underestimation of true needs. Further this variation can be compounded as sweat rate test findings are extrapolated to longer exercise durations. Compounded errors in sweat rate estimates can place athletes at increased risk of hypohydration and hyponatremia. It should be recommended that body weight changes be assessed across multiple sessions even within the same conditions. The closer an athlete can replicate typical conditions (duration, intensity, clothing, environment, time of day) on multiple occasions the more precise the estimated average sweat loss will represent actual losses and provide more insight into hydration strategies to optimize their training.

5. Conclusions

This data highlights interindividual sweat rate during similar exercise is variable even within similar environmental conditions. Therefore, individuals should repeatedly measure and record sweat rate along with environmental conditions along with exercise intensity to have a reliable estimate of actual sweat rate for intensities and conditions.

Author Contributions: Study conceptualization, J.W.S.; methodology, J.W.S. and F.G.P.; formal analysis, J.W.S. and M.L.B.; writing—original draft preparation, J.W.S., M.L.B., and F.G.P.; writing—review and editing, J.W.S., M.L.B., and F.G.P. All authors have read and agreed to the published version of the manuscript.

Funding: This research received no external funding.

Institutional Review Board Statement: The study was conducted according to the guidelines of the Declaration of Helsinki and approved by the Institutional Review Board of Mississippi State University (IRB-19-320 approved 7/26/2019).

Informed Consent Statement: Informed consent was obtained from all subjects involved in the study.

Data Availability Statement: The data presented in this study are available on request from the corresponding author. The data are not publicly available due to participant privacy and confidentiality.

Acknowledgments: The authors thank the participants and graduate students that assisted in data collection.

Conflicts of Interest: The authors declare no conflict of interest.

References

1. Wang, Z.; Deurenberg, P.; Wang, W.; Pietrobelli, A.; Baumgartner, R.N.; Heymsfield, S.B. Hydration of fat-free body mass: Review and critique of a classic body-composition constant. *Am. J. Clin. Nutr.* **1999**, *69*, 833–841. [CrossRef]
2. Shibasaki, M.; Wilson, T.E.; Crandall, C.G. Neural control and mechanisms of eccrine sweating during heat stress and exercise. *J. Appl. Physiol.* **2006**, *100*, 1692–1701. [CrossRef]
3. Armstrong, L.E.; Johnson, E.C.; Casa, D.J.; Ganio, M.S.; McDermott, B.P.; Yamamoto, L.M.; Lopez, R.M.; Emmanuel, H. The American football uniform: Uncompensable heat stress and hyperthermic exhaustion. *J. Athl. Train* **2010**, *45*, 117–127. [CrossRef] [PubMed]
4. Osterberg, K.L.; Horswill, C.A.; Baker, L.B. Pregame urine specific gravity and fluid intake by National Basketball Association players during competition. *J. Athl. Train* **2009**, *44*, 53–57. [CrossRef]

5. Volpe, S.L.; Poule, K.A.; Bland, E.G. Estimation of prepractice hydration status of National Collegiate Athletic Association Division I athletes. *J. Athl. Train* **2009**, *44*, 624–629. [CrossRef] [PubMed]
6. McDermott, B.P.; Casa, D.J.; Yeargin, S.W.; Ganio, M.S.; Lopez, R.M.; Mooradian, E.A. Hydration status, sweat rates, and rehydration education of youth football campers. *J. Sport Rehabil.* **2009**, *18*, 535–552. [CrossRef] [PubMed]
7. Gonzalez-Alonso, J.; Mora-Rodriguez, R.; Below, P.R.; Coyle, E.F. Dehydration reduces cardiac output and increases systemic and cutaneous vascular resistance during exercise. *J. Appl. Physiol* **1995**, *79*, 1487–1496. [CrossRef] [PubMed]
8. McDermott, B.P.; Anderson, S.A.; Armstrong, L.E.; Casa, D.J.; Cheuvront, S.N.; Cooper, L.; Kenney, W.L.; O'Connor, F.G.; Roberts, W.O. National Athletic Trainers' Association position statement: Fluid replacement for the physically active. *J. Athl. Train* **2017**, *52*, 877–895. [CrossRef]
9. Nuccio, R.P.; Barnes, K.A.; Carter, J.M.; Baker, L.B. Fluid balance in team sport athletes and the effect of hypohydration on cognitive, technical, and physical performance. *Sports Med.* **2017**, *47*, 1951–1982. [CrossRef]
10. Montain, S.J.; Sawka, M.N.; Latzka, W.A.; Valeri, C.R. Thermal and cardiovascular strain from hypohydration: Influence of exercise intensity. *Int. J. Sports Med.* **1998**, *19*, 87–91. [CrossRef]
11. Cheuvront, S.N.; Kenefick, R.W.; Montain, S.J.; Sawka, M.N. Mechanisms of aerobic performance impairment with heat stress and dehydration. *J. Appl. Physiol.* **2010**, *109*, 1989–1995. [CrossRef]
12. Walsh, R.M.; Noakes, T.D.; Hawley, J.A.; Dennis, S.C. Impaired high-intensity cycling performance time at low levels of dehydration. *Int. J. Sports Med.* **1994**, *15*, 392–398. [CrossRef] [PubMed]
13. Bardis, C.N.; Kavouras, S.A.; Arnaoutis, G.; Panagiotakos, D.B.; Sidossis, L.S. Mild dehydration and cycling performance during 5-kilometer hill climbing. *J. Athl. Train* **2013**, *48*, 741–747. [CrossRef] [PubMed]
14. Casa, D.J.; Stearns, R.L.; Lopez, R.M.; Ganio, M.S.; McDermott, B.P.; Walker Yeargin, S.; Yamamoto, L.M.; Mazerolle, S.M.; Roti, M.W.; Armstrong, L.E.; et al. Influence of hydration on physiological function and performance during trail running in the heat. *J. Athl. Train* **2010**, *45*, 147–156. [CrossRef]
15. Ebert, T.R.; Martin, D.T.; Bullock, N.; Mujika, I.; Quod, M.J.; Farthing, L.A.; Burke, L.M.; Withers, R.T. Influence of hydration status on thermoregulation and cycling hill climbing. *Med. Sci. Sports Exerc.* **2007**, *39*, 323–329. [CrossRef] [PubMed]
16. Cheuvront, S.N.; Carter, R., 3rd; Castellani, J.W.; Sawka, M.N. Hypohydration impairs endurance exercise performance in temperate but not cold air. *J. Appl. Physiol.* **2005**, *99*, 1972–1976. [CrossRef]
17. Cheuvront, S.N.; Kenefick, R.W. Dehydration: Physiology, assessment, and performance effects. *Compr. Physiol.* **2014**, *4*, 257–285. [CrossRef]
18. Cheuvront, S.N.; Carter, R., 3rd; Sawka, M.N. Fluid balance and endurance exercise performance. *Curr. Sports Med. Rep.* **2003**, *2*, 202–208. [CrossRef]
19. Schrier, R.W.; Fassett, R.G.; Ohara, M.; Martin, P.Y. Pathophysiology of renal fluid retention. *Kidney Int. Suppl.* **1998**, *67*, S127–S132. [CrossRef]
20. Bartsch, P.; Maggiorini, M.; Schobersberger, W.; Shaw, S.; Rascher, W.; Girard, J.; Weidmann, P.; Oelz, O. Enhanced exercise-induced rise of aldosterone and vasopressin preceding mountain sickness. *J. Appl. Physiol.* **1991**, *71*, 136–143. [CrossRef] [PubMed]
21. Hew-Butler, T. Exercise-Associated Hyponatremia. *Front. Horm. Res.* **2019**, *52*, 178–189. [CrossRef] [PubMed]
22. Marino, F.E.; Kay, D.; Cannon, J. Glycerol hyperhydration fails to improve endurance performance and thermoregulation in humans in a warm humid environment. *Pflugers Arch.* **2003**, *446*, 455–462. [CrossRef]
23. Sawka, M.N.; Montain, S.J.; Latzka, W.A. Hydration effects on thermoregulation and performance in the heat. *Comp. Biochem. Physiol. Part A Mol. Integr. Physiol.* **2001**, *128*, 679–690. [CrossRef]
24. Maresh, C.M.; Bergeron, M.F.; Kenefick, R.W.; Castellani, J.W.; Hoffman, J.R.; Armstrong, L.E. Effect of overhydration on time-trial swim performance. *J. Strength Cond. Res.* **2001**, *15*, 514–518. [PubMed]
25. Gigou, P.Y.; Dion, T.; Asselin, A.; Berrigan, F.; Goulet, E.D. Pre-exercise hyperhydration-induced bodyweight gain does not alter prolonged treadmill running time-trial performance in warm ambient conditions. *Nutrients* **2012**, *4*, 949–966. [CrossRef]
26. Goulet, E.D.; Aubertin-Leheudre, M.; Plante, G.E.; Dionne, I.J. A meta-analysis of the effects of glycerol-induced hyperhydration on fluid retention and endurance performance. *Int. J. Sport Nutr. Exerc. Metab.* **2007**, *17*, 391–410. [CrossRef]
27. Monteith, J.L. Latent heat of vaporization in thermal physiology. *Nat. New Biol.* **1972**, *236*, 96. [CrossRef]
28. Baker, L.B. Sweating rate and sweat sodium concentration in athletes: A review of methodology and intra/interindividual variability. *Sports Med.* **2017**, *47*, 111–128. [CrossRef]
29. Baker, L.B.; Barnes, K.A.; Anderson, M.L.; Passe, D.H.; Stofan, J.R. Normative data for regional sweat sodium concentration and whole-body sweating rate in athletes. *J. Sports Sci.* **2016**, *34*, 358–368. [CrossRef]
30. Gonzalez, R.R.; Cheuvront, S.N.; Ely, B.R.; Moran, D.S.; Hadid, A.; Endrusick, T.L.; Sawka, M.N. Sweat rate prediction equations for outdoor exercise with transient solar radiation. *J. Appl. Physiol.* **2012**, *112*, 1300–1310. [CrossRef]
31. Sawka, M.N.; Burke, L.M.; Eichner, E.R.; Maughan, R.J.; Montain, S.J.; Stachenfeld, N.S. American College of Sports Medicine position stand. Exercise and fluid replacement. *Med. Sci. Sports Exerc.* **2007**, *39*, 377–390. [CrossRef] [PubMed]
32. Cheshire, W.P., Jr. Thermoregulatory disorders and illness related to heat and cold stress. *Auton. Neurosci.* **2016**, *196*, 91–104. [CrossRef] [PubMed]
33. Cheuvront, S.N.; Haymes, E.M.; Sawka, M.N. Comparison of sweat loss estimates for women during prolonged high-intensity running. *Med. Sci. Sports Exerc.* **2002**, *34*, 1344–1350. [CrossRef] [PubMed]

34. Convertino, V.A.; Armstrong, L.E.; Coyle, E.F.; Mack, G.W.; Sawka, M.N.; Senay, L.C., Jr.; Sherman, W.M. American College of Sports Medicine position stand. Exercise and fluid replacement. *Med. Sci. Sports Exerc.* **1996**, *28*, i–vii. [CrossRef] [PubMed]
35. Rosner, M.H.; Kirven, J. Exercise-associated hyponatremia. *Clin. J. Am. Soc. Nephrol.* **2007**, *2*, 151–161. [CrossRef]
36. Thomas, D.T.; Erdman, K.A.; Burke, L.M. American College of Sports Medicine joint position statement. Nutrition and athletic performance. *Med. Sci. Sports Exerc.* **2016**, *48*, 543–568. [CrossRef]
37. Baker, L.B.; Stofan, J.R.; Hamilton, A.A.; Horswill, C.A. Comparison of regional patch collection vs. whole body washdown for measuring sweat sodium and potassium loss during exercise. *J. Appl. Physiol.* **2009**, *107*, 887–895. [CrossRef]
38. Hayden, G.; Milne, H.C.; Patterson, M.J.; Nimmo, M.A. The reproducibility of closed-pouch sweat collection and thermoregulatory responses to exercise-heat stress. *Eur. J. Appl. Physiol.* **2004**, *91*, 748–751. [CrossRef]
39. Twerenbold, R.; Knechtle, B.; Kakebeeke, T.H.; Eser, P.; Muller, G.; von Arx, P.; Knecht, H. Effects of different sodium concentrations in replacement fluids during prolonged exercise in women. *Br. J. Sports Med.* **2003**, *37*, 300–303. [CrossRef]
40. Hew-Butler, T.; Loi, V.; Pani, A.; Rosner, M.H. Exercise-associated hyponatremia: 2017 update. *Front. Med.* **2017**, *4*, 21. [CrossRef]
41. Hew-Butler, T.; Rosner, M.H.; Fowkes-Godek, S.; Dugas, J.P.; Hoffman, M.D.; Lewis, D.P.; Maughan, R.J.; Miller, K.C.; Montain, S.J.; Rehrer, N.J.; et al. Statement of the third international exercise-associated hyponatremia consensus development conference, Carlsbad, California, 2015. *Clin. J. Sport Med.* **2015**, *25*, 303–320. [CrossRef]
42. Hubbard, R.W.; Sandick, B.L.; Matthew, W.T.; Francesconi, R.P.; Sampson, J.B.; Durkot, M.J.; Maller, O.; Engell, D.B. Voluntary dehydration and alliesthesia for water. *J. Appl. Physiol. Respir. Environ. Exerc. Physiol.* **1984**, *57*, 868–873. [CrossRef]
43. Baker, L.B. Physiology of sweat gland function: The roles of sweating and sweat composition in human health. *Temperature* **2019**, *6*, 211–259. [CrossRef]
44. Filingeri, D.; Havenith, G. Human skin wetness perception: Psychophysical and neurophysiological bases. *Temperature* **2015**, *2*, 86–104. [CrossRef]
45. McLellan, T.M.; Daanen, H.A.; Cheung, S.S. Encapsulated environment. *Compr. Physiol.* **2013**, *3*, 1363–1391. [CrossRef]
46. Mathews, D.K.; Fox, E.L.; Tanzi, D. Physiological responses during exercise and recovery in a football uniform. *J. Appl. Physiol.* **1969**, *26*, 611–615. [CrossRef]
47. Cheung, S.S. *Advanced Environmental Exercise Physiology*; Human Kinetics: Champaign, IL, USA, 2010.
48. Nielsen, B.; Hales, J.R.; Strange, S.; Christensen, N.J.; Warberg, J.; Saltin, B. Human circulatory and thermoregulatory adaptations with heat acclimation and exercise in a hot, dry environment. *J. Physiol.* **1993**, *460*, 467–485. [CrossRef]
49. Nielsen, B.; Strange, S.; Christensen, N.J.; Warberg, J.; Saltin, B. Acute and adaptive responses in humans to exercise in a warm, humid environment. *Pflugers Arch.* **1997**, *434*, 49–56. [CrossRef] [PubMed]
50. Rollo, I.; Randell, R.K.; Baker, L.; Leyes, J.Y.; Medina Leal, D.; Lizarraga, A.; Mesalles, J.; Jeukendrup, A.E.; James, L.J.; Carter, J.M. Fluid balance, sweat Na+ losses, and carbohydrate intake of Elite male soccer players in response to low and high training intensities in cool and hot environments. *Nutrients* **2021**, *13*, 401. [CrossRef] [PubMed]
51. Fortney, S.M.; Wenger, C.B.; Bove, J.R.; Nadel, E.R. Effect of hyperosmolality on control of blood flow and sweating. *J. Appl. Physiol. Respir. Environ. Exerc. Physiol.* **1984**, *57*, 1688–1695. [CrossRef] [PubMed]
52. Montain, S.J.; Latzka, W.A.; Sawka, M.N. Control of thermoregulatory sweating is altered by hydration level and exercise intensity. *J. Appl. Physiol.* **1995**, *79*, 1434–1439. [CrossRef] [PubMed]
53. Montain, S.J.; Cheuvront, S.N.; Lukaski, H.C. Sweat mineral-element responses during 7 h of exercise-heat stress. *Int. J. Sport Nutr. Exerc. Metab.* **2007**, *17*, 574–582. [CrossRef] [PubMed]
54. Falk, B.; Bar-Or, O.; Calvert, R.; MacDougall, J.D. Sweat gland response to exercise in the heat among pre-, mid-, and late-pubertal boys. *Med. Sci. Sports Exerc.* **1992**, *24*, 313–319. [CrossRef] [PubMed]
55. Falk, B.; Bar-Or, O.; MacDougall, J.D. Thermoregulatory responses of pre-, mid-, and late-pubertal boys to exercise in dry heat. *Med. Sci. Sports Exerc.* **1992**, *24*, 688–694. [CrossRef]
56. Lee, H.; Petrofsky, J.; Shah, N.; Awali, A.; Shah, K.; Alotaibi, M.; Yim, J. Higher sweating rate and skin blood flow during the luteal phase of the menstrual cycle. *Tohoku J. Exp. Med.* **2014**, *234*, 117–122. [CrossRef]
57. Garcia, A.M.; Lacerda, M.G.; Fonseca, I.A.; Reis, F.M.; Rodrigues, L.O.; Silami-Garcia, E. Luteal phase of the menstrual cycle increases sweating rate during exercise. *Braz. J. Med. Biol. Res.* **2006**, *39*, 1255–1261. [CrossRef]
58. Janse, D.E.J.X.A.; Thompson, M.W.; Chuter, V.H.; Silk, L.N.; Thom, J.M. Exercise performance over the menstrual cycle in temperate and hot, humid conditions. *Med. Sci. Sports Exerc.* **2012**, *44*, 2190–2198. [CrossRef]
59. Luetkemeier, M.J.; Allen, D.R.; Huang, M.; Pizzey, F.K.; Parupia, I.M.; Wilson, T.E.; Davis, S.L. Skin tattooing impairs sweating during passive whole body heating. *J. Appl. Physiol.* **2020**, *129*, 1033–1038. [CrossRef]
60. Luetkemeier, M.J.; Hanisko, J.M.; Aho, K.M. Skin tattoos alter sweat rate and Na+ concentration. *Med. Sci. Sports Exerc.* **2017**, *49*, 1432–1436. [CrossRef]
61. Beliveau, J.; Perreault-Briere, M.; Jeker, D.; Deshayes, T.A.; Duran-Suarez, A.; Baker, L.B.; Goulet, E.D.B. Permanent tattooing has no impact on local sweat rate, sweat sodium concentration and skin temperature or prediction of whole-body sweat sodium concentration during moderate-intensity cycling in a warm environment. *Eur. J. Appl. Physiol.* **2020**, *120*, 1111–1122. [CrossRef]
62. Rogers, E.; Irwin, C.; McCartney, D.; Cox, G.R.; Desbrow, B. Tattoos do not affect exercise-induced localised sweat rate or sodium concentration. *J. Sci. Med. Sport* **2019**, *22*, 1249–1253. [CrossRef]
63. Pandolf, K.B.; Gange, R.W.; Latzka, W.A.; Blank, I.H.; Kraning, K.K., 2nd; Gonzalez, R.R. Human thermoregulatory responses during heat exposure after artificially induced sunburn. *Am. J. Physiol.* **1992**, *262*, R610–R616. [CrossRef] [PubMed]

64. Fealey, R.D.; Low, P.A.; Thomas, J.E. Thermoregulatory Sweating Abnormalities in Diabetes Mellitus. *Mayo Clin. Proc.* **1989**, *64*, 617–628. [CrossRef]
65. Price, M.J. Thermoregulation during exercise in individuals with spinal cord injuries. *Sports Med.* **2006**, *36*, 863–879. [CrossRef] [PubMed]
66. Price, M.J.; Campbell, I.G. Thermoregulatory responses of paraplegic and able-bodied athletes at rest and during prolonged upper body exercise and passive recovery. *Eur. J. Appl. Physiol. Occup. Physiol.* **1997**, *76*, 552–560. [CrossRef]
67. Cheshire, W.P.; Fealey, R.D. Drug-induced hyperhidrosis and hypohidrosis: Incidence, prevention and management. *Drug Saf.* **2008**, *31*, 109–126. [CrossRef] [PubMed]
68. Baker, L.B.; Lang, J.A.; Kenney, W.L. Change in body mass accurately and reliably predicts change in body water after endurance exercise. *Eur. J. Appl. Physiol.* **2009**, *105*, 959–967. [CrossRef]
69. Maughan, R.J.; Shirreffs, S.M. Development of individual hydration strategies for athletes. *Int. J. Sport Nutr. Exerc. Metab.* **2008**, *18*, 457–472. [CrossRef]

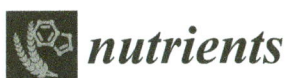

Article

Contribution of Dietary Composition on Water Turnover Rates in Active and Sedentary Men

Alice E. Disher [1], Kelly L. Stewart [1], Aaron J. E. Bach [1,2] and Ian B. Stewart [1,*]

[1] School of Exercise and Nutrition Sciences, Queensland University of Technology, Brisbane 4059, Australia; a.disher@qut.edu.au (A.E.D.); kelly.stewart@qut.edu.au (K.L.S.); a.bach@griffith.edu.au (A.J.E.B.)
[2] National Climate Change Adaptation Research Facility (NCCARF), Griffith University, Gold Coast 4222, Australia
* Correspondence: i.stewart@qut.edu.au

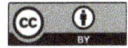

Citation: Disher, A.E.; Stewart, K.L.; Bach, A.J.E.; Stewart, I.B. Contribution of Dietary Composition on Water Turnover Rates in Active and Sedentary Men. *Nutrients* 2021, *13*, 2124. https://doi.org/10.3390/nu13062124

Academic Editors: Douglas J. Casa and Stavros Kavouras

Received: 14 April 2021
Accepted: 16 June 2021
Published: 21 June 2021

Publisher's Note: MDPI stays neutral with regard to jurisdictional claims in published maps and institutional affiliations.

Copyright: © 2021 by the authors. Licensee MDPI, Basel, Switzerland. This article is an open access article distributed under the terms and conditions of the Creative Commons Attribution (CC BY) license (https://creativecommons.org/licenses/by/4.0/).

Abstract: Body water turnover is a marker of hydration status for measuring total fluid gains and losses over a 24-h period. It can be particularly useful in predicting (and hence, managing) fluid loss in individuals to prevent potential physical, physiological and cognitive declines associated with hypohydration. There is currently limited research investigating the interrelationship of fluid balance, dietary intake and activity level when considering body water turnover. Therefore, this study investigates whether dietary composition and energy expenditure influences body water turnover. In our methodology, thirty-eight males (19 sedentary and 19 physically active) had their total body water and water turnover measured via the isotopic tracer deuterium oxide. Simultaneous tracking of dietary intake (food and fluid) is carried out via dietary recall, and energy expenditure is estimated via accelerometery. Our results show that active participants display a higher energy expenditure, water intake, carbohydrate intake and fibre intake; however, there is no difference in sodium or alcohol intake between the two groups. Relative water turnover in the active group is significantly greater than the sedentary group (Mean Difference (MD) [95% CI] = 17.55 g·kg^{-1}·day^{-1} [10.90, 24.19]; $p = <0.001$; g[95% CI] = 1.70 [0.98, 2.48]). A penalised linear regression provides evidence that the fibre intake ($p = 0.033$), water intake ($p = 0.008$), and activity level ($p = 0.063$) predict participants' relative body water turnover ($R^2 = 0.585$). In conclusion, water turnover is faster in individuals undertaking regular exercise than in their sedentary counterparts, and is, in part, explained by the intake of water from fluid and high-moisture content foods. The nutrient analysis of the participant diets indicates that increased dietary fibre intake is also positively associated with water turnover rates. The water loss between groups also contributes to the differences observed in water turnover; this is partly related to differences in sweat output during increased energy expenditure from physical activity.

Keywords: total body water; hydration; physical activity; nutrition

1. Introduction

Body water turnover refers to the movement and replacement of water through the body, typically over a day, and denotes fluid homeostasis [1]. Therefore, accurate assessment of body water turnover can be particularly useful in predicting (and hence, managing) fluid loss in individuals to prevent potential physical [2], physiological [3,4] and cognitive [5] declines associated with hypohydration [6]. The balance of body water, or fluid, is the difference between total fluid gain (influx) and loss (efflux) [1,7]. The majority of the fluid influx in humans is a result of the food and drink consumed, with a minor contribution from water absorbed by the skin or inspired through breathing [8]. Most of the fluid efflux occurs via urine and 'insensible' water loss (i.e., exhaled water vapour, or water lost via the skin, but in the absence of sweating) [1,7]. Minor fluid efflux occurs via human faecal matter [7]. Sweat production can also significantly contribute to an individual's fluid efflux either in times of heightened physical activity and/or in hot climates [9].

Water loss that occurs because of exercise-induced sweating and respiration (non-renal water losses), has been postulated as an important factor separating the water turnover rates of active and inactive individuals [10–13]. Some studies observe that as physical activity increases, thermoregulatory sweat output is primarily responsible for increases in water turnover [11,14–16]. Fluid efflux in active populations resulting from urinary and sweat losses, respiration, and to a lesser extent, substrate oxidation and carbon dioxide removal, has been shown to exceed that of their sedentary equivalents [17,18]. Thus, increased fluid intake in active individuals would be expected to maintain fluid balance.

Ensuring fluid balance can be achieved by consuming adequate fluid volumes, minimising sweat loss (which may not be possible), and/or through diet—by consuming high moisture content foods or by increasing intake of nutrients that improve water retention or reduce its elimination. Currently, there is a small pool of research that has examined the comparison of fluid balance between active and inactive individuals [10–12,14,19,20]; however the contribution of total water intake from both fluid and foods has not been consistently investigated, with just one study of young swimmers that accounted for the moisture content of food [12]. While this study of eight swimmers and six controls identified that water turnover was greater in the swimmers, due to sweat losses, the seven-day weighed dietary records were only assessed for the contribution of total moisture content of the food to daily water intake. The contribution of key nutrients within moisture-containing foods or involved with water retention was not reported.

Thus, this research aims to investigate the relationship between not only energy balance and water turnover, but also the dietary composition and water turnover in both active and sedentary individuals. It was hypothesised that relative body water turnover would be faster in active individuals than their sedentary equivalents, relating to a greater fluid intake and higher overall energy expenditure.

2. Materials and Methods

2.1. Participants

A convenience sample of 38 healthy males volunteered to participate in this study; 19 were physically active, and 19 were sedentary. To distinguish between the two groups, participants completed the International Physical Activity Questionnaire (IPAQ) [21] and self-reported an activity level >150 min (moderate to vigorous exercise) per week, or <90 min of low to moderate exercise per week for active and sedentary, respectively. In addition, physically active participants were included to attain a maximal oxygen consumption (VO_{2max}) value ≥ 60 mL·kg^{-1}·min^{-1}. Participants reported being weight stable (≤ 3 kg fluctuation in the previous three months) at the commencement of participation in the study. Each participant gave voluntary and written informed consent to participate in the study, which received ethical approval from the Queensland University of Technology Human Research Ethics Committee.

2.2. Procedures

Before the commencement of the trial (minimum two days), a maximal aerobic capacity (VO_{2max}) test was performed by all active group participants, in the form of an incremental test to exhaustion on a motorised treadmill, as per standard laboratory procedure [22] and as previously described [23]. Given the sedentary participants had been undertaking <90 min of low to moderate exercise per week, a VO_{2max} test was not required, due to safety concerns, as well as its perceived difficulty by the potential participants, resulting in a barrier to the enrolment of this cohort.

Each participant was studied over seven consecutive days, and the study was undertaken over four months between June and September in Brisbane, Australia, when the mean minimum and maximum daytime temperature was 11.5 ± 1.2 and 23.4 ± 0.8 °C, respectively. Total body water and water turnover rate were determined by water-soluble tracer (deuterium oxide) administration, and its elimination rate throughout the study (as determined by the enrichment of the tracer in daily urine samples). Daily body mass changes were monitored on participants' home scales using seven consecutive daily measurements. Body mass changes were also monitored using laboratory scales for three measurements, each separated by 72 h (the time between laboratory visits). Each laboratory visit also involved collecting specimens (i.e., blood and urine) for later analysis. Participants were required to attend three testing sessions over seven days (every third day). The first session involved collecting a baseline urine sample before the administration of a deuterium oxide dose. Baseline body composition analysis was performed for the determination of participants' fat mass and fat-free mass. Walking and running stride length measurements were also taken, to ensure accurate accelerometry tracking. Blood samples were collected via venipuncture from a superficial forearm vein. Following the initial laboratory session, the subsequent two sessions involved discussion surrounding participants' food diaries and accelerometry data that had been recorded by participants, since the preceding laboratory visit.

During the study, participants were requested to maintain their normal pattern of exercise, eating and drinking, and daily lifestyle. It was, therefore, planned during the recruitment phase that participants did not have any atypical sporting activities or social commitments that would elicit unusual activity levels or eating or drinking (alcohol) behaviours. A seven-day test period was agreed upon that suited 'usual' participant activity and dietary habits.

2.3. Measurements and Equipment

Total body water was measured using the stable, non-radioactive, non-toxic isotope deuterium oxide, in the form of water ($2H_2O$) and followed the methodology outlined by Colley and colleagues [24]. Participants provided a baseline urine sample before consuming an oral bolus equating to 0.05 g·kg^{-1} body mass of $2H_2O$, consumed from a cup through a straw. The pre-dosing baseline urine sample was used to correct for background $2H_2O$ concentration values in the post-dose sample. The plastic cup and straw were weighed following oral ingestion of the dose to account for any leftover dose in the cup. This was then subtracted from the weight of the cup, straw, and dose to give the exact amount of dose ingested. A single, mid-stream urine sample was provided six hours later (± 10 min). No void was made between the two collections. Participants were fasted at the time of dosing and were asked to abstain from food or fluid during the equilibrium period to ensure equilibration across participants occurred under similar conditions.

The subsequent methodology followed procedures outlined by Wishart [25]. The enrichment of the local tap water, the dose given and the $2H_2O$ in the pre-dose and post-dose samples were measured using isotope ratio mass spectrometry (Hydra, PDZ Europa, Crew, UK). Each urine sample was pipetted into 10 mL exetainers (Labco Ltd., Califon, NJ, USA) for analysis. A catalyst, approximately 1 mg of platinum on alumina powder (Sigma Aldrich Inc., St. Louis, MO, USA) contained in a 0.5 mL vial (Chromacol Ltd., Herts, UK), was introduced into the exetainer, ensuring no direct contact with the urine. Each sample was evacuated for 5 min before being filled with 99% hydrogen gas for no more than 2 s. The samples were left at room temperature for a minimum of 72 h to equilibrate the deuterium in the urine sample with the hydrogen gas above it. All reference waters were prepared at the same time and in the same manner. Isotopic enrichments were expressed as the difference per unit volume (‰O) from standard mean ocean water. All assays were performed in duplicate with repeat assays in the laboratory, demonstrating coefficients of variance of <2.0% at low enrichment levels and <1.0% for higher values.

Participants reported to the laboratory between 500 and 1000 h after an overnight fast. Nude body mass was measured upon arrival to each laboratory visit and after the first morning void. The scales were accurate to the nearest 0.05 kg (Tanita BWB-600, Wedderburn, Australia). On their first visit to the laboratory, participants were asked to collect a mid-stream urine sample into a specimen cup. Participants thereafter collected a mid-stream urine sample outside of the laboratory, from the second void each morning for the next six days. It was preferable that the sample was the second void of the day, as an earlier sample would be a concentrated overnight sample and not representative of that collection time point. Individual samples were stored together in a polystyrene storage container for each participant until their next laboratory visit.

Whole nude body mass was measured on participants' home bathroom scales (type and measurement precision varied, including both digital and mechanical varieties) daily, and these values were compared to the laboratory scales when ascertaining daily body mass fluctuations. If participants consumed food or fluid or voided before being weighed, the weight of urine produced, or foodstuffs consumed, before measuring body mass was accounted for when calculating the change in body mass between home scales and laboratory scales. Aside from a total of seven forgotten measures, as instructed, participants mostly (97.4%) recorded their 'home' whole nude body mass after their first void, as close to leaving home before travelling to the laboratory as possible; this elicited the most accurate comparison between participants' home scales and the laboratory scales ($r = 0.999$). The second void was then collected once the laboratory nude body mass was recorded. Height was measured to the nearest 0.1 cm, with shoes removed in an upright posture and during inhalation. Body Mass Index (BMI) was then calculated.

Body composition was measured on a participant's first visit via whole-body air displacement plethysmography using the BODPOD body composition system (Life Measurement, Concord, MA, USA) and performed according to the manufacturer's instructions and recommendations. Participants wore tight-fitting underwear or bike pants and a swimming cap. The procedure involved a volume calibration with and without a 50.008 L metal cylinder. Participants entered the BODPOD and sat inside the anterior chamber (450 L), which was connected to a rear measuring chamber (300 L) via oscillating diaphragms and breathed normally (relaxed tidal breathing). The recommended procedure, consisting of two measurements of body volume (30 s each), was adopted [26]. Occasionally body volumes differed by more than 150 mL, in which case a third measurement was performed. The reported body composition result by the BODPOD instrumentation was the mean of the two (or the two closest) measurements.

A 6 mL blood sample was drawn at each laboratory visit, from a vein in the antecubital fossa, into a serum separating vacutainer to determine serum osmolality as an indicator of acute hydration status. This sample was centrifuged after 20 min (4000 rpm for 10 min) (Universal 320R, Hettich, Germany), and the serum refrigerated (at 6 °C) for later analysis (within one week from collection). Serum osmolality was measured in duplicate using the freezing point depression technique (Osmomat 030, Gonotec, Berlin, Germany).

Urine samples were analysed for specific gravity using a digital refractometer (PAL-10 S, ATAGO, Tokyo, Japan) within 24 h of collection, to measure individuals' acute hydration status. Each sample was measured in duplicate. A third reading was taken where these two measures differed. The mean value of the two closest measures was taken as the urine specific gravity.

2.4. Dietary Tracking

The first laboratory session familiarised participants with the iPhone® application, Easy Diet Diary (Xyris Software Pty Ltd., Brisbane, Australia), including its use and function. Examples of daily intake were shown to participants to improve their understanding of quality reporting methods, and any questions were fielded.

Participants kept a daily record of their dietary intake (both food and fluid consumption). The six-day self-reported diet diary was entered into the iPhone® application (the software used was only compatible with iPhone, and in the instance that a participant owned an Android, a loan iPhone® was provided). Participants were trained in providing portion sizes by using measuring cup reference values and/or their personal kitchen weighing scales where possible. FoodWorks commercial software (Professional Edition, version 7.0, Xyris Software, Brisbane, Australia) was used to determine total daily water intake (moisture content of foods, as well as consuming water and other fluids), as well as daily intake of energy (kilojoules), macronutrients (grams), and specific micronutrients (sodium, potassium in milligrams). The accuracy of reporting was clarified during each laboratory visit by an interview with an Accredited Practising Dietitian, with particular emphasis on reported quantities of fluids and high-moisture-content foods, as well as suspected diary omissions. Participants were asked to refrain from consuming alcohol during the test period and were instructed to continue their habitual intake of caffeine, to not produce significant anomalies in hydration measures.

2.5. Physical Activity Tracking

The first laboratory session was also utilised to familiarise participants with the use of their activity trackers: The FitBit® Flex Wireless Activity Tracker (FitBit). The FitBit is lightweight (16 g) and contains a microelectromechanical system (MEMS) triaxial accelerometer. A proprietary algorithm estimates energy expenditure from the triaxial accelerometer (FitBit® Inc., San Francisco, CA, USA). The participants' height and weight information, along with their age and gender, were entered into the FitBit® user website (www.fitbit.com, accessed on 14 April 2021). According to the manufacturer's direction, the FitBit® Flex was worn on the non-dominant wrist to obtain a more accurate step count (activities of daily living typically require higher non-step-related use of the dominant wrist) [27].

Participants were asked to take 20 strides at their normal walking pace along an indoor corridor. This was repeated for participants' typical running pace in the active participant group. Once familiarisation was complete, individual calibration of stride length was undertaken to ensure accurate accelerometery tracking. Calibration involved the measure of distance travelled over 20 average walking stride lengths, as well as 20 average running stride lengths. The total distance was divided by 20, to calculate the average stride length. Every 20 strides were repeated in triplicate, with the average of the three values reported. Stride length was then entered into the user website.

Data from the FitBit® user website (total steps, distance travelled, energy expenditure) was extracted and used to estimate the energy expenditure of participants at 15-min intervals over every 24 h. In conjunction with this data, records of daily activities to account for anomalies in step count data were collected, whereby participants were asked to keep note (written or mental) of unusual activity that might disturb their FitBit® step results (unusually low or high spikes in steps). Examples included: Cycling where physical activity was occurring despite minimal FitBit® activity; driving where minimal physical activity was occurring despite a higher representation in FitBit® activity, due to hand movements at the steering wheel and/or uneven surfaces eliciting hand/wrist movement; or specific tasks that required the FitBit® to be removed altogether, such as 'no jewellery' rules in team sport, or water immersion activity. This information was collected through recall discussions with participants during each laboratory visit.

2.6. Statistical Analysis

All analyses were performed in R (Version 3.5.3) [28] using the RStudio environment (Version 1.0.143). The analysis was completed in four main parts. First, linear regression was used to determine differences in the descriptive variables of age, height, body mass, BMI, and VO_{2max} between active and sedentary participants. Second, a linear mixed-effects model was used to determine the difference between groups for each individual's coefficient of variation of the hydration markers (body mass, serum osmolality and urine specific gravity). The models included a random intercept for each individual to account for the repeated measurements across days. Third, linear regression was used to determine differences in total body water, body composition and body water turnover between active and sedentary participants. Models included activity level as a fixed factor and were implemented using the base R function 'lm'. Hedges' g [29] and 95% confidence intervals (CI) were calculated for the standardised difference between active and sedentary participants using the 'effsize' package [30]. A weighted pooled SD was used as the denominator, and a non-central t-distribution for the 95% CI. Hedges' g values were interpreted as small 0.2, medium 0.5 and large 0.8 [29]. Finally, a penalised regression model was performed to predict water turnover based on the independent predictor variables. A bivariate (Pearson) correlation was used to identify the variables that shared at least a small association (i.e., $r > 0.1$ or < -0.1) with water turnover. The initial model contained group and the following predictor variables: Fibre, sodium, energy expenditure, carbohydrate and water intake that were standardised using the equation: $y' = y - \bar{x}/s$, where '$\bar{x}$' is the sample mean, 's' the sample standard deviation, and 'y'' the observed value. The least absolute shrinkage and selection operator (Lasso) models were used to identify redundant predictors, by shrinking their coefficients to exactly zero [31], using the R package 'glmnet'. In comparison to more traditional variable selection methods, namely, step-forward and step-back selection, the Lasso model identifies the best subset of predictors, while accounting for co-correlation between predictors [32]. Potentially important predictors identified via Lasso were fit in a 'final' linear mixed-effects model. For all models, the assumption of normality was confirmed via histogram plots of model residuals. Evidence of a statistical effect or difference was accepted at an α level of 0.05.

3. Results

3.1. Participant Characteristics

Participants' anthropometric characteristics are as displayed in Table 1. There was statistical evidence of the active group having a lower body mass (mean difference (MD) Hedges' g[95% CI] = -0.72 [-1.39, -0.07]), BMI (g[95% CI] = -0.73 [-1.40, -0.08]), and body fat percentage (g[95% CI] = -2.00 [-2.78, -1.21]) than the sedentary. There was no evidence of a difference in age, height or lean body mass between the groups.

Table 1. Physical and anthropometric descriptors of study participants.

Characteristic	Sedentary (n = 19) Mean ± Standard Deviation	Active (n = 19) Mean ± Standard Deviation	Mean Difference (95% Confidence Interval), p Value
Age (yrs)	25.9 ± 3.6	24.7 ± 3.2	-1.2 [-3.42, 1.02], $p = 0.281$
Height (m)	1.80 ± 0.06	1.79 ± 0.06	-0.01 [-0.05, 0.03], $p = 0.533$
Mass (kg) †	87.6 ± 17.1	77.9 ± 7.2	-9.7 [-18.3, -1.0], $p = 0.029$
BMI (kg·m^{-2}) †	26.9 ± 4.7	24.3 ± 1.5	-2.58 [-4.86, -0.31], $p = 0.027$
LBM (kg)	63.5 ± 9.0	68.3 ± 5.5	-5.6 [-0.12, 9.71], $p = 0.056$
Fat mass (%) †	24.7 ± 9.9	9.9 ± 3.5	-14.9 [-19.7, -10.0], $p < 0.001$
VO$_2$ max (mL·kg^{-1}·min^{-1})	-	61.1 ± 2.6	

† indicates statistical evidence for a difference between groups; LBM, lean body mass.

3.2. Hydration Marker Coefficients of Variation

There was no statistical evidence of a difference in the coefficient of variation between groups for home body mass (β ± SE [95% CI] = 0.14 ± 0.12 [-0.10, 0.38]; $t = 1.16$; $p = 0.251$) laboratory body mass (β ± SE [95% CI] = -0.05 ± 0.26 [-0.55, 0.45]; $t = -0.20$; $p = 0.841$), serum osmolality (β ± SE [95% CI] = -0.14 ± 0.55 [-1.21, 0.92]; $t = -0.26$; $p = 0.794$) or urine specific gravity (β ± SE [95% CI] = 0.14 ± 0.08 [-0.02, 0.30]; $t = 1.75$; $p = 0.084$).

There was statistical evidence of an increase in the coefficient of variation over the days in both home body mass (β ± SE [95% CI] = 0.04 ± 0.01 [0.02, 0.06]; $t = 3.48$; $p < 0.001$) and urine specific gravity (β ± SE [95% CI] = 0.04 ± 0.01 [0.02, 0.34]; $t = 4.99$; $p < 0.001$). This outcome is the result of a few individuals displaying no change in their measurements on the first two or three consecutive timepoints producing a zero percent coefficient of variation. While this scenario occurred in the laboratory body mass (β ± SE [95% CI] = 0.01 ± 0.06 [-0.11, 0.14]; $t = 0.23$; $p = 0.820$) and serum osmolality (β ± SE [95% CI] = 0.06 ± 0.14 [-0.21, 0.34]; $t = 0.46$; $p = 0.651$), these zero percent coefficient of variations influenced each day equally.

3.3. Energy Intake and Expenditure

Participants' energy expenditure and nutrient consumption data are displayed in Table 2. There was statistical evidence of the active group having a higher energy expenditure (MD g[95% CI] = 1.12 [0.44, 1.84]), intake of water (g[95% CI] = 1.21 [0.53, 1.93]), CHO (g[95% CI] = 0.81 [0.16, 1.49]) and fibre (g[95% CI] = 1.28 [0.60, 2.00]), compared with the sedentary. There was no evidence of a difference in sodium or alcohol intake between the groups.

3.4. Water Turnover and Total Body Water

There was statistical evidence the active group had a significantly greater total body water as a percent of body mass (MD g[95% CI] = 1.57 [0.86, 2.33]), but not absolute total body water compared with the sedentary. This reflected the fact that active participants tended to have a lower %FM (Table 1). Participants' relative water turnover is displayed in Table 2 and Figure 1. Relative water turnover in the active group was significantly greater than the sedentary group (MD g[95% CI] = 1.70 [0.98, 2.48]).

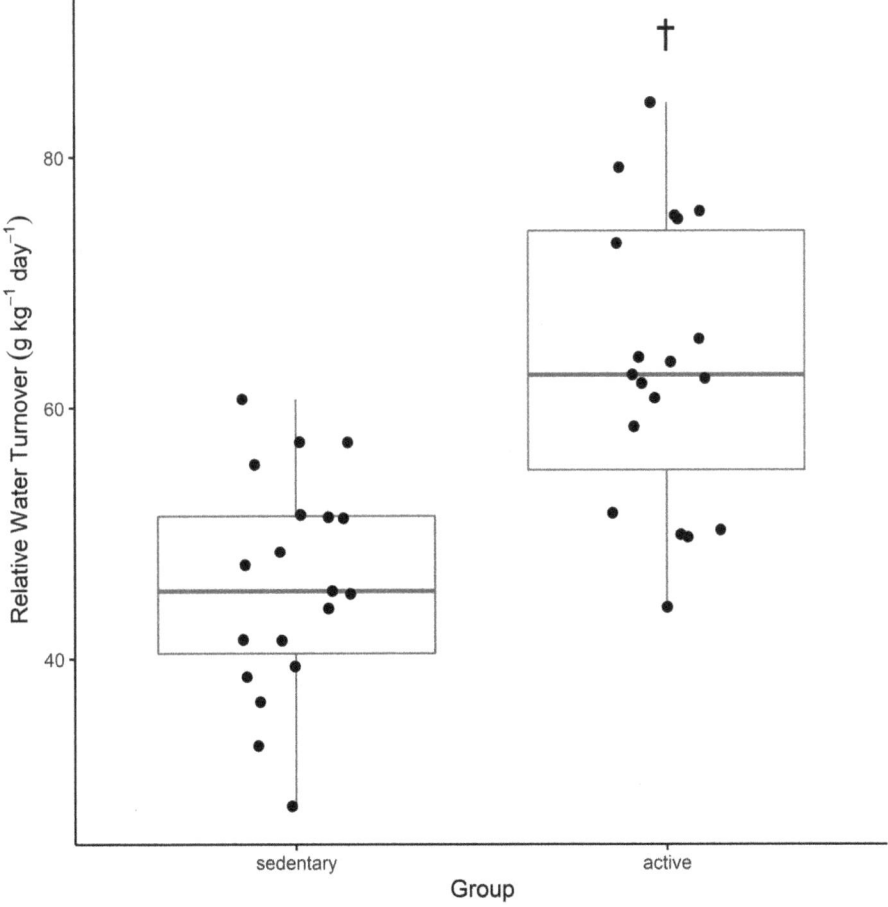

Figure 1. Relative water turnover of active and sedentary participants. † indicates statistical evidence for a difference between groups.

Penalised regression identified potentially important predictors that were included within a final model. The final model provided evidence that the fibre intake ($\beta \pm$ SE [95% CI] = 4.11 $\pm$ 1.85 [0.34, 7.87]; t = 2.22; p = 0.033), water intake ($\beta \pm$ SE [95% CI] = 4.87 $\pm$ 1.74 [1.34, 8.41]; t = 2.81; p = 0.008), sodium intake ($\beta \pm$ SE [95% CI] = −2.0 $\pm$ 1.5 [−5.1, 1.2]; t

$= -1.29$; $p = 0.207$), and activity level ($\beta \pm$ SE [95% CI] = 7.38 ± 3.84 [-0.44, 15.21]; $t = 1.92$; $p = 0.063$) predicted the relative body water turnover (F(4,32) = 13.7, $p < 0.001$; $R^2 = 0.585$).

Table 2. Mean ± standard deviation participant body water turnover, body composition, and dietary influencing factors of water turnover rates.

Characteristic	Sedentary (n = 19) Mean ± Standard Deviation	Active (n = 19) Mean ± Standard Deviation	Mean Difference (95% Confidence Interval), p Value
TBW (kg)	46.4 ± 6.8	48.0 ± 3.8	1.8 [−1.9, 5.4], $p = 0.335$
TBW (%) †	53.7 ± 5.6	61.9 ± 4.9	8.4 [4.9, 11.8], $p < 0.001$
WT (L/d) †	4.0 ± 1.0	5.0 ± 1.0	1.0 [0.3, 1.7], $p = 0.004$
WT (g/kg/d) †	46.0 ± 8.7	63.6 ± 11.3	17.6 [10.9, 24.2], $p < 0.001$
Daily H$_2$O intake (mL) †	3008 ± 683	4105 ± 1050	1097 [514, 1680], $p < 0.001$
Daily Energy Expenditure (kJ) †	11,412 ± 1769	13,265 ± 1452	1853 [775, 2930], $p = 0.001$
Daily CHO intake (g) †	233 ± 58	296 ± 91	63 [12.9, 113.1], $p = 0.015$
Daily Na intake (mg)	3649 ± 973	3487 ± 1299	−162 [−917, 593], $p = 0.666$
Daily EtOH intake (g)	16.7 ± 17.9	11.9 ± 14.6	−4.8 [−15.5, 5.9], $p = 0.368$
Daily Fibre intake (g) †	20.6 ± 6.9	37.2 ± 16.5	17 [8, 25], $p < 0.001$

† indicates statistical evidence for a difference between groups. TBW, total body water; LBM, lean body mass; WT, body water turnover; EtOH, alcohol.

4. Discussion

The main finding of this study was that the daily water turnover rates were faster in active participants undertaking the regular strenuous activity and with greater energy expenditure, than their sedentary counterparts who undertook little to no planned activity during the assessment period. Absolute TBW content of the active group was not significantly greater than that of the sedentary group; however, relative TBW expressed as a percentage of body mass was greater in the active group. Participants in both groups maintained stable body mass measures across the study duration, and therefore, presumably also maintained stable TBW content, as evidenced by stable hydration measures (U$_{SG}$, S$_{Osm}$ and body mass). This suggests that the exercise-induced energy expenditure among active participants promoted greater water losses (renal or non-renal) daily, leading to faster water turnover. Irrespective of this group effect, water turnover in both groups was significantly influenced by increased water and dietary fibre intake.

This study suggests that active young adult men have a water turnover rate that is faster than that of sedentary men of the same age group (Table 2, Figure 1). A comparison of previous water turnover research and the findings from this study indicate that in the active group, water turnover was observed to be 63.6 ± 11.3 g·kg^{-1}·d^{-1} compared with data from other water turnover studies ranging from 47–99.2 g·kg^{-1}·d^{-1} [10–12,14,15,20,33]. In the sedentary group, water turnover was observed to be 46.0 ± 8.7 g·kg^{-1}·d^{-1} compared with data from other water turnover studies ranging from 27.8–53.8 g·kg^{-1}·d^{-1} [10–12,14,15,20,33]. Previous literature emphasises that there are large daily and individual variations in water turnover rates. Water turnovers exceeding 70 g·kg^{-1}·d^{-1} have been seen in individuals undertaking long duration, strenuous activity in harsh environmental conditions, such as firefighters working 12–16 h shifts combatting wildfires across rough terrain in very hot conditions (94.8 g·kg^{-1}·d^{-1}) [15], and in altitude trekking for an average of 7.5 h (over 17 km) per day (78.7 g·kg^{-1}·d^{-1}) [19]. The current study values are more representative of regular physical activity, which at times was strenuous (measured by 'very active minutes' according to FitBit® data), but not on average reflective of lengthy periods or excessively harsh environmental conditions.

An accelerated water turnover can be explained by larger volumes of fluid intake, as well as by increased body fluid losses. Despite the 24 h human water requirement being linked to anthropometric characteristics (i.e., large individuals with a higher body mass require a greater daily total water intake than smaller individuals) [34], increased fluid intake (via food and fluid) was observed in the active participant group (Table 2). This increase may be explained by additional fluid intake associated with the increase in consumption of overall energy (food), which was required to sustain higher levels of energy expenditure in the active group. Increased exercise-associated energy expenditure relates to an increase in energy intake (to maintain energy balance), which could increase water intake as a by-product of increased calorie-containing fluids, or from the moisture content in foods consumed. Several variables affecting fluid gain depend on physical activity levels: Metabolic water production fluctuates depending on metabolic rate (higher metabolic rates produce more water); and sweat volume can sharply increase in very hot weather or during heavy exercise [1]. Fluid intake can also be enhanced by the presence of greater amounts of food in the gastrointestinal tract, due to central nervous system-mediated mechanisms for eating-induced drinking [35]. Urinary output was not measured in this study, and hence, body fluid losses through urine and other mechanisms can only be estimated. Research is mixed on whether urine output differs between active and sedentary individuals despite increased water turnover rates; however, exercise-induced non-renal water losses (skin, respiration, defaecation) appear to be at least partly responsible for increased water turnover [11,12,14,36].

There is evidence that water turnover is influenced by physical activity—in the longer-term (days to weeks), studies have commonly reported that water turnover is more rapid in physically active individuals compared with their sedentary comparisons [14,19,20]. It has also been found that trained status is significantly correlated to an increase in water turnover [19], likely resulting from increased water intake to assist in thermoregulation when physically active, as well as a physiological adaptation of more efficient sweating, due to an early onset and higher sweat rates. In two distinct studies, Leiper and Maughan [11,14] saw a clear difference of increased fluid losses in their exercising cohort, with one study showing non-renal water losses that were almost three times greater, suggesting to some extent that fluid intake in exercising individuals is greater, to counter exercise-associated increased sweat rates and respiratory fluid losses. Given the enhanced water intakes of the active participants in the present study, this suggests is a requirement to balance greater exercise-induced sweat and respiratory water losses than those of the sedentary participants. These differences in fluid intake between active and sedentary groups may be simply due to differences in habitual fluid consumption; however, it is also possible that differences may be seen due to exercise-induced dehydration stimulating thirst, particularly in the absence of adequate electrolyte replacement from sweat losses [37]. Furthermore, although these studies typically did not directly account for metabolic water production, water intake from foods and fluids, respiration, or sweat production, it is postulated that an increased metabolic rate during exercise elevates these factors, and thus, increases water turnover [20].

The more physically active a participant was (measured via energy expenditure), the greater the water turnover. This is perhaps due not only to increased water intake to replace non-renal losses or an increased fluid intake resulting from increased energy intake, but, in part, because of a metabolic water production derived from substrate oxidation. There is a growing body of evidence supporting the production of metabolic water during the oxidation of exogenous fuel sources in the body [18,38–40]; water gains have been reported when glycogen stores are broken down within the muscles and liver [41,42]. Well-trained individuals may have a higher storage capacity for muscle glycogen combined with a higher resting metabolic rate for substrate oxidation. In this situation, if water is endogenously liberated via carbohydrate oxidation, this may explain faster water turnover rates in the active group if this water production does, in fact, contribute to hydration status [19]. As an example, the energy cost of running a marathon for an average 70 kg male is roughly 12,000 kJ (4.18 kJ·kg^{-1}·min^{-1}) [43]. Estimates of carbohydrate oxidation during this event would indicate that an elite male runner would utilise 400 g of glycogen [44]; given the accepted value of 3 g of water per gram of oxidised glycogen [18], this would result in a 1200 mL endogenous water release.

The link between dietary composition and water turnover remains an under-researched area. This study identified that fibre appears to play an independent role in water turnover. There is very limited literature relating to dietary fibre intake and its relationship to TBW or water turnover; however, from the results of this study, it is apparent that increased fibre intake is positively associated with increased water turnover, independent of participants' level of physical activity. The human colon can absorb upwards of 5 L of water per day; water and electrolyte absorption in the colon requires the presence of short-chain fatty acids (SCFAs), which are produced by the fermentation of carbohydrates by colonic bacteria [45]. Microbially-fermentable 'resistant' starch is responsible for generating SCFAs in the colon due to its indigestibility in the small intestine. SCFAs stimulate blood flow in the colon, and importantly, fluid and electrolyte reabsorption. Resistant starch in an acute dose of around 50 g is documented as a common and effective addition to oral rehydration solutions that are delivered for the management of dehydration caused by severe acute diarrhoea [45–48] and more recently has shown promising application in treating exercise-induced fluid deficits [49]. The proposed mechanism of action relates to the ability of the colon to absorb sodium against substantial electrochemical gradients, as well as its considerable reserve capacity to absorb fluid [50]. SCFAs are a potent stimulus for the absorption of sodium and water from the colon, hence dietary fibre intake (specifically resistant starch) may play an important role in promoting body water retention, thus slowing water turnover rates [51,52].

While every effort was made to ensure accurate estimation of energy intake and expenditure throughout the study period, recording and reporting bias were expected given the arduous task of participants keeping food and exercise records for a 7-day period. Another limitation of the current study was that 24-h urine collection was not carried out, and hence, fluid loss origins (renal or non-renal) could not be identified.

5. Conclusions

This study confirms that water turnover is faster in individuals undertaking regular exercise than in their sedentary counterparts, and is, in part, explained by the intake of water from high-moisture containing foods. The nutrient analysis of the participant diets indicated that increased dietary fibre intake was also positively associated with water turnover rates. The water loss between groups also contributes to the differences observed in water turnover; this is partly related to differences in sweat output during increased energy expenditure from physical activity. Appropriate consideration of the dietary composition of food, in conjunction with fluid intake, may give rise to preventative strategies that could be used to positively manipulate hydration status to abate sweat losses, whether in a clinical, occupational or exercise setting.

Author Contributions: Conceptualisation, A.E.D. and I.B.S.; methodology, A.E.D., K.L.S., A.J.E.B. and I.B.S.; formal analysis, A.E.D. and I.B.S.; writing—original draft preparation, A.E.D.; writing—review and editing, A.E.D., K.L.S., A.J.E.B. and I.B.S. All authors have read and agreed to the published version of the manuscript.

Funding: This research received no external funding.

Institutional Review Board Statement: The study was conducted according to the guidelines of the Declaration of Helsinki and approved by the Queensland University of Technology Human Research Ethics Committee (#1400000244).

Data Availability Statement: The data presented in this study are openly available in Dryad at doi:10.5061/dryad.m37pvmd21.

Acknowledgments: The authors would like to thank Connie Wishart for her technical assistance in the analysis of the deuterium oxide urine samples.

Conflicts of Interest: The authors declare no conflict of interest.

References

1. Shimamoto, H.; Komiya, S. The Turnover of Body Water as an Indicator of Health. *J. Physiol. Anthr. Appl. Hum. Sci.* **2000**, *19*, 207–212. [CrossRef]
2. Cheuvront, S.N.; Kenefick, R.W. Dehydration: Physiology, Assessment, and Performance Effects. *Compr. Physiol.* **2014**, *4*, 257–285. [CrossRef]
3. Bardis, C.N.; Kavouras, S.A.; Arnaoutis, G.; Panagiotakos, D.B.; Sidossis, L.S. Mild Dehydration and Cycling Performance During 5 km Hill Climbing. *J. Athl. Train.* **2013**, *48*, 741–747. [CrossRef]
4. Cheuvront, S.N.; Kenefick, R.W.; Montain, S.J.; Sawka, M.N. Mechanisms of aerobic performance impairment with heat stress and dehydration. *J. Appl. Physiol.* **2010**, *109*, 1989–1995. [CrossRef]
5. Nuccio, R.P.; Barnes, K.A.; Carter, J.M.; Baker, L.B. Fluid Balance in Team Sport Athletes and the Effect of Hypohydration on Cognitive, Technical, and Physical Performance. *Sports Med.* **2017**, *47*, 1951–1982. [CrossRef]
6. Lacey, J.; Corbett, J.; Forni, L.; Hooper, L.; Hughes, F.; Minto, G.; Moss, C.; Price, S.; Whyte, G.; Woodcock, T.; et al. A multidisciplinary consensus on dehydration: Definitions, diagnostic methods and clinical implications. *Ann. Med.* **2019**, *51*, 232–251. [CrossRef]
7. Swanson, Z.S.; Pontzer, H. Water turnover among human populations: Effects of environment and lifestyle. *Am. J. Hum. Biol.* **2020**, *32*, e23365. [CrossRef]
8. Raman, A.; Schoeller, D.A.; Subar, A.F.; Troiano, R.P.; Schatzkin, A.; Harris, T.; Bauer, D.; Bingham, S.A.; Everhart, J.E.; Newman, A.B.; et al. Water turnover in 458 American adults 40–79 yr of age. *Am. J. Physiol. Renal Physiol.* **2004**, *286*, F394–F401. [CrossRef]
9. Lieberman, D.E. Human Locomotion and Heat Loss: An Evolutionary Perspective. *Compr. Physiol.* **2015**, *5*, 99–117. [CrossRef]
10. Horiuchi, S.; Miyazaki, M.; Tsuda, A.; Watanabe, E.; Igawa, S. Comparison of Water Turnover Rate between Female Soft Tennis Players and Age-matched Sedentary Individuals during Extensive Summer Training. *J. Hum. Environ. Syst.* **2008**, *11*, 123–127. [CrossRef]
11. Leiper, J.B.; Carnie, A.; Maughan, R.J. Water turnover rates in sedentary and exercising middle aged men. *Br. J. Sports Med.* **1996**, *30*, 24–26. [CrossRef]
12. Leiper, J.B.; Maughan, R.J. Comparison of water turnover rates in young swimmers in training and age-matched non-training individuals. *Int. J. Sport Nutr. Exerc. Metab.* **2004**, *14*, 347–357. [CrossRef]
13. Rush, E.C.; Chhichhia, P.; Kilding, A.E.; Plank, L.D. Water turnover in children and young adults. *Eur. J. Appl. Physiol.* **2010**, *110*, 1209–1214. [CrossRef]
14. Leiper, J.B.; Pitsiladis, Y.; Maughan, R.J. Comparison of Water Turnover Rates in Men Undertaking Prolonged Cycling Exercise and Sedentary Men. *Int. J. Sports Med.* **2001**, *22*, 181–185. [CrossRef]
15. Ruby, B.C.; Schoeller, D.A.; Sharkey, B.J.; Burks, C.; Tysk, S. Water Turnover and Changes in Body Composition during Arduous Wildfire Suppression. *Med. Sci. Sports Exerc.* **2003**, *35*, 1760–1765. [CrossRef]
16. Sawka, M.N. Physiological Consequences of Hypohydration—Exercise Performance and Thermoregulatioin. *Med. Sci. Sports Exerc.* **1992**, *24*, 657–670. [CrossRef]
17. Cheuvront, S.N.; Montain, S.J.; Sawka, M.N. Fluid Replacement and Performance during the Marathon. *Sports Med.* **2007**, *37*, 353–357. [CrossRef]
18. Maughan, R.J.; Shirreffs, S.M.; Leiper, J.B. Errors in the estimation of hydration status from changes in body mass. *J. Sports Sci.* **2007**, *25*, 797–804. [CrossRef]
19. Fusch, C.; Grörer, W.; Dickhuth, H.H.; Moeller, H. Physical fitness influences water turnover and body water changes during trekking. *Med. Sci. Sports Exerc.* **1998**, *30*, 704–708. [CrossRef]
20. Shimamoto, H.; Komiya, S. Comparison of body water turnover in endurance runners and age-matched sedentary men. *J. Physiol. Anthr. Appl. Hum. Sci.* **2003**, *22*, 311–315. [CrossRef]
21. Craig, C.L.; Marshall, A.L.; Sjöström, M.; Bauman, A.E.; Booth, M.L.; Ainsworth, B.E.; Pratt, M.; Ekelund, U.; Yngve, A.; Sallis, J.F.; et al. International Physical Activity Questionnaire: 12-Country Reliability and Validity. *Med. Sci. Sports Exerc.* **2003**, *35*, 1381–1395. [CrossRef]
22. Newburgh, L.H.; Johnston, M.W.; Falcon-Lesses, M. Measurement of Total Water Exchange. *J. Clin. Investig.* **1930**, *8*, 161–196. [CrossRef]
23. Stewart, I.B.; Stewart, K.L.; Worringham, C.J.; Costello, J.T. Physiological Tolerance Times while Wearing Explosive Ordnance Disposal Protective Clothing in Simulated Environmental Extremes. *PLoS ONE* **2014**, *9*, e83740. [CrossRef]
24. Colley, R.C.; Byrne, N.M.; Hills, A.P. Implications of the variability in time to isotopic equilibrium in the deuterium dilution technique. *Eur. J. Clin. Nutr.* **2007**, *61*, 1250–1255. [CrossRef]
25. Wishart, C. *Measurement of Total Body Water (TBW) and Total Energy Expenditure (TEE) Using Stable Isotopes*; Traditional, Queensland University of Technology; Institute of Health and Biomedical Innovation: Brisbane, Australia, 2011.
26. Life Measurement, I.L. *BOD POD Body Composition Tracking System Operator's Manual*; Life Measurement: Conrod, MA, USA, 2004.
27. Chen, M.-D.; Kuo, C.-C.; Pellegrini, C.A.; Hsu, M.-J. Accuracy of Wristband Activity Monitors during Ambulation and Activities. *Med. Sci. Sports Exerc.* **2016**, *48*, 1942–1949. [CrossRef]
28. R Core Team. R: A Language and Environment for Statistical Computing. 2020. Available online: https://www.r-project.org (accessed on 4 March 2020).

29. Hedges, L. Distribution Theory for Glass's Estimator of Effect Size and Related Estimators. *J. Educ. Stat.* **1981**, *6*, 107–128. [CrossRef]
30. Revelle, W. Pysch: Procedures for Personality and Psychological Research. Available online: https://CRAN.R-project.org/package=psychVersion=1.8.12 (accessed on 14 April 2020).
31. Friedman, J.H.; Hastie, T.; Tibshirani, R. Regularization Paths for Generalized Linear Models via Coordinate Descent. *J. Stat. Softw.* **2010**, *33*, 1–22. [CrossRef]
32. James, G.; Witten, D.; Hastie, T.; Tibshirani, R. Linear Model Selection and Regularization. In *An Introduction to Statistical Learning. Springer Texts in Statistics, Vol 103*; Springer: New York, NY, USA, 2013. [CrossRef]
33. Fusch, C.; Gfrörer, W.; Koch, C.; Thomas, A.; Grünert, A.; Moeller, H. Water turnover and body composition during long-term exposure to high altitude (4900–7600 m). *J. Appl. Physiol.* **1996**, *80*, 1118–1125. [CrossRef]
34. Medicine, I.O. *Dietary Reference Intakes for Water, Potassium, Sodium, Chloride, and Sulfate*; Institute of Medicine: Washington, DC, USA, 2004.
35. Kraly, F.S. Effects of eating on drinking. In *Thirst: Physiological and Psychological Aspects*; Ramsay, D.J., Booth, D.A., Eds.; Springer: London, UK, 1990; pp. 297–312.
36. Armstrong, L.E.; Johnson, E.C. Water Intake, Water Balance, and the Elusive Daily Water Requirement. *Nutrients* **2018**, *10*, 1928. [CrossRef]
37. Nadel, E.R.; Mack, G.W.; Takamata, A. Thermoregulation, exercise, and thirst: Interrelationships in humans. In *Perspectives in Exercise Science and Sports Medicine*; Gisolfi, C.V., Lamb, D.R., Nadel, E.R., Eds.; Brown & Benchmark: Dubuque, IA, USA, 1993; pp. 225–257.
38. Pastene, J.; Germain, M.; Allevard, A.M.; Gharib, C.; Lacour, J.-R. Water balance during and after marathon running. *Eur. J. Appl. Physiol. Occup. Physiol.* **1996**, *73*, 49–55. [CrossRef]
39. Sherman, W.M.; Plyley, M.J.; Sharp, R.L.; van Handel, P.J.; McAllister, R.M.; Fink, W.J.; Costill, D.L. Muscle Glycogen Storage and Its Relationship with Water. *Int. J. Sports Med.* **1982**, *3*, 22–24. [CrossRef]
40. Nolte, H.W.; Noakes, T.D.; van Vuuren, B. Protection of total body water content and absence of hyperthermia despite 2% body mass loss ('voluntary dehydration') in soldiers drinking ad libitum during prolonged exercise in cool environmental conditions. *Br. J. Sports Med.* **2011**, *45*, 1106–1112. [CrossRef]
41. King, R.F.G.J.; Cooke, C.; Carroll, S.; O'Hara, J. Estimating changes in hydration status from changes in body mass: Considerations regarding metabolic water and glycogen storage. *J. Sports Sci.* **2008**, *26*, 1361–1363. [CrossRef]
42. Olsson, K.-E.; Saltin, B. Variation in Total Body Water with Muscle Glycogen Changes in Man. *Acta Physiol. Scand.* **1970**, *80*, 11–18. [CrossRef]
43. Harris, C.; Debeliso, M.; Adams, K.J. The effects of running speed on the metabolic and mechanical energy costs of running. *J. Exerc. Physiol. Online* **2003**, *6*, 28–37.
44. Williams, C. Diet and endurance fitness. *Am. J. Clin. Nutr.* **1989**, *49*, 1077–1083. [CrossRef]
45. Ramakrishna, B.S.; Venkataraman, S.; Srinivasan, P.; Dash, P.; Young, G.P.; Binder, H.J. Amylase-Resistant Starch plus Oral Rehydration Solution for Cholera. *N. Engl. J. Med.* **2000**, *342*, 308–313. [CrossRef]
46. Binder, H.J.; Brown, I.; Ramakrishna, B.S.; Young, G.P. Oral Rehydration Therapy in the Second Decade of the Twenty-first Century. *Curr. Gastroenterol. Rep.* **2014**, *16*, 376. [CrossRef]
47. Raghupathy, P.; Ramakrishna, B.S.; Oommen, S.P.; Ahmed, M.S.; Priyaa, G.; Dziura, J.; Young, G.; Binder, H.J. Amylase-Resistant Starch as Adjunct to Oral Rehydration Therapy in Children with Diarrhea. *J. Pediatr. Gastroenterol. Nutr.* **2006**, *42*, 362–368. [CrossRef]
48. Ramakrishna, B.S.; Subramanian, V.; Mohan, V.; Sebastian, B.K.; Young, G.; Farthing, M.J.; Binder, H.J. A Randomized Controlled Trial of Glucose versus Amylase Resistant Starch Hypo-Osmolar Oral Rehydration Solution for Adult Acute Dehydrating Diarrhea. *PLoS ONE* **2008**, *3*, e1587. [CrossRef]
49. O'Connell, S.M.; Woodman, R.J.; Brown, I.L.; Vincent, D.J.; Binder, H.J.; Ramakrishna, B.S.; Young, G.P. Comparison of a sports-hydration drink containing high amylose starch with usual hydration practice in Australian rules footballers during intense summer training. *J. Int. Soc. Sports Nutr.* **2018**, *15*, 46. [CrossRef]
50. Phillips, J.; Muir, J.G.; Birkett, A.; Lu, Z.X.; Jones, G.P.; O'Dea, K.; Young, G.P. Effect of resistant starch on fecal bulk and fermentation-dependent events in humans. *Am. J. Clin. Nutr.* **1995**, *62*, 121–130. [CrossRef] [PubMed]
51. Topping, D.L.; Clifton, P.M. Short-Chain Fatty Acids and Human Colonic Function: Roles of Resistant Starch and Nonstarch Polysaccharides. *Physiol. Rev.* **2001**, *81*, 1031–1064. [CrossRef]
52. Sawka, M.N.; Burke, L.M.; Eichner, E.R.; Maughan, R.J.; Montain, S.J.; Stachenfeld, N.S. American College of Sports Medicine position stand. Exercise and fluid replacement. *Med. Sci. Sports Exerc.* **2007**, *39*, 377–390. [CrossRef]

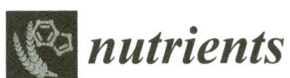

Article

Availability of a Flavored Beverage and Impact on Children's Hydration Status, Sleep, and Mood

Michael R. Szymanski [1,*], Gabrielle E. W. Giersch [1], Margaret C. Morrissey [1], Courteney L. Benjamin [1,2], Yasuki Sekiguchi [1], Ciara N. Manning [1], Rebecca L. Stearns [1] and Douglas J. Casa [1,*]

[1] Department of Kinesiology, Korey Stringer Institute, University of Connecticut, Storrs, CT 06269, USA; gabrielle.giersch@uconn.edu (G.E.W.G.); margaret.morrissey@uconn.edu (M.C.M.); cbenjami@samford.edu (C.L.B.); yasuki.sekiguchi@uconn.edu (Y.S.); ciara.manning@uconn.edu (C.N.M.); rebecca.stearns@uconn.edu (R.L.S.)

[2] Department of Kinesiology, Samford University, Birmingham, AL 35229, USA

* Correspondence: michael.szymanski@uconn.edu (M.R.S.); douglas.casa@uconn.edu (D.J.C.); Tel.: +1-860-486-0265 (M.R.S.)

Citation: Szymanski, M.R.; Giersch, G.E.W.; Morrissey, M.C.; Benjamin, C.L.; Sekiguchi, Y.; Manning, C.N.; Stearns, R.L.; Casa, D.J. Availability of a Flavored Beverage and Impact on Children's Hydration Status, Sleep, and Mood. *Nutrients* 2021, 13, 1757. https://doi.org/10.3390/nu13061757

Academic Editor: Pedro Moreira

Received: 18 March 2021
Accepted: 19 May 2021
Published: 21 May 2021

Publisher's Note: MDPI stays neutral with regard to jurisdictional claims in published maps and institutional affiliations.

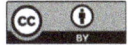

Copyright: © 2021 by the authors. Licensee MDPI, Basel, Switzerland. This article is an open access article distributed under the terms and conditions of the Creative Commons Attribution (CC BY) license (https:// creativecommons.org/licenses/by/ 4.0/).

Abstract: Euhydration remains a challenge in children due to lack of access and unpalatability of water and to other reasons. The purpose of this study was to determine if the availability/access to a beverage (Creative Roots®) influences hydration in children and, therefore, sleep quality and mood. Using a crossover investigation, 46 participants were randomly assigned to a control group (CON) or an intervention group and received Creative Roots® (INT) for two-week periods. We recorded daily first morning and afternoon urine color (Ucol), thirst perception, and bodyweight of the two groups. Participants reported to the lab once per week and provided first morning urine samples to assess Ucol, urine specific gravity (USG), and urine osmolality (Uosmo). Participants also completed the questionnaires Profile of Mood States-Adolescents (POMS-a) and Pittsburgh Sleep Quality Index (PSQI). Dependent t-tests were used to assess the effects of the intervention on hydration, mood, and sleep quality. Uosmo was greater and Ucol was darker in the control group (mean ± SD) [Uosmo: INT = 828 ± 177 mOsm·kg^{-1}, CON = 879 ± 184 mOsm·kg^{-1}, (p = 0.037), [Ucol:INT = 5 ± 1, CON = 5 ± 1, p = 0.024]. USG, POMS-a, and PSQI were not significant between the groups. At-home daily afternoon Ucol was darker in the control group [INT = 3 ± 1, CON = 3 ± 1, p = 0.022]. Access to Creative Roots® provides a small, potentially meaningful hydration benefit in children. However, children still demonstrated consistent mild dehydration based on Uosmo, despite consuming the beverage.

Keywords: euhydration; children; urine; thirst

1. Introduction

There is an increasing body of evidence showing that children are inadequately hydrated [1]. A recent review examining water intake across 19 countries found that about 60% of children aged 4–13 years did not meet water intake guidelines [2]. Specifically, in the United States, Kenny et al. [3] examined the prevalence of insufficient hydration using urine osmolality and found that over 50% of their sample (n = 4134) aged 6–19 years were inadequately hydrated. There are many barriers that may influence the consumption of water among children including, but not limited to, lack of drinking water accessibility while at school, unpalatable water, and the availability of competitive beverages (e.g., sugar-sweetened beverages, 100% fruit and vegetable juices) [4].

The hydration status has been associated with mood state, as well as sleep quality [5–7]. Evidence has demonstrated that dehydration adversely affects mood, with increases in tension and anxiety, as well as fatigue [5,6]. Additionally, Fadda et al. [6] found a negative correlation between hydration status (assessed as urine osmolality) and vigor, indicating that hydration is beneficial in improving vigor. A short sleep duration has also been linked to a poor hydration status, and those with a sleep duration of 6 h were presented higher urine specific gravity and greater odds of being dehydrated [7]. However, the aforementioned study [7] examined adult male participants. There is limited evidence on the hydration status and sleep quality in children.

Water is an essential component for many physiological functions within the human body and plays a critical role in thermoregulation, cardiovascular function, as well as transportation of nutrients and waste production [8]. Inadequate hydration can lead to numerous negative health effects [3,8]. Even mild to moderate dehydration has been associated with sleepiness, headaches, and muscle weakness [8]. Severe dehydration has been associated with irritability and sleepiness, especially in children and infants, low blood pressure, and rapid heartbeat [8]. These negative health effects can be detrimental to the development of children and warrant further access to water, specifically during school hours.

In an attempt to combat the hydration barriers in children, the Kraft Heinz Company (Chicago, IL, USA) developed a coconut water-based beverage. Therefore, the purpose of the present study was to determine if the accessibility to the beverage influences hydration, as well as sleep quality and mood status, in children. We hypothesized that having access to this beverage would improve the hydration status and, therefore, overall mood and sleep quality.

2. Materials and Methods

2.1. Beverage

The Kraft Heinz Company (Chicago, IL, USA) developed an 8.5 oz (251 mL) coconut water-based beverage (15% juice) with one gram of sugar and 11 calories, called Creative Roots®.

Experimental Approach to the Problem

We utilized a randomized crossover study design to guide data collection. All procedures were reviewed and approved by University of Connecticut's Institutional Review Board (H19-212). The participants provided verbal assent, and their parents or guardians provided written consent prior to participation.

2.2. Participants

A sample of 46 children (n = 23 males, n = 23 females) ranging from 7 to 12 years of age (10 ± 2 years old) at the time of consent volunteered for this study. Participants were excluded from the study if they had a history of chronic kidney disease, diabetes, sleep disorder, if used medication that might affect water balance (e.g., diuretics, laxatives, antacids, antihistamines, NSAIDs, blood pressure medication) or mood and anxiety (e.g., antidepressants, anxiolytics, beta-blockers, ADHD medication), as well as other medications that might cause urine color changes (e.g., isoniazid, sulfasalazine, metronidazole, nitrofurantoin, amitriptyline, cimetidine, indomethacin, zaleplon, methocarbamol, metoclopramide, warfarin, rifampin, and phenazopyridine). Participants were also excluded from the study if they did not find any of the drinks palatable.

2.3. Overview of the Study Procedures

Participants reported to the lab once a week over 7 weeks for a total of 7 lab visits. A timeline and overview of the study procedures can be seen in Table 1. Participants began the study with a familiarization visit in which they completed all laboratory procedures and were given detailed instructions by a research team member about how to properly complete data collection at home. The participants returned to the lab at least one week later and, following laboratory procedures, were randomly assigned to either an intervention group or a control group. The intervention group received 40 bottles of Creative Roots© (Kraft Heinz Company, Chicago, IL, USA). The parents/guardians of the participants were instructed to ensure that the participants had the option to drink the beverage at each meal (i.e., breakfast, lunch, and dinner), as well as to allow the participants to drink the beverage ad libitum throughout the day. Participants in the intervention group returned their empty and unused bottles and were given a new batch of 40 bottles each week. The control group did not receive the beverages and were not given any further instructions about fluid or dietary intake.

Table 1. Dependent variables and collection time points.

Variable	Familiarization	Baseline	Daily Data Collection During Weeks 1, 2, 4, 5 (at Home)	Weekly Visit with Researchers (End of Weeks 1–5)
Body mass	X	X	X	X
Urine Sample	X			X
Urine Specific Gravity	X			X
Urine Osmolality	X			X
AM Urine Color		X	X	X
PM Urine Color		X	X	X
Thirst Sensation	X	X	X	X
Sleep Questionnaire	X	X		X
Mood (POMS)	X	X		X

Following this two-week period, both groups (i.e., intervention and control groups) entered a washout week, in which no beverages were given, and participants were instructed to cease the at-home data collection. Following the washout week, participants returned to the lab and were assigned to their new groups (i.e., the intervention group became the control group and vice versa). Both groups were instructed to resume their bi-daily at-home assessments.

2.4. Weekly Lab Visits

Participants reported to the lab once a week over seven weeks for a total of seven lab visits. On the first lab visit, the participants were familiarized with the testing variables and taught how to assess their hydration. First, participants were given an iPod touch (Apple Inc., Cupertino, CA, USA) with the Qualtrics Survey Application (Qualtrics, Provo, UT, USA) to self-assess their daily morning and afternoon urine color, thirst perception, and bodyweight throughout the duration of the study. Additionally, participants tasted the Creative Roots® drink to ensure palatability. If the participant did not like the drink, they were excluded from the study; however, all participants enjoyed the beverage. Weekly lab visits involved a hydration assessment, the completion of the Profile of Mood States adolescent (POMS-a) [9] and of the Pittsburg Sleep Quality Index (PSQI) [10] questionnaires. For the hydration assessments, participants were provided with a urine collection cup, instructed to collect their first morning urine, and bring the sample to the laboratory. Urine color was assessed with the urine color chart that has been validated for children [11]. Urine specific gravity (USG) was assessed using a handheld refractometer (Reichert TS 400, Reichert Inc., Dewpew, NY, USA), and urine osmolality (Uosmo) was assessed using freeze-point depression (OsmoPRO® Multi-Sample Micro-Osmometer; Advanced Instruments, Norwood, MA, USA). Thirst perception was measured using a previously validated [12,13] nine-point (1–9) Likert scale, where 1 is "Not Thirsty at All" and 9 is "Very, Very Thirsty". Additionally, body mass was assessed at this time (Defender R7000 Xtreme; OHAUS Corp., Parsippany, NJ, USA). In order to limit parent and peer influence during the POMS-a and the PSQI, the participants were instructed to direct all questions to a member of the research team.

2.5. At Home Data Collection

Participants were given an iPod touch (Apple Inc., Cupertino, CA, USA) with the Qualtrics Survey Application (Qualtrics, Provo, UT, USA) to self-assess their daily morning and afternoon urine color, thirst perception, and bodyweight throughout the duration of the study. Following urination in the urine collection cup at home, urine color was assessed by the participant with the urine color chart in paper format or as a picture on the iPod. Bodyweight was measured at home with a bodyweight scale (BalanceFrom LLC., Los Angeles, CA, USA), and the perceived level of thirst was assessed immediately upon waking in the morning and upon return home from school in the afternoon (i.e., between 1600 and 1959 h) [14].

2.6. Statistical Analysis

Our sample size calculation was based on the comparison of a low water intake intervention vs. an ad libitum water intake in preadolescent children [1]. To establish an estimate of power and to project a proper sample size, the values for differences in 24 h urine osmolality from a low water intake intervention and an ad libitum water intake were utilized. It was determined that urine osmolality values for low water intake were 912 ± 199 mOsm·kg^{-1}, and those for an ad libitum water intake were 790 ± 257 mOsm·kg^{-1}. For a matched-pairs test with 0.05 alpha level, effect size of 0.52, and desired power level of 0.95, the estimated sample size would be a minimum of 42 participants. We utilized the power calculation software G*power 3.1 to calculate the required sample size needed for this study.

Data are reported as means and standard deviations (M $\pm$ SD). Dependent *t*-tests were used to determine differences between the intervention (INT) and the control (CON) groups for urine color, Uosmo, USG, thirst sensation, PSQI, POMS-a, and daily percent bodyweight changes [(Afternoon bodyweight−morning bodyweight)/morning bodyweight ($\times 100$)]. Alpha level was set a priori at 0.05. All statistical analyses were computed using SPSS (SPSS Statistics version 25, IBM Corp., Armonk, NY, USA).

3. Results

INT samples presented lower Uosmo and lighter urine color compared to CON samples, as shown in Figures 1 and 2, respectively. The afternoon urine color from at-home measures was lighter for the INT group compared to the CON group, as shown in Table 2. INT also had greater percent body mass loss, as shown in Figure 3. For all other measures taken at home, there were no differences, including for morning urine color as well as morning and afternoon thirst sensation, as shown in Table 2. INT did not show any effect on USG, thirst perception, POMS-a total score, or PSQI [USG: INT = 1.023 ± 0.005, CON = 1.024 ± 0.005, $p = 0.091$], [thirst: INT = 4 ± 1.6, CON = 4 ± 1.6, $p = 0.657$], [POMS-a: INT = -1.04 ± 5.6, CON = -0.26 ± 6.6, $p = 0.233$], [PSQI: INT = 2.91 ± 1.8, CON = 3.07 ± 1.5, $p = 0.425$].

Table 2. At-home daily log of morning and afternoon urine color and morning and afternoon thirst perception.

	Morning Urine Color	Afternoon Urine Color	Morning Thirst Perception	Afternoon Thirst Perception
Intervention	4 ± 1	3 ± 1 *	4 ± 1	3 ± 1
Control	4 ± 1	3 ± 1	4 ± 1	3 ± 1

Intervention = flavored beverage. * indicates statistical significance ($p < 0.05$). $n = 46$

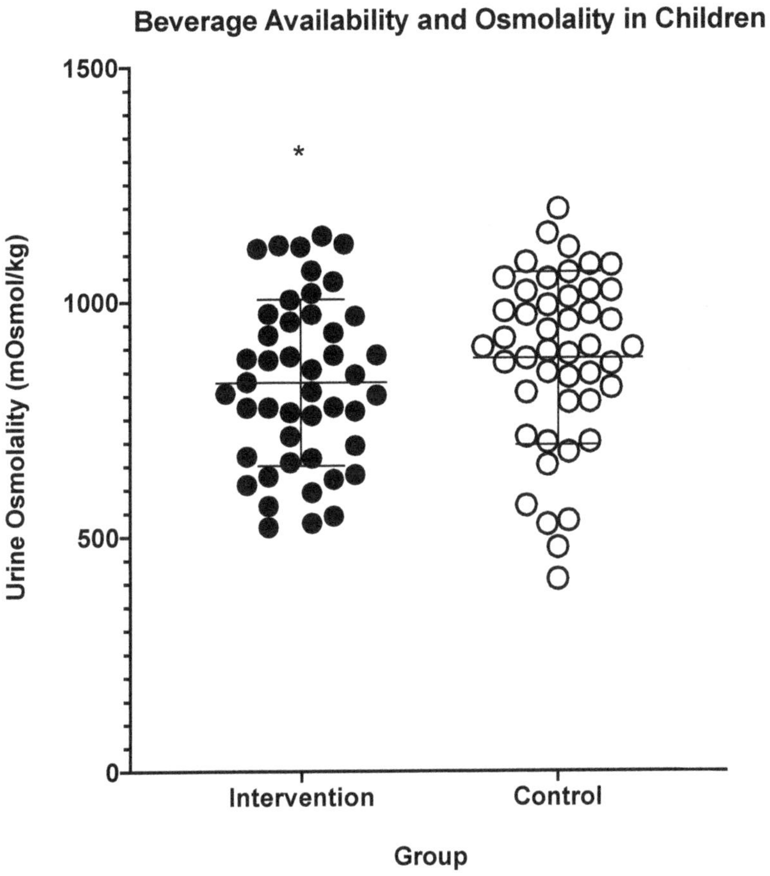

Beverage Availability and Osmolality in Children

Figure 1. Values are averages of lab visit urine osmolality in the intervention and control groups; $n = 46$ after a two-week period. Intervention = flavored beverage. * indicates statistical significance ($p < 0.05$). The lines within the individual data points represent each group's mean and standard deviation.

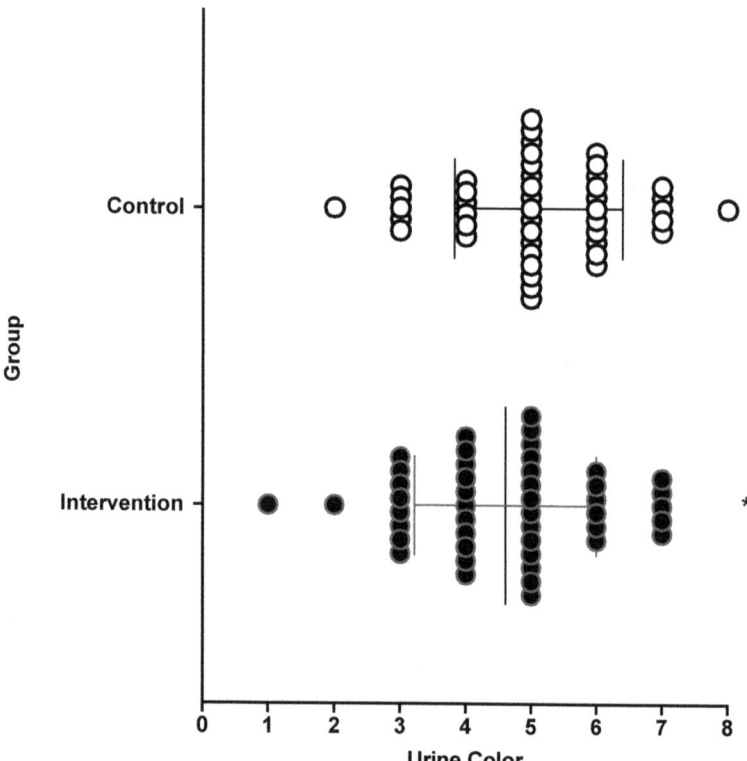

Figure 2. Values are averages of lab visit urine color for the intervention and the control groups; $n = 46$ after a two-week period. Intervention = flavored beverage. * indicates statistical significance ($p < 0.05$). The lines within the individual data points represent each group's mean and standard deviation.

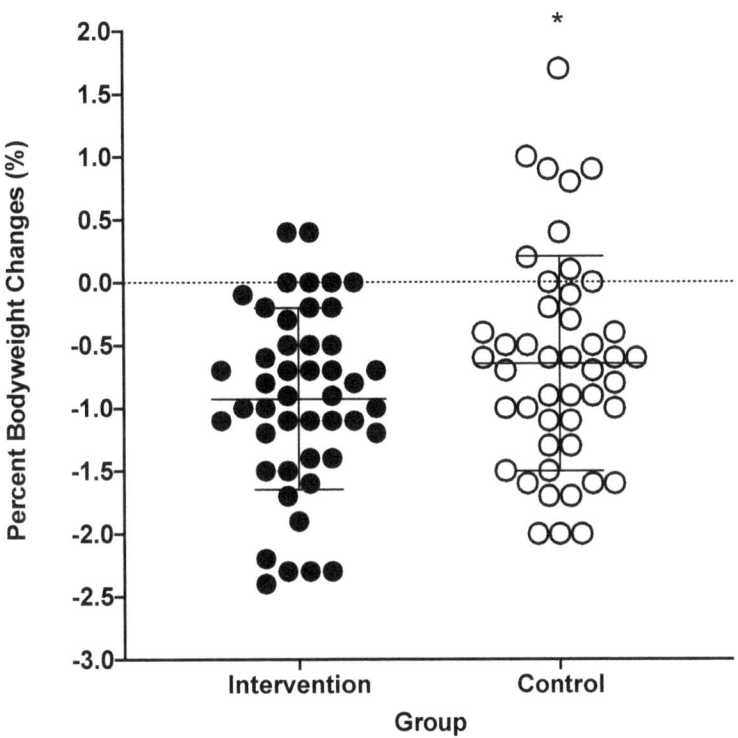

Figure 3. Values are average daily bodyweight percent changes in the intervention and in the control groups; $n = 46$. * indicates statistical significance ($p < 0.05$). The lines within the individual data points represent each group's mean and standard deviation.

4. Discussion

These results suggest that the INT group was able to improve their hydration status based on the decreased Uosmo and urine color from weekly laboratory visits. Although there was an observed decrease of dehydration in the INT group, both groups had clinical signs of dehydration from the spot samples provided (Uosmo > 800mOsm·kg^{-1}). This would suggest that although the INT groups did see improvements to their Uosmo, the INT condition was not sufficient to attain clinical euhydration. Despite being different at a statistically significant level between groups, urine color during the lab visits was similar for both groups, having a value of ~5 and a mean difference of only 0.5. Furthermore, USG and thirst perception during the lab visits were not significantly different between groups, suggesting that having accessibility to the Creative Roots® beverage may only improve Uosmo. However, the improvements in Uosmo may suggest that the Creative Roots® beverage offers a potential benefit for hydration, due to the validity of Uosmo for assessing hydration [15]. The at-home morning urine color and morning and afternoon thirst perception did not show any change in the INT group when the participants were self-assessing their thirst perception and urine color.

Our results are similar to those of Khan et al. [1] who examined hydration markers during a 4-day water intake intervention in children with a prescribed low intake, high intake, and ad libitum intake of fluid. The authors reported Uosmo and urine color values in their ad libitum group that would approach the threshold for clinical dehydration, similar to what we observed in our participants, who were able to consume fluid ad libitum [1]. This similarity may suggest that children with an ad libitum beverage intake may not see improvements in hydration and that a prescribed beverage intake may be more beneficial for improving hydration.

Interestingly, the at-home data (i.e., morning and afternoon urine color, bodyweight, and thirst perception) showed contradictory results. First, the afternoon urine color was lighter for the INT group; however, due to the low reported mean difference, we speculate that it is unlikely that these results have any clinical significance. Additionally, daily percent bodyweight changes were found to be statistically significant between the groups. The intervention group presented greater differences in daily percent bodyweight changes when compared to the control group, suggesting the intervention group was less hydrated than the control group. Bodyweight changes have been noted as one of the more practical markers for hydration, whereas day-to-day bodyweight losses of more than 1% can be an indicator of dehydration [16]. Although the intervention group did not lose over 1% of bodyweight, the group still lost more bodyweight than the control group, which is contradictory with their afternoon urine color measures. However, the bodyweight changes may be related to a reduced consumption of sugary beverages, thus a reduced caloric intake, due to having access to Creative Roots®. Prior research has demonstrated that reducing sugary beverage intake and replacing these beverages with non-caloric ones can result in reduced weight gain [17,18].

Contrary to previous research, we did not find any differences in mood between INT and CON, using the POMS-a. Fadda et al. [6] found that serving children 300–500 mL of water during the school day can improve their mood. This was a prescribed amount, whereas in the present study we utilized ad libitum fluid consumption and only assessed mood in children once per week, which may explain why we did not find any differences between our groups. This may suggest that acute changes in hydration may impact mood, but it is possible that those differences are not observable when only assessed one time per week. We also did not observe any differences in sleep quality, using the PSQI, between the intervention and the control groups despite the intervention group having a lighter urine color in the afternoon. This finding may simply be due to the intervention not changing the hydration status. Further research is warranted, as there is little evidence available regarding hydration status and sleep quality in children.

5. Limitations

There are several limitations to the present study. First, the intervention group was not prescribed a specific amount of fluid. We required the participants to have drinks available and accessible at each meal (i.e., breakfast, lunch, and dinner), as well as ad libitum throughout the day, but did not require them to consume specific amounts. Second, we did not ask the children or their parents to record what was consumed throughout each week. We also used first morning urine samples for hydration analysis (i.e., urine color, USG, Uosmo) in all lab visits in order to reduce scheduling conflicts with the participants and their caretakers. Recent literature suggests that Uosmo of afternoon urine samples is more representative of values observed in 24 h urine collection [14]. Lastly, the daily log data collection was not supervised by the research staff, though research participants were provided detailed instructions to promote compliance.

6. Conclusions

Our results indicate that having access to Creative Roots® seems to produce a small but potentially meaningful benefit in hydration, as indicated by Uosmo and urine color. However, even with the observed improvements, children were still consistently mildly dehydrated regardless of the group. Our data show the intervention group did improve some biomarkers of hydration, but no effect was observed in at-home measures, mood, or sleep. Further research is warranted using a prescribed amount of fluid to determine if the beverage improves the hydration status and monitoring dietary and fluid intake during the entirety of the study.

Author Contributions: Conceptualization, M.R.S., G.E.W.G., M.C.M., C.L.B., Y.S., R.L.S. and D.J.C.; methodology, M.R.S., G.E.W.G., M.C.M., C.L.B., Y.S., R.L.S. and D.J.C.; investigation, M.R.S., G.E.W.G., M.C.M., C.L.B., Y.S., C.N.M. and R.L.S.; data curation, M.R.S., G.E.W.G., M.C.M., C.L.B., Y.S., C.N.M. and R.L.S.; writing—original draft preparation, M.R.S. and G.E.W.G.; writing—review and editing, M.R.S., G.E.W.G., M.C.M., C.L.B., Y.S., C.N.M., R.L.S. and D.J.C.; project administration, D.J.C.; funding acquisition, D.J.C. All authors have read and agreed to the published version of the manuscript.

Funding: This research was funded by the Kraft Heinz Company (Chicago, IL, USA).

Institutional Review Board Statement: The study was conducted according to the guidelines of the Declaration of Helsinki and approved by the Institutional Review Board of the University of Connecticut (H19-212).

Informed Consent Statement: Participants provided verbal assent and their parents or guardians provided written consent prior to participation.

Data Availability Statement: Data available only on request due to ethical restrictions.

Acknowledgments: We would like to thank Fatou Lack, Mark Garcia, Michaela Pruchniki, Jonathan Granata, Radha Patel, Jeb Struder, Erica Filep, Erin Dierickx, and Rachel Katch for their assistance with data collection.

Conflicts of Interest: The authors declare no potential conflict of interest.

References

1. Khan, N.A.; Westfall, D.R.; Jones, A.R.; Sinn, M.A.; Bottin, J.H.; Perrier, E.T.; Hillman, C.H. A 4-d Water Intake Intervention Increases Hydration and Cognitive Flexibility among Preadolescent Children. *J. Nutr.* **2019**, *149*, 2255–2264. [CrossRef] [PubMed]
2. Suh, H.; Kavouras, S.A. Water intake and hydration state in children. *Eur. J. Nutr.* **2019**, *58*, 475–496. [CrossRef] [PubMed]
3. Kenney, E.L.; Long, M.W.; Cradock, A.L.; Gortmaker, S.L. Prevalence of Inadequate Hydration Among US Children and Disparities by Gender and Race/Ethnicity: National Health and Nutrition Examination Survey, 2009–2012. *Am. J. Public Health* **2015**, *105*, e113–e118. [CrossRef] [PubMed]
4. Patel, A.I.; Hampton, K.E. Encouraging consumption of water in school and child care settings: Access, challenges, and strategies for improvement. *Am. J. Public Health* **2011**, *101*, 1370–1379. [CrossRef] [PubMed]
5. Ganio, M.S.; Armstrong, L.E.; Casa, D.J.; McDermott, B.P.; Lee, E.C.; Yamamoto, L.M.; Marzano, S.; Lopez, R.M.; Jimenez, L.; Le Bellego, L.; et al. Mild dehydration impairs cognitive performance and mood of men. *Br. J. Nutr.* **2011**, *106*, 1535–1543. [CrossRef] [PubMed]
6. Fadda, R.; Rapinett, G.; Grathwohl, D.; Parisi, M.; Fanari, R.; Calo, C.M.; Schmitt, J. Effects of drinking supplementary water at school on cognitive performance in children. *Appetite* **2012**, *59*, 730–737. [CrossRef] [PubMed]
7. Rosinger, A.Y.; Chang, A.M.; Buxton, O.M.; Li, J.; Wu, S.; Gao, X. Short sleep duration is associated with inadequate hydration: Cross-cultural evidence from US and Chinese adults. *Sleep* **2019**, *42*. [CrossRef] [PubMed]
8. Jequier, E., Constant, F. Water as an essential nutrient: The physiological basis of hydration. *Eur. J. Clin. Nutr.* **2010**, *64*, 115–123. [CrossRef] [PubMed]
9. Terry, P.C.; Lane, A.M.; Lane, H.J.; Keohane, L. Development and validation of a mood measure for adolescents. *J. Sports Sci.* **1999**, *17*, 861–872. [CrossRef] [PubMed]
10. Buysse, D.J.; Reynolds, C.F.; Monk, T.H., 3rd; Berman, S.R.; Kupfer, D.J. The Pittsburgh Sleep Quality Index: A new instrument for psychiatric practice and research. *Psychiatry Res.* **1989**, *28*, 193–213. [CrossRef]
11. Kavouras, S.A.; Johnson, E.C.; Bougatsas, D.; Arnaoutis, G.; Panagiotakos, D.B.; Perrier, E.; Klein, A. Validation of a urine color scale for assessment of urine osmolality in healthy children. *Eur. J. Nutr.* **2016**, *55*, 907–915. [CrossRef] [PubMed]
12. Adams, W.M.; Vandermark, L.W.; Belval, L.N.; Casa, D.J. The Utility of Thirst as a Measure of Hydration Status Following Exercise-Induced Dehydration. *Nutrients* **2019**, *11*, 2689. [CrossRef] [PubMed]
13. Engell, D.B.; Maller, O.; Sawka, M.N.; Francesconi, R.N.; Drolet, L.; Young, A.J. Thirst and fluid intake following graded hypohydration levels in humans. *Physiol. Behav.* **1987**, *40*, 229–236. [CrossRef]
14. Suh, H.; Summers, L.G.; Seal, A.D.; Colburn, A.T.; Mauromoustakos, A.; Perrier, E.T.; Bottin, J.H.; Kavouras, S.A. Afternoon urine osmolality is equivalent to 24 h for hydration assessment in healthy children. *Eur. J. Clin. Nutr.* **2020**, *74*, 884–890. [CrossRef] [PubMed]
15. Youhanna, S.; Bankir, L.; Jungers, P.; Porteous, D.; Polasek, O.; Bochud, M.; Hayward, C.; Devuyst, O. Validation of Surrogates of Urine Osmolality in Population Studies. *Am. J. Nephrol.* **2017**, *46*, 26–36. [CrossRef] [PubMed]
16. Cheuvront, S.N.; Sawka, M.N. Hydration assessment of athletes. *Sports Sci. Exch.* **2005**, *18*, 1–6.

17. Katan, M.B.; de Ruyter, J.C.; Kuijper, L.D.; Chow, C.C.; Hall, K.D.; Olthof, M.R. Impact of Masked Replacement of Sugar-Sweetened with Sugar-Free Beverages on Body Weight Increases with Initial BMI: Secondary Analysis of Data from an 18 Month Double-Blind Trial in Children. *PLoS ONE* **2016**, *11*, e0159771. [CrossRef] [PubMed]
18. De Ruyter, J.C.; Olthof, M.R.; Seidell, J.C.; Katan, M.B. A trial of sugar-free or sugar-sweetened beverages and body weight in children. *N. Engl. J. Med.* **2012**, *367*, 1397–1406. [CrossRef] [PubMed]

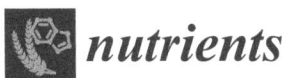

Article

Hydration, Eating Attitudes and Behaviors in Age and Weight-Restricted Youth American Football Players

Susan Yeargin [1,*], Toni M. Torres-McGehee [1], Dawn Emerson [2], Jessica Koller [3] and John Dickinson [4]

1. Exercise Science Department, Arnold School of Public Health University of South Carolina, Columbia, SC 29208, USA; torresmc@mailbox.sc.edu
2. Department of Physical Therapy, Rehabilitation Sciences, and Athletic Training, School of Health Professions University of Kansas Medical Center, Kansas City, KS 66160, USA; demerson@kumc.edu
3. Surgi-Care Inc., Boston, MA 02451, USA; jkoller328@gmail.com
4. Palmetto Health/USC Orthopedic Center, Columbia, SC 29203, USA; johndickinson333@yahoo.com
* Correspondence: syeargin@mailbox.sc.edu

Abstract: There is a paucity of research examining hydration and nutrition behaviors in youth American football players. A potentially unique risk factor are league restrictions based on weight (WR) or age (AR). The purpose of this study was to examine hydration status between WR and AR leagues. The secondary purpose was to describe eating patterns in players. An observational cohort design with 63 youth football players (10 ± 1 yrs, 148.2 ± 9.4 cm, 44.9 ± 15.3 kg) was utilized. Independent variables were league (AR (*n* = 36); WR (*n* = 27)) and activity type (practice (PX = 8); game (GM = 3)). Dependent variables were hydration status (urine osmolality; percent change in body mass (%BM)), eating attitudes (Children's Eating Attitude Test (ChEAT-26)) and self-reported frequency of meals. On average, players arrived activity mildly hypohydrated (830 ± 296 mOsm/kg) and %BM was minimal (−0.1 ± 0.7%) during events. Players consumed 2 ± 1 meals and 1 ± 1 snack before events. The ChEAT-26 survey reported 21.6% (*n* = 8) of players were at risk for abnormal eating attitudes. Among these players, eating binges, vomiting, excessive exercise and drastic weight loss were reported. Youth American football players arrived activity mildly hypohydrated and consumed enough fluid during activity to maintain euhydration. Abnormal eating attitudes and the use of unhealthy weight loss methods were reported by some youth American football players.

Keywords: sweat rate; fluid consumed; pathogenic eating behaviors; hypohydration; American tackle football

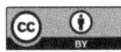

1. Introduction

Pop Warner is the largest youth American football organization in the world and greater than 250,000 children participate per season. Pop Warner football, in an attempt to make the sport safer, sometimes divide their players by age and weight [1]. To ensure these rules are followed, players weigh-in at the beginning of the season and before each game to confirm they are not over the weight limit for that specific team [1]. If they weigh-in at a different weight, then the child may not be allowed to play that day or eventually have to change teams. Leagues without weight restrictions divide their players into teams by age only. However, if there is a larger child on a team (usually greater than 36.3 kg), playing restrictions are typically enforced for that child to ensure safety and encourage fair play.

The National Health and Nutrition Examination Survey, estimated 15.7% of boys 2–19 years old in the US are overweight, 19.1% obese and 6.3% severely obese [2]. When examining boys closer to youth football age range, US boys aged 6–11 years old revealed 20.4% obese [2]. The health risks posed by hypohydration and improper nutrition are heightened for athletes participating in sports that involve weight restrictions. The pressure of these restrictions may lead to unhealthy weight loss methods, which negatively affect the overall function of the body and may predispose athletes for exertional heat illness

(EHI) [3,4]. As mentioned previously, youth weight and age play a major role in the structure of the team composition in youth football. If a youth athlete is overweight, or is in the early maturation stage, it is implied their larger size may put them at higher risk for injury or potentially injuring other athletes. This not only puts an early stigma that being overweight or obese increases higher risk for injury, but may also put a young athlete at higher risk to engage in compensatory behaviors to induce weight loss (e.g., excessive exercise, fasting, self-induced vomiting, use of laxatives, diuretics, appetite suppressants, etc.). These behaviors align with previous research that revealed 12% of adolescent athletes used one or more compensatory behaviors to control weight [5].

When working with youth athletes with weight pressures, it is important to recognize hypohydration and improper diet are predisposing factors of EHI [6–8]. Hypohydration can be intentional when athletes engage in activities that induce passive or active dehydration; using a sauna or exercising in sweat suits were found to be the most common in adolescent athletes [5]. Additionally, poor diet is considered a risk factor for EHI, as low electrolyte levels alter normal muscle/organ function and low energy leads to early muscle fatigue during physical activity [3,9,10]. When examining adolescent male wrestlers and the influence of dietary restriction; a reduction in protein and muscular performance was evident, but there was little effect on linear growth and maturation [11]. There is a robust association between abnormal eating attitudes and behaviors (i.e., disordered eating, eating disorders (ED), pathogenic behaviors) and their contribution to children being overweight and obese [12]. It is important to recognize any association between dietary restraints, dieting and ED risk in the context of pediatric weight management, particularly as the onset of ED risk peaks during adolescence [13]. This early recognition will help in the prevention of unhealthy weight loss methods in this young population.

Youth and adolescent males participating in American football compose the majority of EHI cases that present to United States emergency rooms [14]. Research reveals youth football has the highest EHI rate compared to high school and collegiate teams [15]. Risk factors for EHI in the American football population include uniforms, high body mass index (BMI), environmental conditions, poor physical condition, lack of heat acclimatization and improper work to rest ratio [3,6,7,9]. Beginning physical activity and maintaining a euhydrated state is crucial to support efficient thermoregulation and cardiovascular function [3,9,10]. Studies have concluded high school athletes are hypohydrated before the start of activity and underestimate sweat losses and fluid needs [16,17]. This has been noted in youth football players at summer camp as well [18]. It is unknown if this is true for youth football players during a regular season.

There is a substantial amount of research regarding hypohydration in adult athletics and the effects of unhealthy weight loss methods in weight-restricted sports [11,19–28]. However, there is a scarcity of research in children and in football leagues who utilize weight restricted (WR) or age restricted (AR) guidelines. Therefore, the primary purpose of our study was to examine hydration and eating frequency (number of meals and snacks per/day) among youth football leagues (WR vs. AR) during different activities (practice: PX vs. games: GM). The secondary purpose was to determine the prevalence of ED risk by assessing eating attitudes and compensatory behaviors. We hypothesized that the WR league would have greater hypohydration than the AR league. We also hypothesized ED risk and compensatory behaviors would exist in youth football players.

2. Materials and Methods

2.1. Design

We utilized a cross-sectional research design. The independent variables were football league (age (AR) and weight (WR)) and activity type (practice (PX) or game (GM)). The dependent variables were hydration status (urine osmolality (Uosm), percent change in body mass (%BM)), fluid consumed (FC), sweat rate (SR), eating attitudes (Children's Eating Attitude Test (ChEAT-26)) and self-reported eating frequency.

2.2. Participants

Youth football players ($n = 63$) between the ages of 8–13 years from local recreational leagues in the southeastern region of the United States participated. The convenience sample was recruited during the team parent pre-season meeting. The WR league included participants from 4 teams of specific weight and age categories. Each player within the WR league had to be within the weight range before the season began to be eligible for that division. Additionally, at each game, participants had to weigh in, with full pads and meet requirements to play that day. Players within the AR league were assigned teams by age only. There were no exclusions to participate in the study. The study was approved by the University of South Carolina's Institutional Review Board (Pro00024799) and written assent and informed consent were obtained from participants and their parent/legal guardian prior to baseline testing.

2.3. Instrumentation and Measurements

Hydration Status: A Multi-Sample Osmometer (Advanced Instrument model 2020) was calibrated before each set of urine samples and determined player's pre activity Uosm [29,30]. Samples were run in duplicate. If the values were more than 15 mOsm/kg apart, a triplicate sample was analyzed. The two closest samples were averaged to represent the sample. Each athlete's weight was obtained in kilograms (Tanita TBF 300A, Tokyo, Japan) while wearing only shorts. Percent change in body mass (%BM) was calculated as: [(pre event kg–post event kg)/pre event kg] × 100 [3].

Fluid Consumed and Sweat Rate: Each player was provided a 1 L bottle and could fill it with their normal self-provided drink of choice. FC was tracked throughout PX and GM with fluids added if desired by the player. At the end of activity, the remaining fluid was measured to the nearest 10 mL mark on a graduated cylinder. Sweat rate (SR) was calculated as: [(pre event kg–post event kg) + L of FC)]/hours of exercise [3].

Eating Disorder Attitudes and Compensatory Behaviors: Children's Eating Attitude Test (ChEAT-26) is a modified version of the Eating Attitudes Test (EAT-26) for children between 7 and 14 years old [31–33]. The ChEAT-26 is composed of 26 questions with subscales related to dieting, restricting, purging and food preoccupation and 5 questions related to compensatory behaviors (e.g., binging-eating more than you would normally eat, self-induced vomiting-made yourself throw-up, use of diet pills, excessive exercise, or lost a significant amount of weight in a short period of time). Participants rated their responses using a 6-point Likert scale ranging from 1 to 6 (i.e., never, rarely, sometimes, often, very often, always). A higher score is representative of more problematic or maladaptive eating attitudes and a cut-off score of 20 is indicative of risk for ED pathology. To be considered at risk for ED, we used two criteria: (1) participants scored greater than 20 on the ChEAT-26 and/or (2) participants met the criteria for compensatory behaviors or recent significant weight loss. This instrument does not diagnose an ED, but only aids in identifying characteristics of an ED [33–35]. The ChEAT-26 has an internal consistency of 0.79 and for this study was 0.80 [36].

Self-Reported Eating Frequency: Participants were asked to self-report their eating frequency prior to each observed PX and GM. We measured eating frequency by asking how many meals and snacks were eaten prior to activity (PX and GM) the same day in whole numbers.

2.4. Procedures

An informational meeting explained the study to parents and players before consent/assent was obtained. Basic demographics were collected at this time (age, height, weight). The ChEAT-26 was given to participants to complete after the first PX, but prior to the first GM. Data collection occurred on 7 (AR) or 8 (WR) nonconsecutive practices and the first 3 games of the season for both leagues. The WR had two practices on the last observed day (9:00 am and 6:00 pm). For the most part, practices for both leagues commonly occurred at 6:00 pm. Start times for WR games ranged from 10:00 am–1:00 pm whereas the AR leagues games started at 7:00 pm. Details regarding work to rest ratios of PX and GM have been described previously [37]. When participants arrived at activity (PX and GM) they self-reported their meal/snack frequency and were then given a collection cup to provide a urine sample. Players were weighed before and after activity. There was no intervention by the researchers during PX or GM. Players participated in football as normal and asked to follow their normal hydration behaviors.

2.5. Data Analysis

Statistical Analysis Software (SAS Institute Inc., Cary, NC, USA) was used for hydration behavior variables; and we used SPSS Statistical Software (Version 27; SPSS Inc., Armonk, NY, USA) and alpha < 0.05 for eating behavior variables. G*Power software (version 3.1.9.2., Heinrich Heine University, Dusseldorf, Germany) was used to calculate power for ED risk [38]. Using an alpha of 0.05 and a large effect size (0.7), our power calculation indicated we needed a sample of 34 participants, with estimated power being 0.90. Descriptive statistics were calculated for all dependent and descriptive variables. Differences in Uosm, %BM, FC and SR least square means were assessed between leagues (AR, WR) and activities (PX, GM) with ANOVA or general linear model procedures depending on if the data was complete and balanced, or incomplete and unbalanced, respectively. Frequencies and proportions with 95% confidence intervals were calculated for categorical variables (e.g., ED risk, binge eating, purging, use of diet pills, diuretics and laxatives, excessive exercise and drastic weight loss) along with means and standard deviations for continuous variables (e.g., total ChEAT-26 score and dieting, restricting and purging and food preoccupation subscale scores).

3. Results

A total of 63 youth football players participated in the study. The WR (n = 27, 10 ± 1 years old, 144 ± 9 cm, 37.6 ± 8.0 kg) and AR (n = 36, 11 ± 1 years old, 152 ± 8 cm, 50.1 ± 17.1 kg) players included all positions and levels of experience. Limited data were available for ChEAT-26 (n = 37), whereas 63 participants completed the remaining measures but data were missing at some time points.

3.1. Demographics

Participant demographics are presented in Table 1. Athletes in the WR and AR youth football leagues were within the age range of 9–13 years old, but there was a statistically significant difference in age between leagues (p = 0.003). Although the participants were close in age, the AR players were taller (p = 0.001) and weighed more (p < 0.001) than WR.

Table 1. Descriptive statistics of all participants (n = 63) and by league (WR: n = 27 and AR: n = 36).

	Aggregated			WR			AR			
	M(SD)	Min	Max	M(SD)	Min	Max	M(SD)	Min	Max	p-Value
Age (y)	11(1)	9	13	10(1)	9	12	11(1) [a]	9	13	0.003
Height (cm)	148(9)	127	167	144(9)	127	163	152(8) [a]	133	167	0.001
Weight (kg)	44.7(15.2)	26.2	95.7	37.6(8.0)	26.2	56.3	50.1(17.1) [a]	27.7	95.7	<0.001

All values are represented in mean (SD) and minimum and maximum values. WR: weight-restricted league; AR: age-restricted league.
[a]: AR > WR.

3.2. Hydration Status

Descriptive statistics for Uosm and %BM are presented in Table 2. Uosm ranged from 78 to 1383 mOsm/kg pre activity. There was no interaction between league and activity type (F = 1.35, p = 0.240) for Uosm. The AR league had higher Uosm than the WR league (F = 6.01, p = 0.015), but there was no main effect for activity type (F = 0.52, p = 0.471). Percent body mass change within an activity session ranged from −2.4% to +2.0%. There was a significant interaction between league and activity type for %BM (F = 5.44, p = 0.020) with WR having a greater %BM after games. A main effect existed for league (F = 4.51, p = 0.034), but not activity type (F = 0.18, p = 0.666).

Table 2. Descriptive statistics for pre activity urine osmolality and percent change in body mass.

	Agg			WR			AR		
	Agg	PX	GM	Agg	PX	GM	Agg	PX	GM
Uosm (mOsm/kg)									
Mean (SD)	829 (296)	823 (307)	855 (251)	786 (291)	770 (312)	839 (200)	899 (290)[a]	903 (282)	886 (330)
Min–Max	78–1383	78–1383	184–1262	78–1321	78–1321	184–1262	196–1383	287–1383	196–1215
%BM									
Mean (SD)	+0.1 (0.7)	+0.1 (0.6)	+0.1 (0.9)	+0.1 (0.7)	+0.2 (0.7)	0.0 (1.0)[b]	+0.2 (0.6)	+0.1 (0.6)	+0.4 (0.6)
Min–Max	+2.4−−2.0	+2.4−−2.0	+1.5−−1.8	+2.4−−2.0	+2.4−−2.0	+1.5−−1.8	+2.1−−1.4	+2.1−−1.4	+1.2−−0.9

Agg: Aggregated; WR: Weight-Restricted League; AR: Age-Restricted League; Uosm: pre activity urine osmolality; %BM: percent change in body mass after activity; [a]: AR > WR; [b]: WR > AR.

3.3. Fluid Consumed and Sweat Rate

Descriptive statistics for FC are presented in Table 3. FC between GM and PX was not different (p = 0.272). There was a statistically significant difference in FC between WR and AR during activity (PX and GM) (p = 0.045). There was no difference in FC between WR and AR during GM (p = 0.072) or during PX (p = 0.378). The WR players consumed less fluid during GM than PX (p = 0.048). There was no difference in FC when comparing GM and PX for AR (p = 0.929). There was a positive correlation between FC and SR (r = 0.875).

Table 3. Sweat rate and fluid consumed of all youth football players (n = 63) from weight (n = 27) and age (n = 36) restricted leagues, during combined practices and games.

	Agg			WR			AR		
(L/hr)	Agg	PX	GM	Agg	PX	GM	Agg	PX	GM
SR	0.4 (0.2)	0.5 (0.2)[b]	0.4 (0.2)	0.4 (0.2)	0.4 (0.2)	0.4 (0.2)	0.5 (0.2)[a]	0.5 (0.2)	0.4 (0.2)
FC	0.4 (0.2)	0.4 (0.2)	0.3 (0.2)	0.4 (0.2)	0.4 (0.2)[b]	0.3 (0.2)	0.4 (0.2)	0.4 (0.2)	0.4 (0.2)

All values are represented in mean (SD). Agg: Aggregated; WR: Weight-Restricted League; AR: Age-Restricted League; [a]: AR > WR; [b]: PX > GM.

Descriptive statistics for SR are presented in Table 3. The maximum SR value recorded in a player was 1.3 L/hr during a PX. There was a significant difference in SR between GM and PX (p = 0.013). AR had a greater SR during activity (PX and GM) than WR players (p = 0.028). There was also a statistically significant difference in SR when comparing GM and PX for WR (p = 0.004). There was no difference in SR when comparing GM and PX for AR (p = 0.311).

3.4. Eating Disorder Attitudes and Compensatory Behaviors

Only 37 youth football players completed the ChEAT-26. The estimated prevalence for ED risk for all youth football players was 21.6% (n = 8); of those, 5.4% (n = 2) were at risk based on the ChEAT-26, 13.5% (n = 5) on compensatory behaviors and 2.7% (n = 1) from both the ChEAT-26 and compensatory behaviors. WR league accounted for 87.5% (n = 7) of ED risk and AR for 12.5% (n = 1). Overall, 16.2% (n = 6) of our participants reported use of compensatory behaviors, with 10.8% (n = 4) reporting binge eating where they felt that they may not be able to stop, at least 2–3 times per month; 2.7% (n = 1) had vomited to control their weight or shape at least once a month, 5.4% (n = 2) had exercised more than 60 min a day to lose or to control their weight at least once a day and 2.7% (n = 1) noticed they lost a significant amount of weight in the last 6 months. None of our participants reported use of laxatives, diet pills or diuretics to control their weight. Overall, the player's self-reported current weight and their ideal weight only differed by 1.2 kg as 25% (n = 9) indicated their current weight was their ideal weight. The remaining players indicated both a lower ideal weight (29.7%, n = 11) and a greater ideal weight (43.2%, n = 16).

3.5. Self-Reported Eating Frequency

Overall, youth football players had an average of 2 ± 1 meals and 1 ± 1 snack prior to activity (PX and GM). This also represents the average eating frequency prior to PX. Before GM, players overall self-reported 1 ± 1 meal and 1 ± 1 snack with WR reporting 1 ± 0 and AR reporting 2 ± 1. There were players who reported 0 meals and snacks prior to PX ($n = 2$) and GM ($n = 4$). There were no statistical differences for meals and snacks between leagues ($p > 0.05$)

4. Discussion

The purpose of our study was to examine hydration status and eating frequency in WR and AR youth American football leagues during PX and GM. We found players from both leagues were mildly hypohydrated. We hypothesized that the WR league would have greater hypohydration than the AR league. Contrary to our hypothesis, we found AR players experienced greater hypohydration compared to WR. Our data support our hypotheses that youth football players exhibit ED risk and compensatory behaviors, finding approximately 20% of players self-reported items that indicated ED risk on the ChEAT or compensatory behaviors. Eating frequency seemed more dependent on event type.

4.1. Hydration Status

Urine osmolality indicated that our participants arrived to activity (PX and GM) hypohydrated, with the exception of WR pre PX. According to generally accepted guidelines [29], participants' hypohydration was mild on average. There were individual players with Uosm values that could be described as severe hypohydration at PX and GM (maximum values recorded ranged from 1128–1383 mOsm/kg) [29]. Similar pre-activity hypohydration has been found in youth athletes participating in soccer and other sports [17,39,40]. Specifically in youth football, up to 70% of players arrived to camp and morning practices hypohydrated with individual variances [18,41]. Our study confirms this, as on average 64% of our players arrived at least mildly hypohydrated for a PX or GM.

AR players were more hypohydrated than WR players, particularly before PX. Data collection for WR PX started before school began in August, while school had started when AR began PX in September. The WR players were likely coming to PX from home, while AR may have been coming to PX straight from school or after-school care. This may explain why AR had higher Uosm values, as they may not have had a chance to hydrate sufficiently during school before PX. WR players had higher Uosm values before their GM than PX (not statistically). One explanation may be the start time for WR games, which began at 10:00 am and players may have had less time between waking and the GM to consume food and fluids. It is also possible WR players may have purposely not consumed as much water if they were concerned about passing the weigh-in prior to the game.

Our participants had small changes in %BM during activity (PX and GM). This indicates our participants maintained their pre hydration status throughout activity by matching sweat losses with FC. Our results, coupled with previous research in young athletes [17,18,39,41], solidifies a common theme: dehydration during activity is minimized when fluids are accessible, but athletes do not optimize the time between activity sessions to reach euhydration.

4.2. Fluid Consumed and Sweat Rate

The average FC of our participants was similar to studies with adolescent soccer, volleyball and football players and youth campers [16–18,41,42]. Specifically, previous research in youth football campers participating in three sessions per day recorded an average of 0.76 L of fluid per hour during activity [18]. Campers consumed enough fluid to account for sweat loss during activity [18]. Similarly, high school players consumed fluids equivalent to two-thirds of their sweat loss [16,18]. Our participants, both AR and WR players, consumed enough fluids to make up for their sweat losses during activity. Fluid consumed increased as sweat rate increased as noted by the positive correlation. However, the strong relationship can be partly explained by FC calculated within the SR equation.

Sweat rates in our study were likely affected by a variety of factors including hydration status of the players, intensity of activity and environmental conditions [10]. Age-restricted players were larger than WR; therefore, AR players may have had greater increases in metabolic heat generation resulting in higher SR. However, though there was statistical difference in SR between leagues, any clinical significance in relation to anthropometrics would need to be determined in future research. Practice SR was greater than GM in our results, which is in contrast to McDermott et al. (2009) that reported a larger SR during GM than PX. Differences may exist because of the timing of each activity was different in both studies. SR is a valuable variable to calculate in athletes to determine fluid needs. If players drink the amount of fluid that they are losing through sweat per hour, then hydration status can be maintained.

4.3. Eating Disorder Characteristics and Behaviors

Our study is the first to examine ED risk in American youth tackle football players (boys) who participated in either a WR or AR league. We found approximately 20% of players were at higher risk for ED attitudes and compensatory behaviors compared to previous research that estimated 14.4% of youth male athletes (from various sports) were at risk for Eds [5,43–48]. Additionally, it has been noted in previous research that pediatric EDs are more common than type 2 diabetes and the higher rates of EDs are evident in younger children, boys and minority groups [49–51]. However, generally speaking, male athletes typically have lower scores than their female counterparts, as well as their non-athlete controls [43]. In our study, regardless of WR or AR league, we also found low ChEAT-26 scores in our youth football players. Of those who were, the majority were in the WR league. Youth football players who were at risk for an ED may find themselves in a vulnerable developmental period in which they are faced with a range of general as well as sport-specific risk factors. For example, adolescence is characterized by growth, physical changes and personality development [5]; and/or adolescent athletes' frequent drive to "be their best" combined with performance pressures from coaches and/or parents can create an overly competitive environment contributing to increase risk for ED attitudes and use of compensatory behaviors [44].

Boys involved in sports that necessitate weight restrictions include not only wrestlers, but also youth football players, gymnast, runners, swimmers, etc. In these sports, "cutting weight" may provide an edge to qualify for competition, reduce restrictions for competition, or to enhance performance. Vomiting, eating binges and excessive exercise to manipulate weight was self-reported by a small number of youth football players in our study. These behaviors have also been observed in high school wrestlers [23,25]. In approximately 2500 high school wrestlers during a single season, most took part in at least one unhealthy weight loss method per week [23]. Findings across multiple youth sport revealed ~ 8% of youth athletes reported they were trying to lose weight and 12% reported use of one or more compensatory behaviors; with the most common behaviors included activities inducing passive or active dehydration (e.g., sauna, exercise in sweat suite, etc.) [5]. Our study revealed ~16% reported use of compensatory behaviors, with the most common compensatory behaviors being binge eating and excessive exercise. Our participants who reported use of unhealthy weight loss methods may have been utilizing these methods to lose weight for football. Unhealthy weight loss methods cause hypohydration and electrolyte imbalances, which alters normal thermoregulatory system and organ function. In combination with exercise, this can lead to EHI and other health related risks [4,6,7]. Unhealthy compensatory behaviors in sport may commonly be perceived as a method to "cut weight"; however, these behaviors may also be used to "gain weight". Sports, such as football, may unintentionally portray the message that "bigger is better" to enhance performance for certain positions. Thus, in turn, possibly putting pressures on athletes to binge eat to gain weight. Future research should examine if pressures related to eating are position specific. Our results indicated that some youth football players wanted a lower ideal weight, while others wanted a greater weight.

4.4. Self-Reported Eating Frequency

Intensive physical training and participation in competitive sports during childhood/adolescence may affect athletes' pubertal development. Contrarily, maturational timing, early or late, may impact the athletes' development and the selection of their sport and/or sport position. Therefore, it is important to assure that youth athletes are appropriately fueling. Although our study did not examine daily dietary intake and actual number of consumed, calories, we identified the frequency of meals and snacks per day. We reported general differences in self-reported eating behaviors between PX and GM. This may have been due to the time-of-day PX and GM took place. Practices started at 6 pm for both leagues and GM for AR were at 7 pm. However, GM started at 10 am, 11:30 am and 1 pm for WR; therefore, WR players would not have eaten as many meals and snacks as they would have eaten before PX. Food intake findings could have also been influenced by WR players purposely not eating as much on game days because of the weigh-in prior to the GM. Similar to WR youth football, wrestling also has weight restrictions and limiting food consumption is sometimes used by wrestlers as a weight control method to ensure participation [23]. Studies have shown that during high school wrestling season, there is a decrease in protein consumption, body protein and fat stores in wrestlers [26]. In addition, wrestlers' weight and muscular strength and power significantly increase during the post season when compared to mid-season [20,26]. Not eating enough nutrients prior to activity can decrease energy levels and performance and it is a predisposing factor for EHI [4,7,52]. It is recommended parents and coaches familiarize themselves with the energy/nutritional requirements (incorporating total energy expenditure, plus exercise energy expenditure/physical activity levels and energy deposits of growing tissues) for youth populations which have been previously published [53]. This will provide parents and coaches a better understanding not only of the fueling needs of youth athletes but how to plan the frequency of meals when schedules do not align with standard mealtimes.

4.5. Strengths and Limitations

We are the first study to examine hydration status of American tackle football players younger than high school during a regular practice and competition season. We are also the first to examine eating attitudes in this population. A limitation included that PX and GM started at different times during the day, confining the comparisons of hydration status and eating behaviors of players between PX and GM. Environmental conditions were different on each day of data collection which has the potential to impact sweat rates. Variables were self-reported data and questions could have been answered untruthfully. There was also inconsistency with participation due to the young age of the players, parents not getting their children to PX and GM early enough and participants playing at different field locations at the same time resulting in some datasets being incomplete or unbalanced. These reasons also explain the low numbers of players completing the ChEAT questionnaire. Future research should focus on evaluating hydration and nutrition knowledge of youth football parents and coaches. It would also be beneficial to repeat this study with youth football players for an entire season. Examining specifically what types of food youth football players are eating and reasons for their eating behaviors would provide additional insight into the patterns presented in our study.

5. Conclusions

Overall, youth football players arrived to PX and GM slightly hypohydrated, although players in the AR league were more hypohydrated than WR. It seems that the players understood the importance of hydrating during physical activity and consumed enough fluids during PX and GM to match SR. Meal and snack frequency were adequate for practices but could be considered limited for game days. As we hypothesized, we observed the existence of ED risk and compensatory eating behaviors in this group of youth football players. This was noted in both leagues, but particularly in the WR league. This may be a result of players trying to alter their weight for football. The incorporation of hydration guidelines (similar to wrestling) and nutrition education for athletes and their parents should be considered for youth football leagues to help prevent the use of unhealthy weight loss methods.

Author Contributions: Conceptualization, S.Y., T.M.T.-M., D.E. and J.K.; Data curation, T.M.T.-M., D.E., J.K. and J.D.; Formal analysis, T.M.T.-M.; Methodology, S.Y., T.M.T.-M., D.E., J.K. and J.D.; Project administration, S.Y.; Supervision, S.Y.; Writing—original draft, S.Y., T.M.T.-M., D.E. and J.D.; Writing—review & editing, S.Y., T.M.T.-M., D.E., J.K. and J.D. All authors have read and agreed to the published version of the manuscript.

Funding: This work was supported in part by the University of South Carolina's College of Education Internal Grant Program. The study was also supported in part by the Master's Grant program of the Datalys Center for Sports Injury Prevention and Research. Funding sources did not influence the study design, data collection, analysis, or writing of the manuscript.

Institutional Review Board Statement: The study was conducted according to the guidelines of the Declaration of Helsinki, and approved by the Institutional Review Board of University of South Carolina (protocol code 00024799).

Informed Consent Statement: Informed consent and assent were obtained from all participants involved in the study.

Data Availability Statement: The data presented in this study are openly available in openICPSR at [https://www.doi.org/], accessed on 25 July 2021, reference number openicpsr-146124.

Acknowledgments: We would like to acknowledge the hard work and significant time commitment of all the research assistants who helped during data collection. We would also like to thank the players and their parents for their willingness to participate in the study and patience during data collection. Last, we recognize Ross Hayden for his help with statistical analysis.

Conflicts of Interest: The authors declare no conflict of interest.

References

1. Pop Warner Little Scholars. Pop Warner Little Scholars Rule Handbook. Available online: https://www.popwarner.com/Default.aspx?tabid=2676344 (accessed on 17 March 2021).
2. Fryar, C.D.; Carroll, M.D.; Ogden, C.L. *Prevalence of Overweight, Obesity, and Severe Obesity Among Children and Adolescents Aged 2–19 Years: United States, 1963–1965 through 2015–2016*; Centers for Disease Control and Prevention: Washington, DC, USA, 2018.
3. Sawka, M.N.; Burke, L.M.; Eichner, E.R.; Maughan, R.J.; Montain, S.J.; Stachenfeld, N.S. American College of Sports Medicine position stand. Exercise and fluid replacement. *Med. Sci. Sports Exerc.* **2007**, *39*, 377–390.
4. Turocy, P.S.; DePalma, B.F.; Horswill, C.A.; Laquale, K.M.; Martin, T.J.; Perry, A.C.; Somova, M.J.; Utter, A.C. National Athletic Trainers' Association position statement: Safe weight loss and maintenance practices in sport and exercise. *J. Athl. Train.* **2011**, *46*, 322–336. [CrossRef]
5. Giel, K.E.; Hermann-Werner, A.; Mayer, J.; Diehl, K.; Schneider, S.; Thiel, A.; Zipfel, S.; Group, G.S. Eating disorder pathology in elite adolescent athletes. *Int. J. Eat. Disord.* **2016**, *49*, 553–562. [CrossRef]
6. Armstrong, L.E.; Casa, D.J.; Millard-Stafford, M.; Moran, D.S.; Pyne, S.W.; Roberts, W.O. American College of Sports Medicine position stand. Exertional heat illness during training and competition. *Med. Sci. Sports Exerc.* **2007**, *39*, 556–572. [CrossRef]
7. Casa, D.J.; DeMartini, J.K.; Bergeron, M.F.; Csillan, D.; Eichner, E.R.; Lopez, R.M.; Ferrara, M.S.; Miller, K.C.; O'Connor, F.; Sawka, M.N.; et al. National Athletic Trainers' Association Position Statement: Exertional Heat Illnesses. *J. Athl. Train.* **2015**, *50*. [CrossRef] [PubMed]
8. Rav-Acha, M.; Hadad, E.; Epstein, Y.; Heled, Y.; Moran, D.S. Fatal exertional heat stroke: A case series. *Am. J. Med. Sci.* **2004**, *328*, 84–87. [CrossRef]
9. Bergeron, M.F.; Devore, C.; Rice, S.G. Policy statement-Climatic heat stress and exercising children and adolescents. *Pediatrics* **2011**, *128*, e741–e747. [PubMed]
10. McDermott, B.P.; Anderson, S.A.; Armstrong, L.E.; Casa, D.J.; Cheuvront, S.N.; Cooper, L.; Kenney, W.L.; O'Connor, F.G.; Roberts, W.O. National Athletic Trainers' Association Position Statement: Fluid Replacement for the Physically Active. *J. Athl. Train.* **2017**, *52*, 877–895. [CrossRef]
11. Roemmich, J.N.; Sinning, W.E. Weight loss and wrestling training: Effects on growth-related hormones. *J. Appl. Physiol.* **1997**, *82*, 1760–1764. [CrossRef]

12. Edition, F. *Diagnostic and Statistical Manual of Mental Disorders*; American Psychiatric Association: Washington, DC, USA, 2013; Volume 21.
13. De Girolamo, G.; McGorry, P.D.; Sartorius, N. *Age of Onset of Mental Disorders: Etiopathogenetic and Treatment Implications*; Springer: New York, NY, USA, 2018.
14. Nelson, N.G.; Collins, C.L.; Comstock, R.D.; McKenzie, L.B. Exertional heat-related injuries treated in emergency departments in the U.S., 1997–2006. *Am. J. Prev. Med.* **2011**, *40*, 54–60. [CrossRef]
15. Yeargin, S.W.; Kerr, Z.Y.; Casa, D.J.; Djoko, A.; Hayden, R.; Parsons, J.T.; Dompier, T.P. Epidemiology of Exertional Heat Illnesses in Youth, High School, and College Football. *Med. Sci. Sports Exerc.* **2016**, *48*, 1523–1529. [CrossRef]
16. Yeargin, S.W.; Casa, D.J.; Judelson, D.A.; McDermott, B.P.; Ganio, M.S.; Lee, E.C.; Lopez, R.M.; Stearns, R.L.; Anderson, J.M.; Armstrong, L.E.; et al. Thermoregulatory responses and hydration practices in heat-acclimatized adolescents during preseason high school football. *J. Athl. Train.* **2010**, *45*, 136–146. [CrossRef]
17. Silva, R.P.; Mundel, T.; Natali, A.J.; Bara Filho, M.G.; Lima, J.R.; Alfenas, R.C.; Lopes, P.R.; Belfort, F.G.; Marins, J.C. Fluid balance of elite Brazilian youth soccer players during consecutive days of training. *J. Sports Sci.* **2011**, *29*, 725–732. [CrossRef]
18. McDermott, B.P.; Casa, D.J.; Yeargin, S.W.; Ganio, M.S.; Lopez, R.M.; Mooradian, E.A. Hydration status, sweat rates, and rehydration education of youth football campers. *J. Sport Rehabil.* **2009**, *18*, 535–552. [CrossRef]
19. Abraham, S. Eating and weight controlling behaviours of young ballet dancers. *Psychopathology* **1996**, *29*, 218–222. [CrossRef]
20. Buford, T.W.; Rossi, S.J.; Smith, D.B.; O'Brien, M.S.; Pickering, C. The effect of a competitive wrestling season on body weight, hydration, and muscular performance in collegiate wrestlers. *J. Strength Cond. Res.* **2006**, *20*, 689–692. [CrossRef] [PubMed]
21. Burckhardt, P.; Wynn, E.; Krieg, M.A.; Bagutti, C.; Faouzi, M. The effects of nutrition, puberty and dancing on bone density in adolescent ballet dancers. *J. Danc. Med. Sci.Off. Publ. Int. Assoc. Danc. Med. Sci.* **2011**, *15*, 51–60.
22. Gibbs, A.E.; Pickerman, J.; Sekiya, J.K. Weight management in amateur wrestling. *Sports Health* **2009**, *1*, 227–230. [CrossRef]
23. Kiningham, R.B.; Gorenflo, D.W. Weight loss methods of high school wrestlers. *Med. Sci. Sports Exerc.* **2001**, *33*, 810–813. [CrossRef]
24. Lakin, J.A.; Steen, S.N.; Oppliger, R.A. Eating behaviors, weight loss methods, and nutrition practices among high school wrestlers. *J. Community Health Nurs.* **1990**, *7*, 223–234. [CrossRef]
25. Oppliger, R.A.; Landry, G.L.; Foster, S.W.; Lambrecht, A.C. Bulimic behaviors among interscholastic wrestlers: A statewide survey. *Pediatrics* **1993**, *91*, 826–831. [PubMed]
26. Roemmich, J.N.; Sinning, W.E. Weight loss and wrestling training: Effects on nutrition, growth, maturation, body composition, and strength. *J. Appl. Physiol. (1985)* **1997**, *82*, 1751–1759. [CrossRef] [PubMed]
27. Weissinger, E.H.T.; Johnson, G.O.; Evans, S.A. Weight Loss Behavior in HIgh School Wrestling: Wrestler and Parent Perceptions. *Pediatric Exerc. Sci.* **1991**, *3*, 64–73. [CrossRef]
28. Ziegler, P.; Sharp, R.; Hughes, V.; Evans, W.; Khoo, C.S. Nutritional status of teenage female competitive figure skaters. *J. Am. Diet. Assoc.* **2002**, *102*, 374–379. [CrossRef]
29. Armstrong, L.E.; Pumerantz, A.C.; Fiala, K.A.; Roti, M.W.; Kavouras, S.A.; Casa, D.J.; Maresh, C.M. Human hydration indices: Acute and longitudinal reference values. *Int. J. Sport Nutr. Exerc. Metab.* **2010**, *20*, 145–153. [CrossRef] [PubMed]
30. Chadha, V.; Garg, U.; Alon, U.S. Measurement of urinary concentration: A critical appraisal of methodologies. *Pediatric Nephrol.* **2001**, *16*, 374–382. [CrossRef] [PubMed]
31. Bonci, C.M.; Bonci, L.J.; Granger, L.R.; Johnson, C.L.; Malina, R.M.; Milne, L.W.; Ryan, R.R.; Vanderbunt, E.M. National athletic trainers' association position statement: Preventing, detecting, and managing disordered eating in athletes. *J. Athl. Train.* **2008**, *43*, 80–108. [CrossRef]
32. Garner, D.M.; Garfinkel, P.E. The Eating Attitudes Test: An index of the symptoms of anorexia nervosa. *Psychol. Med.* **1979**, *9*, 273–279. [CrossRef] [PubMed]
33. Garner, D.; Garfinkel, P. Eating attitudes test (EAT-26): Scoring and interpretation. *EAT-26 Self-Test*, 1979.
34. Smolak, L.; Murnen, S.K.; Ruble, A.E. Female athletes and eating problems: A meta-analysis. *Int. J. Eat. Disord.* **2000**, *27*, 371–380. [CrossRef]
35. Loucks, A.B.; Kiens, B.; Wright, H.H. Energy availability in athletes. *J. Sports Sci.* **2011**, *29* (Suppl. 1), S7–S15. [CrossRef]
36. Lommi, S.; Viljakainen, H.T.; Weiderpass, E.; de Oliveira Figueiredo, R.A. Children's Eating Attitudes Test (ChEAT): A validation study in Finnish children. *Eat. Weight Disord. Stud. Anorex. Bulim. Obes.* **2020**, *25*, 961–971. [CrossRef]
37. Yeargin, S.W.; Dickinson, J.J.; Emerson, D.M.; Koller, J.; Torres-McGehee, T.M.; Kerr, Z.Y. Exertional heat illness risk factors and physiological responses of youth football players. *J. Sport Health Sci.* **2021**, *10*, 91–98. [CrossRef]
38. Faul, F.; Erdfelder, E.; Lang, A.-G.; Buchner, A. G* Power 3: A flexible statistical power analysis program for the social, behavioral, and biomedical sciences. *Behav. Res. Methods* **2007**, *39*, 175–191. [CrossRef]
39. Arnaoutis, G.; Kavouras, S.A.; Kotsis, Y.P.; Tsekouras, Y.E.; Makrillos, M.; Bardis, C.N. Ad libitum fluid intake does not prevent dehydration in suboptimally hydrated young soccer players during a training session of a summer camp. *Int. J. Sport Nutr. Exerc. Metab.* **2013**, *23*, 245–251. [CrossRef]
40. Arnaoutis, G.; Kavouras, S.A.; Angelopoulou, A.; Skoulariki, C.; Bismpikou, S.; Mourtakos, S.; Sidossis, L.S. Fluid Balance During Training in Elite Young Athletes of Different Sports. *J. Strength Cond. Res. Natl. Strength Cond. Assoc.* **2015**, *29*, 3447–3452. [CrossRef] [PubMed]

41. Decher, N.R.; Casa, D.J.; Yeargin, S.W.; Ganio, M.S.; Levreault, M.L.; Dann, C.L.; James, C.T.; McCaffrey, M.A.; Oconnor, C.B.; Brown, S.W. Hydration status, knowledge, and behavior in youths at summer sports camps. *Int. J. Sports Physiol. Perform.* **2008**, *3*, 262–278. [CrossRef] [PubMed]
42. Cleary, M.A.; Hetzler, R.K.; Wasson, D.; Wages, J.J.; Stickley, C.; Kimura, I.F. Hydration behaviors before and after an educational and prescribed hydration intervention in adolescent athletes. *J. Athl. Train.* **2012**, *47*, 273–281. [CrossRef]
43. Fortes Lde, S.; Kakeshita, I.S.; Almeida, S.S.; Gomes, A.R.; Ferreira, M.E. Eating behaviours in youths: A comparison between female and male athletes and non-athletes. *Scand. J. Med. Sci. Sports* **2014**, *24*, e62–e68. [CrossRef] [PubMed]
44. Mancine, R.; Kennedy, S.; Stephan, P.; Ley, A. Disordered Eating and Eating Disorders in Adolescent Athletes. *Spartan Med. Res. J.* **2020**, *4*, 11595. [PubMed]
45. Martinsen, M.; Bratland-Sanda, S.; Eriksson, A.K.; Sundgot-Borgen, J. Dieting to win or to be thin? A study of dieting and disordered eating among adolescent elite athletes and non-athlete controls. *Br. J. Sports Med.* **2010**, *44*, 70–76. [CrossRef] [PubMed]
46. Martinsen, M.; Sundgot-Borgen, J. Higher prevalence of eating disorders among adolescent elite athletes than controls. *Med. Sci. Sports Exerc.* **2013**, *45*, 1188–1197. [CrossRef] [PubMed]
47. Muise, A.M.; Stein, D.G.; Arbess, G. Eating disorders in adolescent boys: A review of the adolescent and young adult literature. *J. Adolesc. Health* **2003**, *33*, 427–435. [CrossRef]
48. Nagata, J.M.; Ganson, K.T.; Murray, S.B. Eating disorders in adolescent boys and young men: An update. *Curr. Opin. Pediatrics* **2020**, *32*, 476–481. [CrossRef] [PubMed]
49. Dominé, F.; Berchtold, A.; Akré, C.; Michaud, P.-A.; Suris, J.-C. Disordered eating behaviors: What about boys? *J. Adolesc. Health* **2009**, *44*, 111–117. [CrossRef] [PubMed]
50. Pinhas, L.; Morris, A.; Crosby, R.D.; Katzman, D.K. Incidence and age-specific presentation of restrictive eating disorders in children: A Canadian Paediatric Surveillance Program study. *Arch. Pediatrics Adolesc. Med.* **2011**, *165*, 895–899. [CrossRef]
51. Smink, F.R.; Van Hoeken, D.; Hoek, H.W. Epidemiology of eating disorders: Incidence, prevalence and mortality rates. *Curr. Psychiatry Rep.* **2012**, *14*, 406–414. [CrossRef] [PubMed]
52. O'Connor, F.G.; Casa, D.J.; Bergeron, M.F.; Carter, R., 3rd; Deuster, P.; Heled, Y.; Kark, J.; Leon, L.; McDermott, B.; O'Brien, K.; et al. American College of Sports Medicine Roundtable on exertional heat stroke-return to duty/return to play: Conference proceedings. *Curr. Sports Med. Rep.* **2010**, *9*, 314–321. [CrossRef]
53. Torun, B. Energy requirements of children and adolescents. *Public Health Nutr.* **2005**, *8*, 968–993. [CrossRef]

MDPI
St. Alban-Anlage 66
4052 Basel
Switzerland
Tel. +41 61 683 77 34
Fax +41 61 302 89 18
www.mdpi.com

Nutrients Editorial Office
E-mail: nutrients@mdpi.com
www.mdpi.com/journal/nutrients

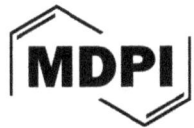

www.ingramcontent.com/pod-product-compliance
Lightning Source LLC
LaVergne TN
LVHW070046120526
838202LV00101B/650